ORTHOPAEDICS
for
Physician
Assistants

ORTHOPAEDICS
for
Physician Assistants,
First Edition

Sara D. Rynders, MPAS, PA-C
Physician Assistant
University of Virginia Hand Center
Department of Orthopaedic Surgery
Division of Hand and Upper Extremity Surgery
Charlottesville, Virginia

Jennifer A. Hart, MPAS, PA-C
Physician Assistant
University of Virginia
Department of Orthopaedic Surgery
Charlottesville, Virginia

ELSEVIER
SAUNDERS

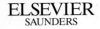

1600 John F. Kennedy Blvd.
Ste 1800
Philadelphia, PA 19103-2899

ORTHOPAEDICS FOR PHYSICIAN ASSISTANTS

ISBN: 978-1-4557-2531-1

Library of Congress Cataloging-in-Publication Data

Orthopaedics for physician assistants / [edited by] Sara D. Rynders, Jennifer A. Hart.
     p. ; cm.
Includes bibliographical references and index.
ISBN 978-1-4557-2531-1 (pbk. : alk. paper)
I. Rynders, Sara D. II. Hart, Jennifer A. (Jennifer Adele), 1974-
[DNLM: 1. Musculoskeletal Diseases—therapy—Handbooks. 2. Orthopedic Procedures—methods—Handbooks. 3. Musculoskeletal System—injuries—Handbooks. 4. Physician Assistants—Handbooks. WE 39]

     617.4'7—dc23

                                                                    2012047502

Senior Content Strategist: Kate Dimock
Senior Content Development Specialist: Anne Snyder
Publishing Services Manager: Julie Eddy/Hemamalini Rajendrababu
Senior Project Manager: Richard Barber
Project Manager: Anitha Sivaraj
Design Direction: Steven Stave

Printed in China

Last digit is the print number: 9   8   7   6   5   4   3   2   1

Dedication

This book is dedicated to my teachers and mentors who have encouraged my professional development and believed in me long before I believed in myself. It is also dedicated to my hard-working support staff and PA colleagues whom I have had the true honor of working with—I could not do it without you. I am grateful to Dr. Bobby Chhabra, Jennifer Hart MPAS, PA-C, and Elsevier, Inc., for the opportunity to be a PA editor and author. Thank you to my best friend, Corey Rynders, for our exciting life together. And thank you to my parents for getting me off to a great start.—SDR

This book is for my PA colleagues who go to work each day to deliver exemplary medical care to their patients without fanfare or acclaim. I am thankful for great supervising physicians, Dr. Lloyd Dennis, Dr. David Diduch, and Dr. Mark Miller, who took a leap of faith in me as their first PA hire, giving me the knowledge and the confidence for this project. And to my husband, Joe Hart, who has been there from the beginning of this great PA ride.—JAH

Contributors

Deana Bahrman, PA-C
Physician Assistant
Department of Orthopaedic Surgery
University of Virginia
Charlottesville, Virginia

Damond A. Cromer, BA
Orthopaedic Technologist Certified
University of Virginia Hand Center
University of Virginia
Charlottesville, Virginia

Gregory Domson, MD
Physician Assistant
University of Virginia
Charlottesville, Virginia

Suzanne Eiss, PA
Physician Assistant
Orthopaedic Surgery
University of Michigan Health System
Ann Arbor, Michigan
University of Michigan South Main
    Orthopaedics
Huron Valley Professional Center
Ann Arbor, Michigan

Cara B. Garrett, MA, MPAS
Physician Assistant
Department of Orthopaedic Surgery
Sports Medicine Division
University of Virginia
Charlottesville, Virginia

Jennifer A. Hart, MPAS, PA-C
Physician Assistant
University of Virginia
Department of Orthopaedic Surgery
Charlottesville, Virginia

Adam Katz, MD
Associate Professor of Plastic Surgery
    and Biomedical Engineering
Department of Plastic and Maxillofacial
    Surgery
University of Virginia
Charlottesville, Virginia

Ian W. Marks, MSc
Medical Officer
Deployable Operations Group
United States Coast Guard
Co-mentor
School of Medicine
University of Virgnia
Charlottesville, Virginia

Amy Radigan, MPAS, PA-C
Physician Assistant
University of Virginia Hand Center
Department of Orthopaedic Surgery
Division of Hand and Upper Extremity
    Surgery
Charlottesville, Virginia

Sara D. Rynders, MPAS, PA-C
Physician Assistant
University of Virginia Hand Center
Department of Orthopaedic Surgery
Division of Hand and Upper Extremity
    Surgery
Charlottesville, Virginia

Margaret Schick, PA
Physician Assistant
University of Michigan Health System
Ann Arbor, Michigan
University of Michigan Orthopaedics
Ann Arbor, Michigan

Katherine Sharpe
Physician Assistant
Department of Orthopaedic Surgery
University of Virginia
Charlottesville, Virginia

Shruti Tannan, MD
Resident Physician
Department of Plastic Surgery
University of Virginia
Charlottesville, Virginia

Scott Yang, MD
Resident Physician
Department of Orthopaedic Surgery
University of Virginia Health System
Charlottesville, Virginia

Preface

Orthopaedics for Physician Assistants is designed for those PAs who at some point find themselves alone in the vast world of musculoskeletal care and need a fast, reliable source to make it through the day. This text is the first of its kind. It is written for PAs by PAs or PA advocates. Its format is made for quick reading and referencing. Its small size is meant for storage in a pocket or at a clinic workstation. Its content and depth of knowledge are meant to appeal to the level of orthopaedic care provided by PAs working in the emergency department, primary care office, urgent care office, or orthopaedic clinic. This text is a reference and meant to be part of every PA student's library upon graduation.

The topics covered in this text are some of the most common orthopaedic conditions organized by body location. Each chapter begins with an overview of anatomy with beautiful, detailed anatomic illustrations. The chapter is then subdivided into specific orthopaedic conditions. Each condition has an overview of the history and presentation, the pertinent physical examination findings, suggestions on what imaging or tests to order, and a treatment guide. Surgical indications and contraindications are also reviewed, and an overview of a common surgical treatment is outlined with pertinent surgical risks and expected recovery course. Also included is a beautifully photographed chapter that provides step-by-step guidance for splinting and casting. It really is a complete orthopaedic resource.

We sincerely thank all of our contributors, who range from physicians to residents, PAs, and cast technicians who are truly masters in their specialty areas. We appreciate your time and effort and support of PAs in medicine and orthopaedic surgery.

—*Sara D. Rynders*

—*Jennifer A. Hart*

Contents

ANATOMY
Bones: Figure 1-1

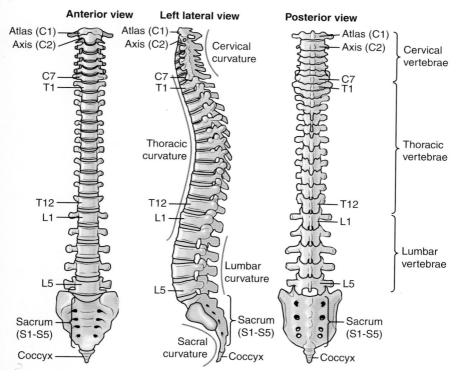

Figure 1-1. The bony anatomy and alignment of the spine. *(From Miller MD, Hart JA, MacKnight JM, editors:* Essential orthopaedics: *Philadelphia, 2010, Saunders, p 454.)*

■ Cervical: Figures 1-2 and 1-3

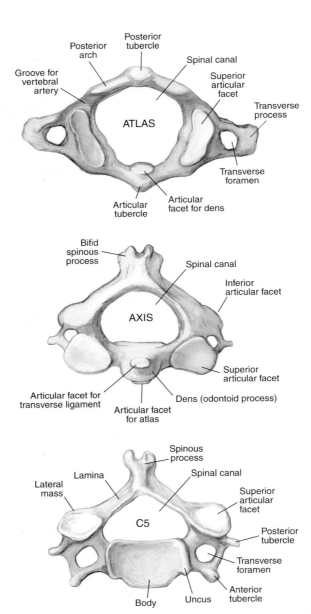

Figure 1-2. Bony anatomy of the cervical vertebrae (C1, C2, and C5). *(From Miller MD, Chhabra AB, Hurwitz S, et al, editors:* Orthopaedic surgical approaches: *Philadelphia, 2008, Saunders, p 213.)*

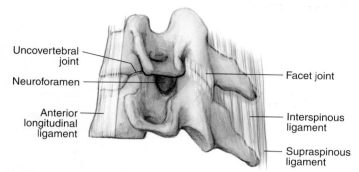

Figure 1-3. Anatomy of the cervical spine, lateral view. *(From Miller MD, Chhabra AB, Hurwitz S, et al, editors:* Orthopaedic surgical approaches: *Philadelphia, 2008, Saunders, p 217.)*

■ Thoracic: Figures 1-4 and 1-5

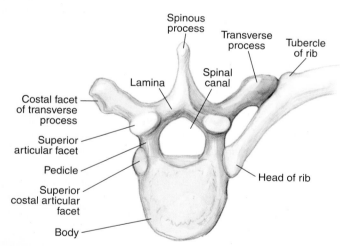

Figure 1-4. Bony anatomy of a thoracic vertebra (shown with rib). *(From Miller MD, Chhabra AB, Hurwitz S, et al, editors:* Orthopaedic surgical approaches: *Philadelphia, 2008, Saunders, p 215.)*

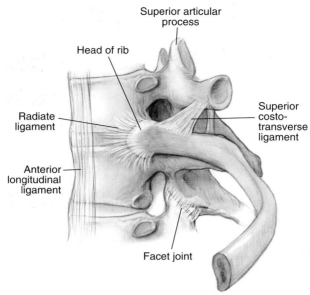

Figure 1-5. Anatomy of the thoracic spine, lateral view. *(From Miller MD, Chhabra AB, Hurwitz S, et al, editors:* Orthopaedic surgical approaches: *Philadelphia, 2008, Saunders, p 218.)*

■ Lumbar: Figures 1-6 and 1-7

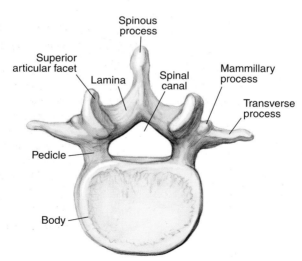

Figure 1-6. Bony anatomy of a lumbar vertebra. *(From Miller MD, Chhabra AB, Hurwitz S, et al, editors:* Orthopaedic surgical approaches: *Philadelphia, 2008, Saunders, p 215.)*

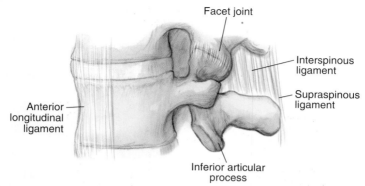

Figure 1-7. Anatomy of the lumbar spine, lateral view. *(From Miller MD, Chhabra AB, Hurwitz S, et al, editors:* Orthopaedic surgical approaches: *Philadelphia, 2008, Saunders, p 218.)*

Muscles and Soft Tissue:
Figures 1-8 through 1-11

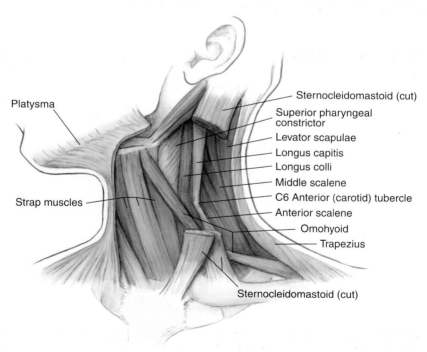

Figure 1-8. Anterior cervical spine muscles. *(From Miller MD, Chhabra AB, Hurwitz S, et al, editors:* Orthopaedic surgical approaches: *Philadelphia, 2008, Saunders, p 219.)*

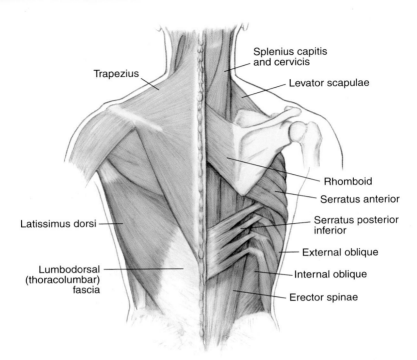

Figure 1-9. Posterior view of the spine musculature, superficial and intermediate layers. *(From Miller MD, Chhabra AB, Hurwitz S, et al, editors:* Orthopaedic surgical approaches: *Philadelphia, 2008, Saunders, p 222.)*

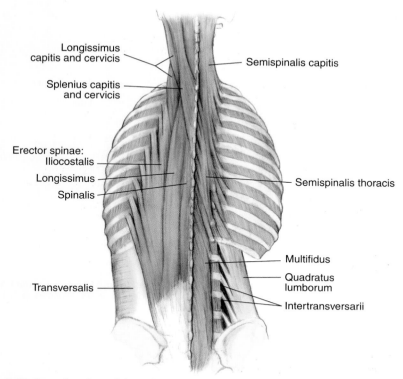

Longissimus capitis and cervicis

Semispinalis capitis

Splenius capitis and cervicis

Erector spinae:
Iliocostalis
Longissimus
Spinalis

Semispinalis thoracis

Multifidus

Quadratus lumborum

Transversalis

Intertransversarii

Figure 1-10. Posterior view of the spine musculature, deep view. *(From Miller MD, Chhabra AB, Hurwitz S, et al, editors: Orthopaedic surgical approaches: Philadelphia, 2008, Saunders, p 223.)*

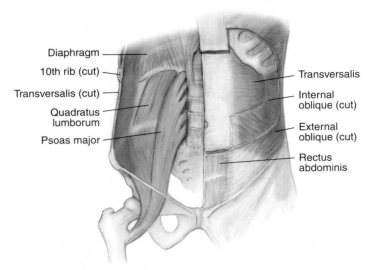

Figure 1-11. Anterior view of the lumbar spine musculature. *(From Miller MD, Chhabra AB, Hurwitz S, et al, editors:* Orthopaedic surgical approaches: *Philadelphia, 2008, Saunders, p 221.)*

Nerves and Arteries: Figures 1-12 through 1-14

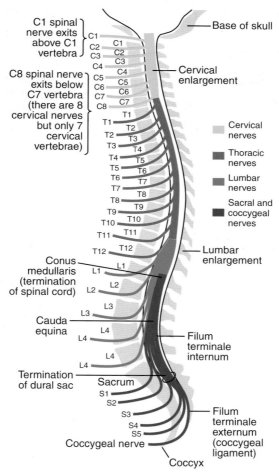

Figure 1-12. The spinal cord and nerve root orientation. (*From Miller MD, Hart JA, MacKnight JM, editors: Essential orthopaedics: Philadelphia, 2010, Saunders, p 457.*)

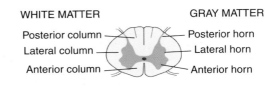

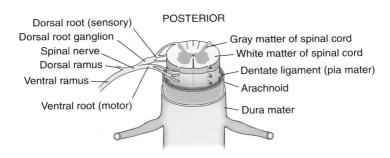

Figure 1-13. The cross-sectional anatomy of the spinal cord. *(From Miller MD, Chhabra AB, Hurwitz S, et al, editors: Orthopaedic surgical approaches: Philadelphia, 2008, Saunders, p 225.)*

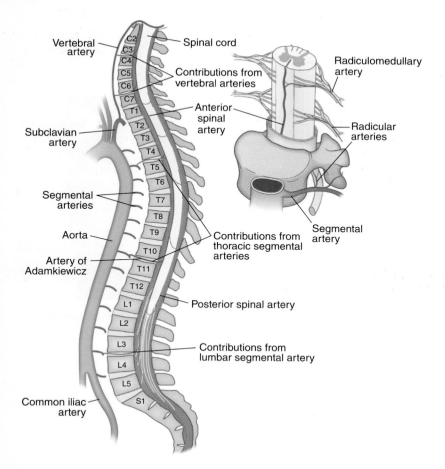

Figure 1-14. The vasculature of the vertebral column. *(From Miller MD, Chhabra AB, Hurwitz S, et al, editors:* Orthopaedic surgical approaches: *Philadelphia, 2008, Saunders, p 227.)*

Surface Anatomy: Figure 1-15

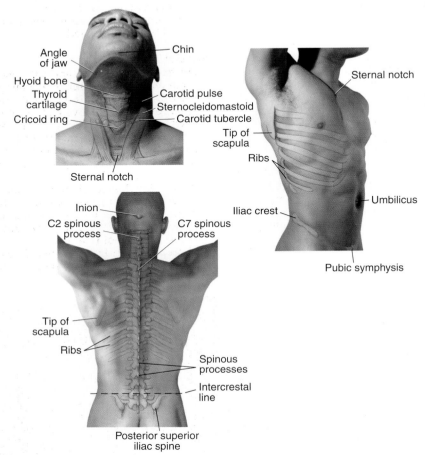

Figure 1-15. The surface anatomy of the spine. *(From Miller MD, Chhabra AB, Hurwitz S, et al, editors:* Orthopaedic surgical approaches, *Philadelphia, 2008, Saunders, p 231.)*

Normal X-Ray Appearance:
Figures 1-16 and 1-17

PHYSICAL EXAMINATION
Inspect for edema, rash, or deformity.
Inspect gait for:
- Forward leaning or cane, walker, shopping cart use: spinal stenosis
- Trendelenburg gait: hip disease
- Wide stance: cervical myelopathy

Palpate specific structures to evaluate complaint:
- Spinous processes
- Musculature of trunk or spine
- Sacroiliac (SI) joints
- Greater trochanters

Percuss costovertebral angles (CVAs).
Normal range of motion (ROM): Table 1-1
Neurovascular examination: Figure 1-18
- Cervical reflexes include biceps (C5), triceps (C7), and brachioradial (C6).
- Lumbar reflexes include patella (L4) and Achilles (S1).

- Pulses to be checked include radial, dorsalis pedis, and posterior tibialis.
- Sensation of gross soft touch in the dermatomal pattern is assessed.
- Pinprick and point discrimination is tested as needed.

Special Tests
- **Hoffman reflex:** Hoffmann reflex most often reflects the presence of an upper motor neuron lesion from spinal cord compression. **A positive test** result is elicited by flicking either the volar or dorsal surfaces of the middle finger and observing the reflex contraction of the thumb and index finger to form an "OK" sign (Fig. 1-19).
- **Babinski reflex:** Involuntary dorsiflexion of the hallux and spreading of the lesser toes occur in response to forceful scratching of the plantar or lateral aspect of the foot (Fig. 1-20).
- **Clonus:** Involuntary repetitive dorsiflexion of ankle occurs in response to

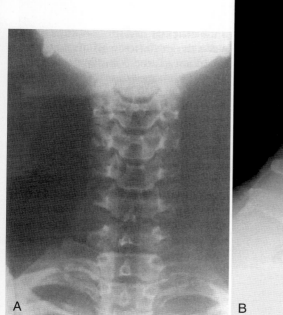
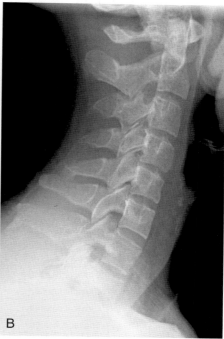

A   B

Figure 1-16. Normal cervical spine x-ray studies. **A,** Anteroposterior view. **B,** Lateral view. (**A,** *From Schwartz AJ: Imaging of degenerative cervical disease,* Spine State Art Rev *14:545-569, 2000;* **B,** *from Pretorious ES, Solomon JA, editors:* Radiology secrets, *ed 2, Philadelphia, 2006, Mosby.*)

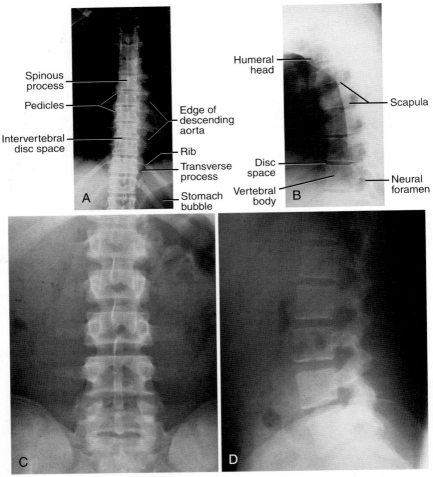

Figure 1-17. Normal spine x-ray studies. A, Anteroposterior (AP) view of the thoracic spine. **B,** Lateral view of the thoracic spine. **C,** AP view of the lumbar spine. **D,** Lateral view of the lumbar spine. (*A* and *B, From Mettler F:* Essentials of radiology, *ed 2, Philadelphia, 2005, Saunders;* **C** *and* **D,** *from Mercier L:* Practical orthopedics, *ed 6, Philadelphia, 2008, Mosby.*)

Table 1-1. Normal Range of Motion	
Motion	**Range (Degrees)**
Cervical extension	60
Cervical flexion	75
Cervical lateral flexion	45
Cervical rotation	80
Thoracic flexion	50
Thoracic rotation	30
Lumbar extension	60
Lumbar flexion	25

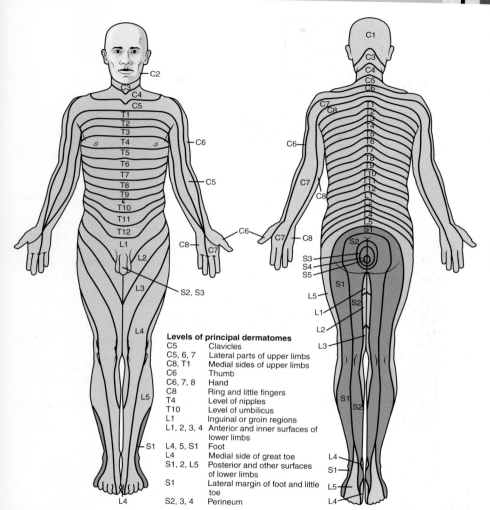

Figure 1-18. The dermatomes. *(From Miller MD, Hart JA, MacKnight JM, editors:* Essential orthopaedics, *Philadelphia, 2010, Saunders, p 458.)*

Levels of principal dermatomes

C5	Clavicles
C5, 6, 7	Lateral parts of upper limbs
C8, T1	Medial sides of upper limbs
C6	Thumb
C6, 7, 8	Hand
C8	Ring and little fingers
T4	Level of nipples
T10	Level of umbilicus
L1	Inguinal or groin regions
L1, 2, 3, 4	Anterior and inner surfaces of lower limbs
L4, 5, S1	Foot
L4	Medial side of great toe
S1, 2, L5	Posterior and other surfaces of lower limbs
S1	Lateral margin of foot and little toe
S2, 3, 4	Perineum

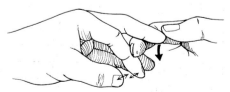

Figure 1-19. Hoffman reflex. *(From Fong W, et al. Evaluation of cervical spine disorders. In Devlin VJ, editor:* Spine secrets plus, *ed 2, St. Louis, 2012, Mosby, p 38.)*

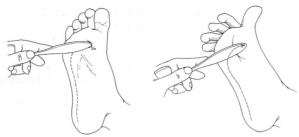

Figure 1-20. Babinski reflex. *(From Fong W, et al. Evaluation of cervical spine disorders. In Devlin VJ, editor: Spine secrets plus, ed 2, St. Louis, 2012, Mosby, p 38.)*

one-time forceful dorsiflexion of the ankle by the examiner (Fig. 1-21).

- **Bulbocavernosus reflex:** This refers to anal sphincter contraction in response to squeezing the glans penis or tugging on the Foley catheter tube carefully and involves the S1-S3 nerve roots. This is a spinal cord–mediated reflex. Following spinal cord trauma, the presence or absence of this reflex carries prognostic significance; in cases of cervical or thoracic spinal cord injury (SCI), absence of this reflex documents continuation of spinal shock or spinal injury at the level of the reflex arc. Return of the reflex signals the end of spinal shock. In lumbar injuries below the level of the spinal

cord, absence of the reflex may reflect cauda equina injury.

- **Straight leg raise:** The test is performed by passively raising the leg while the patient is supine. **A positive test** result is indicated by reproduction if radicular symptoms on the involved side (Fig. 1-22).
- **Waddell signs:** These are tests for nonorganic low back pain:
  1) Tenderness that is not anatomic
  2) Axial loading (should not cause low back pain)
  3) Distraction on straight leg raise
  4) Nonanatomic or breakaway weakness
  5) Overreaction (the most important Waddell sign)

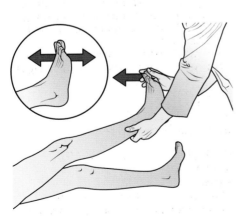

Figure 1-21. Clonus. *(From Miller MD, Hart JA, MacKnight JM, editors: Essential orthopaedics, Philadelphia, 2010, Saunders, p 460.)*

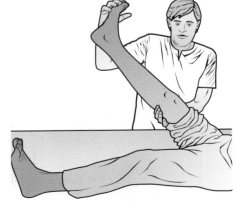

Figure 1-22. Straight leg raise. *(From Miller MD, Hart JA, MacKnight JM, editors: Essential orthopaedics, Philadelphia, 2010, Saunders, p 462.)*

Differential Diagnosis: Table 1-2

LUMBAR STRAIN
History
- Bending, twisting, and lifting reproduce pain.
- Pain in back occurs with movement, coughing, or sneezing.
- Leg pain or weakness is lacking.
- Injury can be minor or mild.

Physical Examination
- Slow gait
- Tenderness to palpation over muscular structures
- Pain with flexion, extension, and/or rotation of the trunk
- Normal neurologic examination

Imaging
- Anteroposterior (AP) or lateral views are obtained initially only if the mechanism warrants. Persistent pain for more than 1 week should be explored with bone scan.

Table 1-2. Differential Diagnosis

Low back pain	Lumbar muscle pain
	Degenerative disc disease
	Lumbar facet disease
	Nephrolithiasis
	Lumbar compression fracture
	Osteomyelitis
	Malingering
	Ovarian cyst
Lumbar radiculopathy	Herniated disc
	Foraminal stenosis
	Spinal stenosis
	Neuropathy
Cervical or thoracic pain	Muscle strain
	AAA
	Fracture
	Facet disease
	Degenerative disc disease
	Ankylosing spondylitis
Regional or dermatomal pain	Shingles
Deformity	Scoliosis
	Kyphosis

Initial Treatment
Patient Education
- Back pain, one of the most common medical problems, affects 8 out of 10 people at some point during their lives. Most back pain goes away on its own, although it may take a while. However, staying in bed for more than 1 or 2 days can make it worse.

Treatment Options
Nonoperative Management
- A short 1- to 2-day rest period for severe pain is prescribed.
- Over-the-counter nonsteroidal anti-inflammatory drugs (NSAIDs) or acetaminophen is recommended.
- Skeletal muscle relaxants are used sparingly.
- Physical therapy and "back school" can be beneficial for persistent pain.
- Advanced imaging is used only in the most refractory cases.
- Long-term prevention with core strengthening and ROM exercises is indicated.

Differential Diagnosis
- Compression fracture
- Intra-abdominal or pelvic disease such as nephrolithiasis, pyelonephritis, abdominal aortic aneurysm, intra-abdominal, intrapelvic, or spinal mass, or metastasis
- SI joint instability
- Occult vertebral body fracture: Bone scan or magnetic resonance imaging (MRI) will identify injury in cases of persistent pain.
- Malingering: Secondary gain must be considered. Assess with Waddell signs.

ICD-9 Codes
724.2 Back pain
V65.2 Malingerer
847.2 Lumbar strain

VERTEBRAL COMPRESSION FRACTURE
History
- Low-velocity fall occurs in older adults; injury could be very minor in this population.
- Higher-velocity injury may occur in younger patients.

- Patients complain of back pain.
- Injury can occur with motor vehicle crash (MVC).
- Look for pathologic causes.

Physical Examination
- Slow gait
- Tenderness to palpation over muscular structures
- Pain with flexion, extension, and/or rotation of the trunk
- Normal neurologic examination

Imaging
- AP or lateral views (with possible flexion or extension views) may show depressed or wedged end plates.
- Look for other injury such as spinous process fracture in higher-velocity injury.
- MRI is indicated if radiculopathy is present or for planning a cement procedure. Use contrast if concern exists for pathologic fracture.

Initial Treatment
- Short-duration narcotics
- Lumbar bracing for comfort (lumbosacral orthosis [LSO] or lumbar corset)

Patient Education
- Early ambulation is essential. Avoid flexion activities until pain-free.

Treatment Options
Nonoperative Management
- A short 1- to 2-day rest period is indicated for severe pain.
- Narcotic pain medications are prescribed.
- Use skeletal muscle relaxants sparingly.
- LSO brace or lumbar corset is recommended.
- Physical therapy and "back school" can be beneficial for persistent pain.
- MRI is used for evaluation for pathologic fracture or cement procedure.

Operative Management
Codes
ICD-9 codes: 805.2 Closed fracture of dorsal thoracic vertebra without mention of spinal cord injury
805.4 Closed fracture of dorsal lumbar vertebra without mention of spinal cord injury

CPT codes: 22520 Percutaneous vertebroplasty, 1 vertebral body; thoracic
22521 Percutaneous vertebroplasty, 1 vertebral body; lumbar
22522 Each additional thoracic or lumbar vertebral body
22523 Percutaneous vertebral augmentation, including cavity creation using mechanical device, 1 vertebral body; thoracic
22524 Percutaneous vertebral augmentation, including cavity creation using mechanical device, 1 vertebral body; lumbar
22525 Each additional thoracic or lumbar vertebral body
72291 Radiological supervision and interpretation
72292 Under CT guidance

Operative Indications
- Compression fracture or endplate fracture without neural injury
- Intractable pain
- Pathologic fracture for palliative care

Informed Consent and Counseling
- May not improve pain
- Not likely to improve fracture height

Anesthesia
- Local with sedation an option in those not able to tolerate general anesthesia
- General anesthesia

Patient Positioning
- The patient is prone on a Jackson frame or other similar radiopaque table.
- Space is left in the operating room (OR) for fluoroscopy.
- Many surgeons like two fluoroscopy machines, for a 360-degree view.

Surgical Procedures
- Cement augmentation (vertebroplasty)
  - Approach depends on lesion location, with the classic approach being transpedicular (can also be anterolateral, posterolateral, or parapedicular).
  - A trocar and cannula are introduced into the bone, one or two transpedicular needles are placed using fluoroscopy, and cement is introduced per the manufacturer's instructions.

- Caution is used to prevent and/or address any potential leaks of the cement outside the bony cavity.
■ Cement augmentation with cavity preparation (kyphoplasty)
  - The procedure is as described earlier, except that first a balloon tamp is inserted and inflated to restore vertebral body height.
  - The balloon is then removed, and cement is introduced as with vertebroplasty.

Estimated Recovery Course
■ Postoperative 2 to 4 weeks: Return for wound check, and obtain AP or lateral x-ray studies.
■ Postoperative 2 months: Return for a final evaluation.

Suggested Readings
Herkowitz HN, Garfin SR, Eismont FJ, et al: *Rothman-Simeone the spine,* ed 6, Philadelphia, 2011, Saunders.
Shen FH, Shaffrey CI: *Arthritis and arthroplasty: the spine,* Philadelphia, 2010, Saunders.
Yue JJ, Guyer RD, Johnson JP, et al: *The comprehensive treatment of the aging spine: minimally invasive and advanced techniques,* Philadelphia, 2011, Saunders.

DEGENERATIVE DISORDERS OF THE SPINE
History
■ The patient has insidious onset of neck or lumbar pain.
■ Often no precipitating injury is reported.
■ If neural impingement is present, patients likely will have spine and radicular pain to arms or legs that correlates to the location of neural compression or injury.

Physical Examination
■ Slow gait, possible shopping cart sign with central stenosis: Patients report that leaning forward while walking improves lower extremity symptoms; they may also report that they can ambulate only short distances without having to sit to relieve symptoms.
■ Antalgia: Pain with flexion and extension and radicular pain with stenosis occur.
■ Wide stance gait occurs with cervical central stenosis.

■ Focal weakness with lateral neural impingement: Upper extremity weakness occurs with central spinal cord syndrome.
■ Focal reflex loss with lateral impingement is noted.
■ Hyperreflexia or clonus occurs in cases of myelopathy.
■ Check Hoffman sign for evidence of spinal cord compression.
■ Dysesthesia in extremities is common.
■ Palpable step-off occurs in cases of high-grade spondylolisthesis.
■ Patients may have thoracolumbar degenerative scoliosis in severe cases.

Imaging
■ Standing plain film: AP, lateral, and flexion or extension views
■ Disc height loss, instability (retrolisthesis, anterolisthesis), obvious deformity identified
■ May need full-length spine AP
■ MRI for cases with radiculopathy
■ MRI with contrast with lumbar radiculopathy if prior uninstrumented spine surgery or if infection or tumor suspected
■ Computed tomography (CT) or myelogram if previous instrumented spine surgery or if MRI contraindicated
■ Discogram rarely indicated

Initial Treatment
Patient Education
■ Short-duration narcotics can be used if necessary. NSAIDs, activity modification, and physical therapy are often effective in the first 6 weeks of symptom onset.

Treatment Options
Nonoperative Management
■ If initial care is not effective, then advanced imaging is indicated, especially in cases of radicular symptoms or weakness in extremities. Patients with suspected cases of cauda equina syndrome or myelopathy need urgent MRI.
■ Bracing is rarely helpful.
■ If noninvasive measures are not helpful to improve symptoms, then epidural spine injections can give good relief of symptoms, particularly for radicular pain. Facet blocks and median branch ablation can follow up facet blocks if effective.

Operative Management

Codes
ICD-9 codes: 724.4 Lumbar radiculopathy
723.0 Cervical stenosis
724.0 Thoracolumbar spine stenosis
722.10 Lumbar herniated disc
722.0 Cervical herniated disc
722.52 Lumbar degenerative disc
CPT codes: 22318 to 22328 Fracture-dislocation treatment codes
22532 to 22634 Arthrodesis codes
22554 Anterior cervical discectomy and fusion (ACDF)
63001 to 63048 Posterior extradural laminotomy or laminectomy for exploration/decompression of neural elements or excision of herniated intervertebral discs

Operative Indications
- Failed all conservative measures
- Instability
- Myelopathy

Informed Consent
- Failure to improve symptoms
- Need for further surgery
- Infection
- New back and/or leg pain
- Nerve injury
- Bowel or bladder difficulties
- Anesthesia complications

Anesthesia
- General via endotracheal tube
- Some procedures possible under local or regional block

Patient Positioning
This is based on the type of approach indicated.
- Supine for anterior cervical
  - May need traction or bolstering
  - Tongs common
  - Arm traction or taping with sleds
- Prone with neck flexed for posterior cervical
  - Watch shaving of hair; infection is a major risk.
  - Watch draping.
- Supine for anterior lumbar
- Lateral decubitus for thoracolumbar lateral procedures
- Prone for thoracolumbar spine posterior procedures
  - Various different frames used
  - Flexed or extended position critical for each procedure

Surgical Procedures
Numerous procedures are used for degenerative spine problems. Choice of procedure is based on the type and severity of degenerative changes and the surgeon's preference.
- Lumbar laminectomy or hemilaminectomy
- Microdiscectomy
- Foraminotomy
- Interspinous spacer placement
- Discectomy or fusion
- Cervical laminoplasty

Special Considerations
- Every surgeon has very specific needs for table and position.
- Neuromonitoring is common for all cervical or thoracic cases and many lumbar procedures.
- Fluoroscopy is common because many procedures are done with minimally invasive techniques.

Suggested Readings
Herkowitz HN, Garfin SR, Eismont FJ, et al: *Rothman-Simeone the spine,* ed 6, Philadelphia, 2011, Saunders.
Shen FH, Shaffrey CI: *Arthritis and arthroplasty: the spine,* Philadelphia, 2010, Saunders.
Yue JJ, Guyer RD, Johnson JP, et al: *The comprehensive treatment of the aging spine: minimally invasive and advanced techniques,* Philadelphia, 2011, Saunders.

SPINAL DEFORMITY

History
- Important to determine cause of curve initially
- Four general types of scoliosis:
  - Congenital: malformation of vertebrae
  - Neuromuscular: cerebral palsy, polio, tethered spinal cord, neurofibromatosis
  - Idiopathic: unknown, more common in girls
    - Degenerative
  - Kyphosis
    - Rounded or "hunch" back

Symptoms
- Backache or low back pain
- Fatigue
- Uneven appearance of shoulders, shoulder blades, or hips
- Abnormal spinal curvature
- May be noted by teacher or parent first
- May have neurologic or radiculopathy signs in cases of impingement

Physical Examination
- Progressive curve of the spine is noted.
- Curve changes can be subtle and require consistent measurement over time.
- Shoulder and pelvis height is often uneven.
- Severe curves can cause respiratory restriction; pulmonary function testing is needed in these cases.
- Check for skin changes or hairy patches on the back, signs of neurofibromatosis.
- Complete neuromuscular examination includes strength, Hoffman and Babinski reflexes, and clonus.

Imaging
- Standing full-length spine x-ray studies include AP and lateral views.
- Lateral bending films while standing may be needed as well.
- MRI is used to evaluate for tethered spinal cord and is useful in potential surgical cases.
- CT is used for evaluation of congenital deformity such as hemivertebra.
- Check the Cobb angle, which is the angle between two lines, drawn perpendicular to the upper endplate of the uppermost involved vertebrae and the lower endplate of the lowest involved vertebrae. For patients with two curves, Cobb angles are followed for both curves (Fig. 1-23).
  - In some patients, lateral-bending x-ray studies are obtained to assess the flexibility of the curves or the primary and compensatory curves.

Initial Treatment
Patient Education
- Often curves that are identified early require only monitoring. Bracing for immature idiopathic scoliosis is

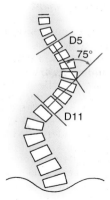

Figure 1-23. Cobb angle. *(From Canale ST, Beaty JH, editors:* Campbell's operative orthopaedics, *ed 11, Philadelphia, 2008, Mosby, p 1934.)*

poorly tolerated but, used with intensive exercise programs, has shown some improvement of outcome.

First Treatment Step
- Determine the type of deformity, as well as the cause, to determine further management.

Treatment Options
Nonoperative Management
- Close follow-up with x-ray studies is indicated to determine whether the curve is accelerating. In a growing adolescent, consider monitoring every 3 to 4 months after diagnosis, then at 6 months, and a year. An adult or skeletally mature patient can be monitored yearly. Progression of the curve is generally defined as a change of 5 degrees or more on consecutive x-ray studies.
- Symptomatic care is indicated for resulting pain or neural impingement if present.
- A brace and exercise program may be initiated. A brace may be indicated in a skeletally immature individual with 35 to 40 degrees of curvature. If the patient has reached skeletal maturity, a brace is not indicated.

Operative Management

Stabilization of the curve takes priority over correction. If correction is attempted, it may involve osteotomy (pedicle subtraction, Smith-Peterson, vertebrectomy) to correct sagittal or coronal deformity. Long or short segment instrumented fusions are used to stabilize these corrections. Growing rods in immature spines are commonly used, and pedicle screw and rod constructs placed posteriorly have replaced Harrington rod and wiring techniques for the most part. Anterior procedures are less common because lateral procedures are becoming more common.

Codes

ICD-9 codes: 737.0 to 737.9 Curvature of spine
    737.30 Scoliosis [and kyphoscoliosis], idiopathic
    737.40 Curvature of spine associated with other conditions
CPT codes: 22800 to 22819 Spinal fusion codes
    22840 to 22855 Spinal instrumentation codes

Operative Indications

- Failed bracing or exercise
- Curve acceleration
- Respiratory difficulty resulting from high-degree thoracic curve
- Cosmetic improvement
- Poor seating balance in patients with neuromuscular disorders

Informed Consent

- Nerve injury
- Paralysis
- Infection
- Scar
- Need for further surgery
- Failure to correct deformity
- Nonunion of fusion
- New deformity

Anesthesia

- General endotracheal anesthesia
- Long procedures, coordinate with anesthesia team for predicted blood loss and neuromonitoring. **Wake-up tests** should be planned for (postoperative neurologic examination; they can be conducted while in the OR when anesthesias is reduced and the patient can respond to commands).
- For anterior and posterior procedures, prepare for patient flip or repositioning. These procedures may be staged over several days.

Patient Positioning

This is based on the type of procedure and approach.

- Jackson table or similar radiolucent table
- Prone position with neck flexed for the posterior cervical approach
  - Watch shaving of hair; infection is a major risk.
  - Watch draping.
- Supine position for the anterior lumbar approach
- Lateral decubitus position for thoracolumbar lateral procedures
- Prone position for thoracolumbar spine posterior procedures
- Neuromonitoring very likely and recommended, with wires placed out of the way

Surgical Procedures

- Numerous procedures may be performed, based on the type and severity of deformity and the surgeon's preference. In general, spinal fusion with instrumentation is the treatment of choice.

Special Considerations

- Every surgeon has very specific needs for table, draping, and position.
- Neuromonitoring is common for all scoliosis cases.
- Fluoroscopy is common, and intraoperative CT is becoming more common.
- Ensure that staged cases are planned with all members of the team, especially anesthesia.

Suggested Readings

DeWald RL: *Spinal deformities: the comprehensive text,* New York, 2003, Thieme.
Herkowitz HN, Garfin SR, Eismont FJ, et al: *Rothman-Simeone the spine,* ed 6, Philadelphia, 2011, Saunders.
Shen FH, Shaffrey CI: *Arthritis and arthroplasty: the spine,* Philadelphia, 2010, Saunders.

TRAUMA AND SPINE FRACTURES
History
- Mechanism of injury is very important. Patients may have multiple other injuries, so planning surgical procedures and treatments may require coordination with other services.
- Often, patients have high-energy injuries such as falls from a height or MVC. Low-velocity injury can result in severe injury in patients with underlying osteoporosis or tumor.
- Thoracolumbar spine fractures are four times more common in men.
- In cases of neurologic complaints after a high-velocity injury, ensure spinal cord health.

Physical Examination
- Complete examination is critical for determining the injury extent and prognosis, especially in the case of an SCI.
- In addition to standard examinations and reflexes discussed in the beginning of the chapter, perform a rectal examination for tone in all suspected cases of SCI.

Cervical Clearance
- An alert, asymptomatic patient without a distracting injury or neurologic deficit and who is able to complete a functional ROM examination may safely be cleared from cervical spine immobilization without radiographic evaluation.
- If cross-table x-ray studies of the cervical spine from the skull to T1 are negative and the patient has cervical spine tenderness, leave the collar in place until voluntary flexion and extension radiographs or MRI can be performed.
- An initial CT scan during trauma evaluation is ideal and may discover occult injuries, especially with high-velocity mechanisms.
- Cervical spine injuries in patients with altered mental status are more difficult to evaluate. Recommendations for evaluation include removal of the cervical collar after 24 hours in patients with normal radiographs, indefinite immobilization in a cervical collar, CT scan evaluation, and more recently cervical flexion-extension examinations using dynamic fluoroscopy. CT may be more beneficial in that it allows for examination of the skull and cervical spine during same examination.

American Spinal Injury Association Examination: Figure 1-24
Imaging
- During initial trauma evaluation, CT is becoming more common to evaluate a head injury. Cervical spine or other isolated cuts can be done with little risk to the patient but a high yield in the ability to clear spine injury.
- X-ray study is used for cervical clearance as noted earlier, as well as to evaluate possible bony injury in the thoracolumbar spine.
- CT is useful for evaluation of fracture at all levels of the spine.
- MRI without contrast is used for evaluation of ligamentous structures, as well as for occult fracture of the spinal column.

Fracture Types
Cervical Fracture
- Rule of 3s:
  - The predentate space should be less than 3 mm.
  - The prevertebral soft tissue at C3 is usually 3 mm.
  - Anterior wedging of 3 mm or more suggests a fracture.

Atlantoaxial Dislocation
- Head slipped anteriorly on C1
- Usually fatal
- Children more commonly affected then adults

Neural Arch Fracture of C1
- Most common fracture of C1

Jefferson Fracture: Figure 1-25
- Compression or burst-type fracture to the atlas or C1 vertebrae
- Rare neural injury
- Seen on an open-mouth (odontoid view) x-ray study as a bilateral offset of C1-C2

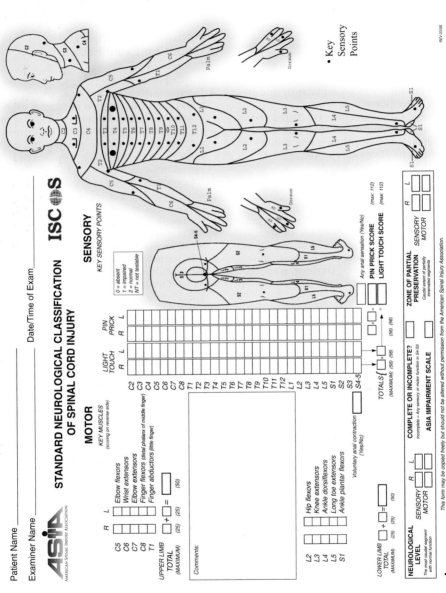

MUSCLE GRADING

0 Total paralysis

1 Palpable or visible contraction

2 Active movement, full range of motion, gravity eliminated

3 Active movement, full range of motion, against gravity

4 Active movement, full range of motion, against gravity and provides some resistance

5 Active movement, full range of motion, against gravity and provides normal resistance

5* Muscle able to exert, in examiner's judgment, sufficient resistance to be considered normal if identifiable inhibiting factors were not present

NT, [?] not testable. Patient unable to reliably exert effort or muscle unavailable for testing due to factors such as immobilization, pain on effort, or contracture.

ASIA IMPAIRMENT SCALE

☐ **A = Complete:** No motor or sensory function is preserved in the sacral segments S4-S5.

☐ **B = Incomplete:** Sensory but not motor function is preserved below the neurological level and includes the sacral segments S4-S5.

☐ **C = Incomplete:** Motor function is preserved below the neurological level, and more than half of key muscles below the neurological level have a muscle grade less than 3.

☐ **D = Incomplete:** Motor function is preserved below the neurological level, and at least half of key muscles below the neurological level have a muscle grade of 3 or more.

☐ **E = Normal:** Motor and sensory function are normal.

CLINICAL SYNDROMES (OPTIONAL)

☐ Central Cord
☐ Brown-Séquard
☐ Anterior Cord
☐ Conus Medullaris
☐ Cauda Equina

STEPS IN CLASSIFICATION

The following order is recommended in determining the classification of individuals with SCI.

1. Determine sensory levels for right and left sides.

2. Determine motor levels for right and left sides.
   Note: in regions where there is no myotome to test, the motor level is presumed to be the same as the sensory level.

3. Determine the single neurological level.
   This is the lowest segment where motor and sensory function is normal on both sides, and is the most cephalad of the sensory and motor levels determined in steps 1 and 2.

4. Determine whether the injury is Complete or Incomplete. (sacral sparing).
   If voluntary and contraction = **No** AND all S4-5 sensory scores = **0** AND any anal sensation = **No**, then injury is COMPLETE.
   Otherwise injury is incomplete.

5. Determine ASIA Impairment Scale (AIS) Grade:

   Is injury Complete? If **YES**, AIS=A Record ZPP
   (For ZPP record lowest dermatome or myotome on each side with some (non-zero score) preservation)

   NO ↓

   Is injury motor incomplete? If **NO**, AIS=B
   (Yes=voluntary anal contraction OR motor function more than three levels below the motor level on a given side.)

   YES ↓

   Are at least half of the key muscles below the (single) neurological level graded 3 or better?

   NO ↓ → AIS=C   YES ↓ → AIS=D

   If sensation and motor function is normal in all segments, AIS=E
   Note: AIS E is used in follow up testing when an individual with a documented SCI has recovered normal function. If at initial testing no deficits are found, the individual is neurologically intact; the ASIA Impairment Scale does not apply.

B

Figure 1-24. A and **B,** Standard neurologic classification of spinal cord injury from the American Spinal Injury Association (ASIA). *(From Canale ST, Beaty JH (eds) Campbell's operative orthopaedics. Vol 2. Mosby/Elsevier. 2008. fig 35-3, page 1765)*

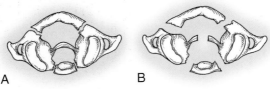

Figure 1-25. A and **B,** Jefferson fracture. *(From Canale ST, Beaty JH, editors:* Campbell's operative orthopaedics, *ed 11, Philadelphia, 2008, Mosby, p 1787.)*

Hangman's Fracture: Figure 1-26
- Fractures through the pedicles of C2 with anterior slippage of C2 on C3
- Most common cervical spine fracture
- Hyperextension or compression fracture

Clay Shoveler's Fracture
- C6, C7, or T1 spinous process fracture
- Stable
- Managed with collar, nonoperative care

Odontoid Fractures: Figure 1-27
- Hyperextension injury
- High nonunion rate
- Open mouth x-ray study or CT

Flexion-Compression Fracture: Figure 1-28
- High-velocity injury
- Large number of neural injuries
- Comminuted bone fragments in the spinal canal

Thoracolumbar Fractures
- Three-column evaluation for stability is performed (Fig. 1-29).

- If the middle column is intact, the fracture is stable.

Vertebral Compression Fracture: Figure 1-30
- Stable
- Often pathologic

Burst Fracture: Figure 1-31
- Axial loading injury
- Stable injury without neural component that can often be treated conservatively
- Advanced imaging critical for determining stability

Chance Fracture: Figure 1-32
- Horizontal fracture through the vertebra, lamina, pedicles, or spinous process
- Flexion-distraction mechanism of injury
- High-velocity injury
- Neural injury likely

Fracture-Dislocation: Figure 1-33
- SCI common
- High-velocity injury

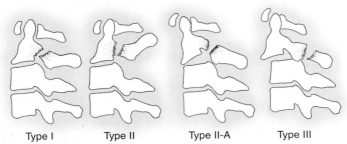

Type I   Type II   Type II-A   Type III

Figure 1-26. Hangman's fracture. *(From Canale ST, Beaty JH, editors:* Campbell's operative orthopaedics, *ed 11, Philadelphia, 2008, Mosby, p 1796.)*

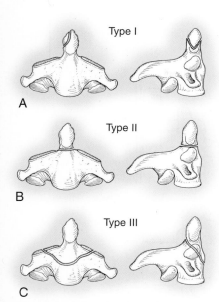

Figure 1-27. A to C, The three types of odontoid fractures. *(From Canale ST, Beaty JH, editors:* Campbell's operative orthopaedics, *ed 11, Philadelphia, 2008, Mosby, p 1791.)*

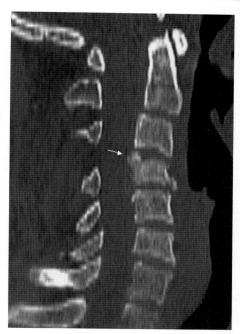

Figure 1-28. Teardrop fracture of C4 *(arrow)* as seen on sagittal computed tomography with retropulsed fragment. *(From Kim DH, Ludwig SC, Vaccaro AR, et al:* Atlas of spine trauma: adult and pediatric, *Philadelphia, 2008, Saunders, p 242.)*

Initial Treatment

- Determine the extent of injuries, and perform lifesaving procedures first. Unstable fractures may need immediate surgery in coordination with the rest of the trauma team. Consider SCI without radiographic abnormality (SCIWORA) in a young athlete or child with a likely mechanism, neural injury signs or symptoms, and normal radiographs.

Patient Education

- Many stable fracture patterns can be treated with bracing and cervical collars, but the clinician must ensure patient compliance. Frequent radiographic follow-up to ensure healing and proper alignment is important.

Treatment Options
Nonoperative Management

- Rigid cervical collars have been shown to be effective for low-velocity odontoid fractures when compared with operative care or halo placement.

- Reduction of cervical perched or jumped facets followed by evaluation of stability can be accomplished with closely supervised traction. These injuries are often unstable following reduction and require stabilization. Traction should be applied with a gradual increase in weight using a halo or tongs. Serial neurologic examinations, should be done and the procedure should be halted if neurologic status worsens.
- Bracing of thoracolumbar spine fractures includes rigid LSO, thoracolumbosacral orthosis (TLSO), or cervicothoracolumbar sacral orthosis (CTLSO). Ensure that the brace maintains alignment above and below the fracture.

Operative Management

- Stabilization procedures of the spine are commonly instrumented. Constructs vary by surgeon training and

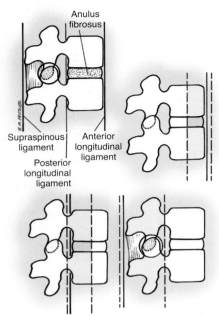

Figure 1-29. The three-column classification of spinal instability. *(From Canale ST, Beaty JH, editors:* Campbell's operative orthopaedics, *ed 11, Philadelphia, 2008, Mosby, p 1812.)*

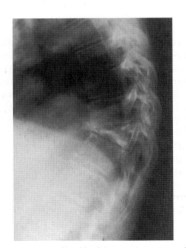

Figure 1-30. Radiographic appearance of **T11 compression fracture.** *(From Barr JD, Barr MS, Lemley TJ, et al: Percutaneous vertebroplasty for pain relief and spinal stabilization,* Spine *25:923, 2000.)*

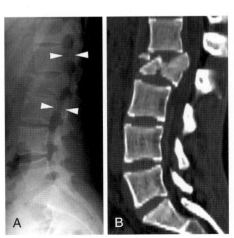

Figure 1-31. Burst fracture. **A,** X-ray appearance. **B,** Computed tomography appearance (note retropulsed fragment). *(From Czervionke LF, Fenton DS:* Imaging painful spinal disorders, *Philadelphia, 2011, Saunders, p 97.)*

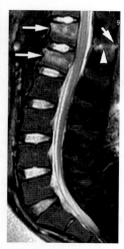

Figure 1-32. Chance fracture (flexion-distraction injury). The arrows indicate the fractures to the vertebral bodies and spinous process. *(From Czervionke LF, Fenton DS:* Imaging painful spinal disorders, *Philadelphia, 2011, Saunders, p 100.)*

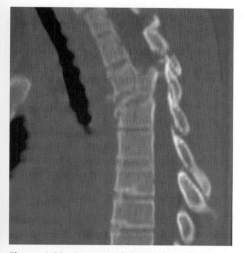

Figure 1-33. Fracture-dislocation appearance on sagittal computed tomography reconstructions. *(From Kim DH, Ludwig SC, Vaccaro AR, et al:* Atlas of spine trauma: adult and pediatric, *Philadelphia, 2008, Saunders, p 353.)*

fracture pattern. Alignment by manipulation or ligamentum taxis, as well as decompression of bone fragments, disc material, and ligament, should be accomplished in cases of neural impingement.

- Common procedures include:
  - Posterior instrumented decompression and fusion
  - Lateral thoracolumbar decompression and fusion

ICD-9 Codes
805 Fracture of vertebral column without mention of spinal cord injury. This code includes the neural arch, spine, spinous process, transverse process, and vertebra.
805.0 Cervical vertebra fracture, closed
805.1 Cervical vertebra fracture, open
805.2 Dorsal [thoracic] vertebra fracture, closed
805.3 Dorsal [thoracic] vertebra fracture, open
805.4 Lumbar vertebra fracture, closed
805.5 Lumbar vertebra fracture, open
839.0 Cervical vertebra dislocation, closed
- The following fifth-digit subclassification is for use with codes 805.0 to 805.1 and 839.01:
0 Cervical vertebra fracture, unspecified level
1 First cervical vertebra fracture
2 Second cervical vertebra fracture
3 Third cervical vertebra fracture
4 Fourth cervical vertebra fracture
5 Fifth cervical vertebra fracture
6 Sixth cervical vertebra fracture
7 Seventh cervical vertebra fracture
8 Multiple cervical vertebrae fracture
806 Fracture of vertebral column with spinal cord injury, that is, any condition classifiable to 805 with a complete or incomplete transverse lesion (of the spinal cord): hematomyelia, cauda equina, nerve paralysis, paraplegia, quadriplegia, spinal concussion.
806.0 Cervical, closed
806.1 Cervical, open
806.2 Dorsal [thoracic], closed
806.3 Dorsal [thoracic], open
806.4 Lumbar, closed
806.5 Lumbar, open

Surgical Procedures
- Anterior cervical discectomy and fusion
- Posterior instrumented decompression and fusion
- Lateral thoracolumbar decompression and fusion

CPT Codes

22035 Closed treatment of vertebral process fracture

22318 to 22328 Fracture-dislocation treatment codes

22532 to 22634 Arthrodesis codes

22554 Anterior cervical discectomy and fusion (ACDF)

63001 to 63048 Posterior extradural laminotomy or laminectomy for exploration or decompression of neural elements or excision of herniated intervertebral discs

Anterior Cervical Discectomy and Fusion (Similar for Cervical Disc Replacement)

Indications
- Cervical fracture
- Cervical stenosis or herniated nucleus pulposus (HNP)
- May be combined with posterior procedure

Approach
- A right-sided approach is common to avoid the recurrent laryngeal nerve. Use a transverse incision from the anterior edge of the sternocleidomastoid muscle to near the midline through the fascia to the platysma.
- Avoid damage to the esophagus with all retractor systems. Fluoroscopy is commonly used to ensure proper placement of retractors and instrumentation if used.
- Closure is typically with resorbable braided suture to the platysma and resorbable monofilament for subcuticular closure of skin. Dermabond may also be used. Dress with tape and gauze. A rigid or soft collar may be used, depending on the surgeon's technique. A drain may be used for a day.

Postoperative Course
- For patients without trauma or tumor, the procedure is typically outpatient or requires a 23-hour stay. Patients with trauma or neoplasm often stay longer because of other conditions. Redress the wound before discharge, and remove the drain if appropriate.

- Postoperative days 14 to 30
  - Return to the office for a wound check. An x-ray study of the cervical spine should be done as well. No therapy is given. The brace comes off if it was given for comfort and not stability.
- Postoperative days 60 to 90
  - X-ray studies, neurologic examination; increased activity, but activity limitations taught per surgeon's preference; physical therapy if needed for ROM
- Postoperative days 160 to 365
  - X-ray studies, functional evaluation

Thoracolumbar Procedures

Lumbar Decompression
- Could include microdiscectomy, laminectomy, hemilaminectomy

Indications
- Herniated disc
- Lumbar stenosis
- Rarely, tumor or infection

Approach
- For discectomy or hemilaminectomy, the approach is often slightly off the midline on the affected side. For laminectomy, the approach is at the midline at the affected level. Following skin incision, electrocautery is used to cut or dissect through the fascia for open procedures, and wire placement under fluoroscopy is followed by tube retractor placement.

Microdiscectomy (Removal of Herniated Disc Material)

1) Microscope
   Table or frame
   Retractor system (tube or McCulloch)
2) Typically an outpatient procedure or 23-hour stay; patient positioned in flexion; closure with absorbable braided stitch followed by subcuticular stitch and/or skin cement
3) Dressing removed as soon as no drainage
4) Follow-up on postoperative days 14 to 30 in office and again 6 to 12 weeks later; x-ray studies needed

only if concerns for destabilization (rare)
5) No physical therapy needed in most cases

Laminectomy (Decompression of Spinal Canal or Foramina Following Removal of Laminar Bone)
1) Table or frame
   Retractor system
   Fluoroscopy
   Neuromonitoring for thoracic spine
2) A 23-hour stay up to 2 days, depending on number of levels operated on; patient positioned in flexion; closure with suture or staples
3) Dressing change postoperative day 1 and then redressed until wound no longer draining
4) Follow-up postoperative days 14 to 30, 90 days and again 6 to 12 weeks later; x-ray studies taken at the first postoperative visit
5) Physical therapy after the first postoperative visit only if needed

Thoracolumbar Fusion (Posterior, Anterior, with or without Interbody)
This is used for instability, fracture, tumor or infection deformity reconstruction, and indirect decompression with interbody.
1) Radiopaque table
   Retractors (blade type for open, expandable tube for minimally invasive procedure)
   Fluoroscopy
   Neuromonitoring
2) Hospital stay determined by health of patient and disorder
3) Patients often needing home health care for dressings, nursing care, physical therapy in postoperative period, except after single level decompression-fusion or total disc replacement
4) Postoperative day 1: dressing change, out of bed to chair minimum except in cases of poor health. In-office follow-up for wound check 14 to 30 days postoperatively. Follow-up at 3, 6, and 12 months after the procedure, with goals of increasing activity and a return to the premorbid state

5) Patients with a deformity often need outpatient patient therapy only, depending on age and degree of surgery

Other Surgical Procedures
Transforaminal Interbody Fusion (TLIF) and Posterior Lumbar Interbody Fusion (PLIF)
- Patients with single-level cases performed with minimally invasive techniques may have 23-hour stays. Most patients stay 3 days total, including the day of surgery.
- Positioning is prone, and closure is done with two deep layers and subcuticular closure or Steri-strips, skin cement, or staples.

Total Disc Replacement (TDR)
- A regular OR table is in a lithotomy position. The surgeon is positioned between the patient's legs, and the assistant is to the side. The abdominal incision is similar to that used in anterior lumbar interbody fusion (ALIF), on the left side of the abdomen and 3 to 5 inches in length. After both these procedures, remember to watch bowel function or ileus.

Bone Graft Collection and Use
- Allograft (donor) bone is often used to pack interbody devices and to augment local bone and bone taken from the patient iliac rest (autograft) that contains stem cells and bone morphogenic proteins.
- The donor site for most spine surgery requiring autograft is the iliac crest. Significant morbidity and mortality from this site led to decreased use and increased use of allograft and bone alternative.
- Anterior: Make an incision on the anterior crest just below the anterior wing. Dissect to the periosteum to make a window in the cortex with a small osteotome or other instrument. Use a curette or rongeur to remove some cancellous bone from between the inner and outer cortical tables. Closure may require drains, and patients should be watched closely for infection.

■ Posterior: Make an incision longitudinally over the posterior crest. Dissect
using elevators to the periosteum.
Avoid cluneal nerves, ligaments of the
sacroiliac joint, and the superior gluteal
artery. A Taylor retractor is commonly
used at this time. An osteotome is used
to breach the cortex, followed by
gouges and curettes to collect the graft.
Drains are often needed following this
technique. The posterior procedure
has the advantage of significantly
more bone availability and proximity

to the lumbar spine for draping and
positioning.

Suggested Readings

DeWald RL: *Spinal deformities: the comprehensive
text,* New York, 2003, Thieme.
Herkowitz HN, Garfin SR, Eismont FJ, et al:
Rothman-Simeone the spine, ed 6,
Philadelphia, 2011, Saunders.
Kim DH, Ludwig SC, Vaccaro AR, et al: *Atlas of
spine trauma: adult and pediatric,* Philadelphia,
2008, Saunders.
Shen FH, Shaffrey CI: *Arthritis and arthroplasty:
the spine,* Philadelphia, 2010, Saunders.

Shoulder and Humerus 2
Jennifer A. Hart

ANATOMY OF JOINT
Bones: Figures 2-1 through 2-3

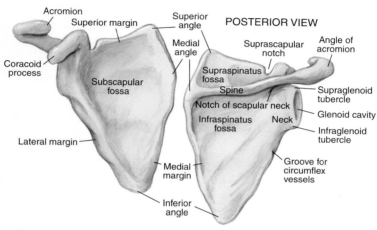

Figure 2-1. The scapula. *(From Miller MD, Chhabra AB, Hurwitz SR, et al, editors:* Orthopaedic surgical approaches, *Philadelphia, 2008, Saunders, p 8.)*

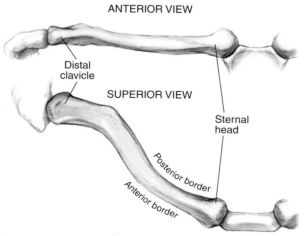

Figure 2-2. The clavicle. *(From Miller MD, Chhabra AB, Hurwitz SR, et al, editors:* Orthopaedic surgical approaches, *Philadelphia, 2008, Saunders, p 9.)*

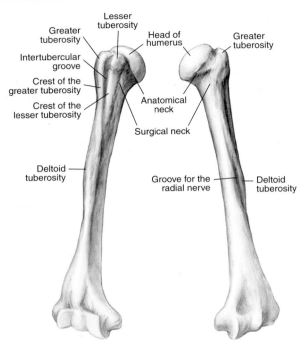

Figure 2-3. The humerus. *(From Miller MD, Chhabra AB, Hurwitz SR, et al, editors:* Orthopaedic surgical approaches, *Philadelphia, 2008, Saunders, p 11.)*

Ligaments: Figures 2-4 and 2-5

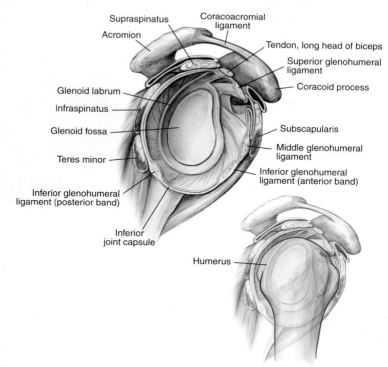

Figure 2-4. The glenohumeral joint. *(From Miller MD, Chhabra AB, Hurwitz SR, et al, editors: Orthopaedic surgical approaches, Philadelphia, 2008, Saunders, p 13.)*

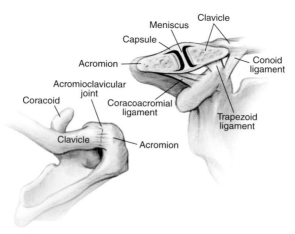

Figure 2-5. The acromioclavicular (AC) joint. *(From Miller MD, Chhabra AB, Hurwitz SR, et al, editors: Orthopaedic surgical approaches, Philadelphia, 2008, Saunders, p 13.)*

Muscles and Tendons:
Figure 2-6

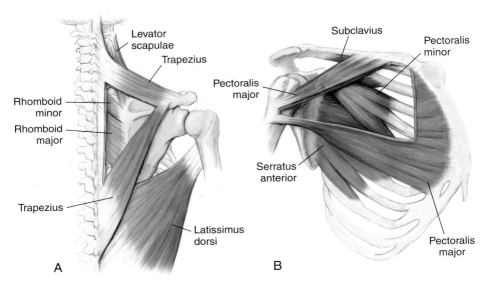

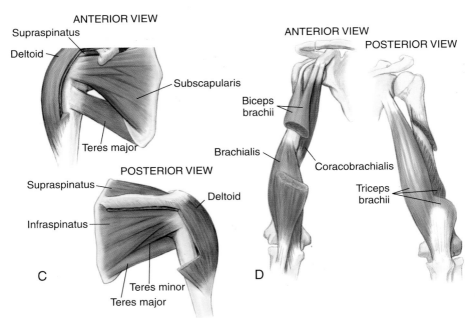

Figure 2-6. A to **D,** The muscles of the shoulder and upper arm. *(From Miller MD, Chhabra AB, Hurwitz SR, et al, editors:* Orthopaedic surgical approaches, *Philadelphia, 2008, Saunders, p 15.)*

Nerves and Arteries:
Figures 2-7 through 2-9

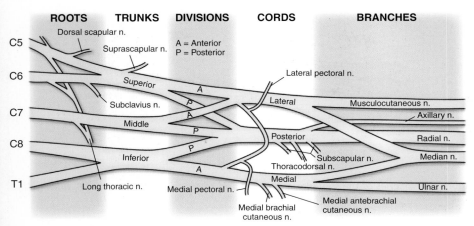

Figure 2-7. The brachial plexus. *(From Miller MD, Chhabra AB, Hurwitz SR, et al, editors: Orthopaedic surgical approaches, Philadelphia, 2008, Saunders, p 16.)*

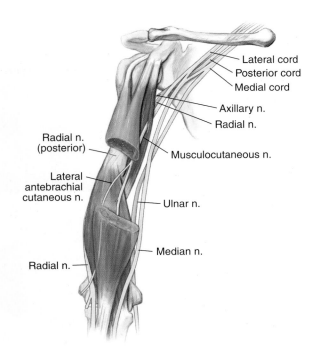

Figure 2-8. Major branches of the brachial plexus in the upper arm. *(From Miller MD, Chhabra AB, Hurwitz SR, et al, editors:* Orthopaedic surgical approaches, *Philadelphia, 2008, Saunders, p 17.)*

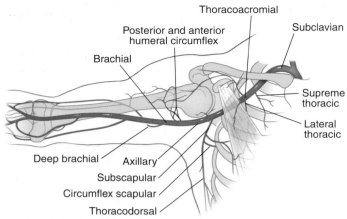

Figure 2-9. Arteries of the shoulder and upper arm. (*From Miller MD, Chhabra AB, Hurwitz SR, et al, editors:* Orthopaedic surgical approaches, *Philadelphia, 2008, Saunders, p 18.*)

Surface Anatomy: Figure 2-10

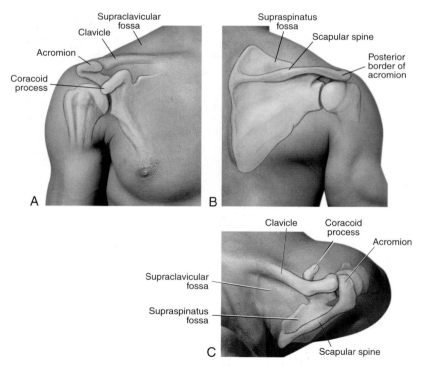

Figure 2-10. A to C, Surface landmarks and underlying anatomy of the shoulder. (*From Miller MD, Chhabra AB, Hurwitz SR, et al, editors:* Orthopaedic surgical approaches, *Philadelphia, 2008, Saunders, p 20.*)

Normal Radiographic Appearance: Figure 2-11 A-C

PHYSICAL EXAMINATION

Inspect for deformity or muscle atrophy.
Palpate the specific structures to evaluate for deformity or tenderness:
- Acromioclavicular (AC) joint
- Glenohumeral joint
- Scapula body
- Coracoid process
- Biceps tendon/bicipital groove

Normal range of motion (ROM):
Table 2-1

Special Tests

Neer Impingement Sign
- *Tests for* shoulder impingement
- *Performed by* fully passively forward flexing the shoulder
- *Positive test* indicated by pain in this position

Table 2-1. Normal Shoulder Range of Motion

Forward Flexion	180 degrees
Abduction	180 degrees
External Rotation	90 degrees
Internal Rotation	90 degrees

Hawkins Impingement Sign
- *Tests for* shoulder impingement
- *Performed by* passively forward flexing the shoulder to 90 degrees and internally rotating with the elbow flexed.
- *Positive test* indicated by pain in this position

Cross-body Adduction Test
- *Tests for* AC joint dysfunction (e.g., osteolysis, shoulder separation, arthritis)

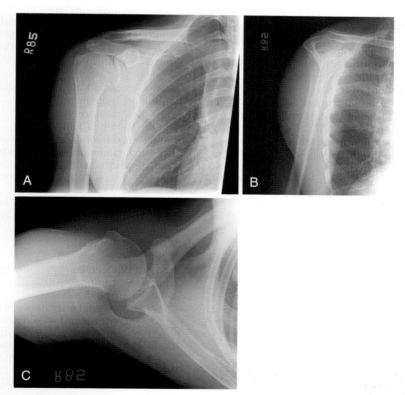

Figure 2-11. Normal shoulder radiographs. **A,** Anteroposterior view. **B,** Outlet view. **C,** Axillary view.

- *Performed by* passively moving the arm into maximum adduction across the body
- *Positive test* indicated by pain over the AC joint in this position

Supraspinatus Stress Test
- *Tests for* rotator cuff abnormality (e.g., impingement or tear)
- *Performed by* having the patient hold the arm in 90 degrees of abduction and the thumb pointed down to the floor while holding against downward resistance by the examiner
- *Positive test* indicated by weakness and/or pain

Drop Arm Sign
- *Tests for* rotator cuff tear, usually massive
- *Performed by* having the patient hold the arms with the shoulder abducted to 90 degrees with the thumbs down
- *Positive test* indicated by an inability to hold the arm in this position

External Rotation Strength
- *Tests for* rotator cuff tear (infraspinatus)
- *Performed by* asking the patient to hold the arm against the side with the elbow in 90 degrees of flexion and externally rotating against resistance from the examiner
- *Positive test* indicated by weakness

Lift-off Test
- *Tests for* rotator cuff tear (subscapularis)
- *Performed by* asking the patient to internally rotate the arm to allow the dorsum of the hand to rest just off the back and then to hold that position against resistance by the examiner
- *Positive test* indicated by weakness

Belly Press Test
- *Tests for* rotator cuff tear (subscapularis); alternative to lift-off test for patients unable to position their arm behind their back
- *Performed by* asking the patient to use the heel of the hand and press it into his or her abdomen while holding the elbow forward

- *Positive test* indicated by an inability to hold the elbow forward, thus allowing it to drift back to the side

Sulcus Sign
- *Tests for* general shoulder laxity
- *Performed by* applying downward force on the humerus
- *Positive test* indicated by the appearance of a "gap" between the humeral head and the acromion

Apprehension Test
- *Tests for* shoulder instability (anterior)
- *Performed by* asking the patient to lie supine while the examiner passively moves the shoulder into an abducted and externally rotated position
- *Positive test* indicated by "apprehension" on the part of the patient as he or she feels the shoulder slide anteriorly

Relocation Test
- *Tests for* shoulder instability
- *Performed by* first doing an apprehension test and, after obtaining a positive response, applying a posterior force to the humeral head with the examiner's other hand
- *Positive test* indicated by relief of the "apprehension"

Jerk Test
- *Tests for* posterior shoulder instability
- *Performed by* abducting the arm to 90 degrees, internally rotating it, and applying an axial load to the shoulder while adducting the arm
- *Positive test* indicated by a sudden jerk as the humeral head slides over the edge of the glenoid

O'Brien Test
- *Tests for* superior labrum anterior to posterior (SLAP) tear
- *Performed by* having the patient hold the arm in 90 degrees of forward flexion and 10 to 20 degrees of adduction with the thumb down then resisting a downward force to the arm applied by the examiner; test repeated with the thumb up
- *Positive test* indicated by pain, which should be worse with the "thumb

down" position; if pain present also in the "thumb up" position, may indicate an AC joint problem

Differential Diagnosis: Table 2-2

SHOULDER IMPINGEMENT
History
- Overuse, repetitive activity
- Shoulder pain, worse with overhead lifting or reaching, can radiate to lateral upper arm (deltoid area)

Physical Examination
- May be tender anteriorly
- ROM typically normal (if not, suspect adhesive capsulitis)
- Positive Hawkins and/or Neer impingement signs
- May have weakness secondary to pain with abduction or supraspinatus strength testing

Imaging
- Anteroposterior (AP), axillary, outlet commonly used "standard" radiographic views

Radiographic Image: Figure 2-12A and B

Table 2-2. Differential Diagnosis

Anterior shoulder pain	Shoulder impingement Biceps tendinitis Arthritis Rotator cuff tear Instability Labral tear
Posterior shoulder pain	Periscapular muscle pain Posterior instability Cervical radiculopathy Posterior labral tear Subscapular bursitis Scapula fracture
Superior shoulder pain	Acromioclavicular joint osteolysis Acromioclavicular joint arthritis Clavicle fracture Shoulder (AC) separation Superior labral tear
Arm pain	Humerus fracture Rotator cuff tear Shoulder impingement Cervical radiculopathy

Initial Treatment
Patient Education
- Shoulder impingement is part of the spectrum of rotator cuff injury. Generally, in the early stages this involves inflammation (bursitis and rotator cuff

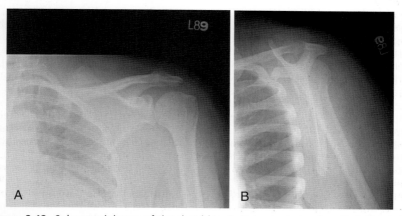

Figure 2-12. Subacromial spur of the shoulder. **A,** Anteroposterior view. **B,** Outlet view.

tendinitis) without actual tearing of the tendon. Partial tears can develop over time and can progress to a full-thickness tear. If symptoms do not improve with early treatment, call the office because a magnetic resonance imaging (MRI) scan may be necessary to evaluate for a rotator cuff tear.

First Treatment Steps
- Begin general antiinflammatory measures including nonsteroidal antiinflammatory drugs (NSAIDs), ice, and activity modification.
- Perform subacromial steroid injection.
- Begin physical therapy that emphasizes rotator cuff strengthening exercises.
- If symptoms persist despite injection and physical therapy, consider ordering an MRI scan with an arthrogram of the shoulder to evaluate the integrity of the rotator cuff.
- Use of a sling is generally discouraged because this can lead to shoulder stiffness and adhesive capsulitis.

Treatment Options
Nonoperative Management
- Nonoperative management is indicated if the patient has pain without evidence of a full-thickness rotator cuff tear (night pain, weakness on examination, history of recent shoulder dislocation in patient over the age of 40 years).
- Treatment generally begins with the addition of NSAIDs and/or subacromial steroid injection.
- Physical therapy and/or a home program with Thera-Bands should be started to focus on rotator cuff strengthening.
- Work restrictions may be necessary if the patient has a job that involves repetitive activity or overhead reaching with the affected arm, to prevent repeat aggravation of the inflammation.
- Prognosis for shoulder impingement is good with these nonsurgical treatment options.
- Generally the patient should be reevaluated in 6 weeks to check ROM and strength.
- Failure to improve at that point may warrant further evaluation of rotator cuff integrity with an MRI arthrogram.

- Generally, failure to improve with one to two subacromial injections and a minimum of 6 weeks of physical therapy should prompt referral to a surgeon to consider surgical options for shoulder impingement.

Operative Management: Subacromial Decompression
Codes
ICD-9 code: 726.10 Shoulder impingement, disorders of the bursae and tendons in the shoulder region, unspecified

CPT codes: 29826 Arthroscopic acromioplasty (Shoulder arthroscopic decompression of the subacromial space with partial acromioplasty, with or without coracoacromial release) 23130 Open acromioplasty (acromioplasty or acromionectomy, partial with or without coracoacromial ligament release)

Operative Indications
- Shoulder pain that has failed to improve with nonoperative treatment including subacromial injection and physical therapy
- Absence of other potential causes of shoulder pain such as cervical radiculopathy

Informed Consent and Counseling
- Routine surgical risks should be discussed with the patient (infection, bleeding, bruising, surgical pain, continued symptoms, and anesthesia complications).
- If your institution routinely uses nerve blocks as part of postoperative pain management, the expected duration of action of these blocks should be discussed.
- Generally, the patient is expected to be in a sling for up to 2 weeks, and use of the sling is discontinued based on patient comfort.
- Physical therapy is generally expected after surgery for approximately 6 weeks.
- Informed consent should include the possibility of rotator cuff repair if an unexpected tear is discovered at the time of surgery because this could lead to a longer recovery time

(6 weeks in a sling and an average of 12 weeks of physical therapy).

Anesthesia
- General anesthesia with or without nerve block

Patient Positioning
- Beach chair or lateral decubitus (surgeon preference)

Surgical Procedures
- Arthroscopic acromioplasty
- Open acromioplasty

Arthroscopic Acromioplasty
- The posterior portal is first created as the primary viewing portal for the arthroscope, followed by the anterior portal (working portal) for instruments.
- Diagnostic arthroscopy should be performed before the initiation of any procedure, with careful evaluation of the glenohumeral joint, labrum, biceps tendon, rotator cuff, and joint capsule.
- Placing the camera in the posterior portal and directing it superiorly allows visualization of the subacromial space.
- A lateral portal can be made to pass instruments for the acromioplasty.
- Electrocautery or radiofrequency devices may be superior to routine arthroscopic shavers because they help to control bleeding as the highly vascular bursa is débrided.
- After the bursa is adequately débrided, the coracoacromial ligament is cut, and an arthroscopic bur is used to remove impinging bone from the inferior surface of the acromion.
- Adequate bony resection should be confirmed before removing the arthroscope and closing the portals.

Estimated Postoperative Course
- Initial postoperative visit (7 to 14 days)
  - Suture removal
  - Physical therapy orders
  - Pain medication refill, if necessary
  - Discontinuation of sling as tolerated
  - Review of work status, light duty desk work generally for 6 weeks

- 6-week postoperative visit
  - Evaluate wound healing, ROM, and strength.
  - Determine the need for additional physical therapy.
  - Review the return to work plan.
- 12-week postoperative visit (optional)
  - Generally only if pain is persistent, motion is limited, or reevaluation of work status is needed

Suggested Readings
Mazzocca AD, Alberta FG, Cole BJ, et al: Shoulder: patient positioning, portal placement, and normal arthroscopic anatomy. In Miller MD, Cole BJ, editors: *Textbook of arthroscopy,* Philadelphia, 2004, Saunders.
Miller MD, Hart JA, MacKnight JM, editors: *Essential orthopaedics,* Philadelphia, 2010, Saunders.
Willenborg MD, Miller MD, Safran MR: Shoulder arthroscopy. In Miller MD, Chhabra AB, Safran MR, editors: *Primer of arthroscopy,* Philadelphia, 2010, Saunders.

ROTATOR CUFF TEARS
History
- Pain is located in the anterior and lateral shoulder.
- Pain frequently radiates to the deltoid area, but not usually below elbow.
- Tears are generally atraumatic, with progression of pain and weakness over time.
- They may be related to an acute trauma (e.g., fall on the outstretched hand).
- Waking at night is one of the frequently described symptoms.
- The patient may or may not complain of weakness in that arm.

Physical Examination
- Active ROM may be limited, but passive ROM is generally full.
- Hawkins and Neer impingement signs may or may not be present.
- The drop arm sign (inability to hold the arm in an abducted position against gravity) indicates a likely massive rotator cuff tear.
- The supraspinatus stress test (weak with resisted abduction) is positive.
- Weakness with resisted external rotation indicates involvement of the infraspinatus.

- A positive lift-off or belly press sign indicates involvement of the subscapularis.
- A positive O'Brien sign indicates involvement of the biceps tendon.

Imaging
- Plain radiography should include AP, axillary, and outlet views.
- An MRI scan with arthrogram is the "gold standard" for diagnosing and evaluating the extent of rotator cuff disease (Fig. 2-13).
- A computed tomography (CT) arthrogram may be necessary for patients who are unable to undergo MRI (e.g., patients with a pacemaker).

Classification System
- Rotator cuff tears are typically described by the number of tendons involved, the size of the tear, the amount of tendon retraction, and the degree of fatty atrophy of the rotator cuff muscles.
- Partial tears are commonly seen in patients who are more than 40 years old and may or may not be symptomatic. It is helpful to determine the

percentage of involved tendon with MRI to determine treatment.
- Complete rotator cuff tears should be described by the number of involved tendons and the amount of retraction.
- Massive tears are generally defined as those involving two or more tendons and retracted more than 5 cm.
- Rotator cuff arthropathy denotes massive, retracted, chronic rotator cuff tears that are generally considered irreparable.
  - These patients are significantly weak on examination and may demonstrate a drop arm sign.
  - Diagnosis can be made by plain radiographs when proximal migration of the humeral head relative to the glenoid is seen (Fig. 2-14).
- At the time of arthroscopy, rotator cuff tears can further be described by the shape of the tear (e.g., U-shaped tear).

Initial Treatment
- Initial treatment is determined by the size of the rotator cuff tear.
- Partial rotator cuff tears involving less than 50% of the total tendon area may respond well to conservative treatment including NSAIDs, subacromial steroid injections, and physical therapy.
- High-grade partial rotator cuff tears (involving >50% of the total tendon

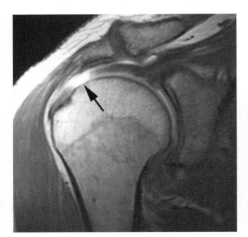

Figure 2-13. Complete tear of the supraspinatus tendon *(arrow)*. *(From Miller MD, Sanders TG, editors:* Presentation, imaging, and treatment of common musculoskeletal conditions: MRI-arthroscopy correlation, *Philadelphia, 2012, Saunders, p 41.)*

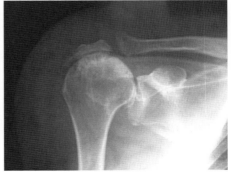

Figure 2-14. Radiologic appearance of rotator cuff arthropathy. Note superior migration of the humeral head.

area) may be treated conservatively but may require surgical repair. This decision is determined by the degree of the patient's pain and dysfunction and the severity of the tear (for a 60% tear, an attempt at conservative treatment is more likely, whereas a 90% tear may suggest the need for earlier operative intervention).

- Complete rotator cuff repairs should be treated with surgery in most cases.

Patient Education

- Rotator cuff tears occur as a spectrum of injury ranging from tendinitis to partial tearing to complete tear to irreparable tear.
- Complete tears of the rotator cuff require surgery to repair the tendon.
- Patients should use the shoulder normally to maintain ROM but avoid repetitive overhead activities and heavy lifting.

First Treatment Steps

- Complete rotator cuff tears should be referred to a shoulder surgeon.
- Although surgical treatment is not urgent, ideally surgery occurs in the first 1 to 3 months of diagnosis because of the risk of tendon retraction with longer delays.
- The use of a sling should be avoided because this can lead to the development of adhesive capsulitis.

Treatment Options
Nonoperative Management

- Nonoperative management typically is reserved for partial, low-grade rotator cuff tears.
- NSAIDs, subacromial steroid injections, and physical therapy effective in managing pain and improving function.
- Patients should be instructed to follow up for a new evaluation if conservative treatment does not improve symptoms in 6 to 8 weeks.
- MRI arthrogram, if not already performed, may be necessary at that point to evaluate for a full-thickness rotator cuff tear.

Operative Management: Rotator Cuff Repair
Codes
ICD-9 code: 727.61 Complete rupture of the rotator cuff
CPT code: 29827 Arthroscopy, shoulder, with rotator cuff repair

Operative Indications
- Complete tear of the rotator cuff
- High-grade partial tear of the rotator cuff
- Partial rotator cuff tear that has failed to improve with conservative treatment

Informed Consent and Counseling
- Routine surgical risks should be discussed with the patient (infection, bleeding, bruising, surgical pain, continued symptoms, and anesthesia complications).
- If your institution routinely uses nerve blocks as part of the postoperative pain management, the expected duration of action of these blocks should be discussed.
- Generally, the patient is expected to be in a sling for approximately 6 weeks postoperatively.
- Physical therapy is generally started after the first postoperative appointment and continued for 12 weeks.
- Return to full function can take 6 to 12 months.

Anesthesia
- General, often with accompanying nerve block

Patient Positioning
- Beach chair or lateral decubitus (surgeon's preference)

Surgical Procedures
- Arthroscopic rotator cuff repair
- Open rotator cuff repair (may be used based on the surgeon's experience or because of massive tears in which adequate repair cannot be obtained arthroscopically)

Rotator Cuff Repair
- For arthroscopic repair, the posterior portal is first created as the primary

viewing portal for the arthroscope, followed by the anterior portal (working portal) for instruments.

- Diagnostic arthroscopy should be performed before the initiation of any procedure, with careful evaluation of the glenohumeral joint, labrum, biceps tendon, rotator cuff, and joint capsule.
- For open repair, an incision is made in the anterior aspect of the shoulder lateral to the acromion along the Langer lines; access to the joint capsule is gained through the deltoid either by splitting the fibers (traditional open approach) or detaching it from the acromion (mini-open approach).
- Acromioplasty is typically performed as described earlier.
- The rotator cuff is evaluated to determine the degree of tear, the shape of the tear, and retraction.
- Partial-thickness tears of less than 50% can be débrided with the shaver rather than repaired.
- Full-thickness tears and high-grade partial tears must be mobilized and repaired.
- Arthroscopic repair is performed by passing sutures through the cuff tissue and directly repairing it to the bone by suture anchors.
- Margin convergence may be necessary before direct repair of tendon back to bone in the case of L-shaped or U-shaped tears (Fig. 2-15).
- Sutures are then passed either in antegrade or retrograde fashion and are secured to suture anchors placed in the footprint (single row, double row, suture bridge technique, as preferred by the surgeon).

- In open repair, direct suture repair to bone is performed by passing sutures through bone tunnels and then tying knots.
- Sutures are tensioned, and the repair is examined before irrigation and closure of the portals and/or incision.

Estimated Postoperative Course
- Initial postoperative visit (7 to 14 days)
  - Suture removal
  - Physical therapy orders given to focus on passive ROM of the shoulder only
  - Pain medication refill, if necessary
  - Continued use of sling removing only for pendulum exercises and elbow motion
  - Review of work status; light duty desk work begun as tolerated by patient, with no use of surgical arm
- 6-week postoperative visit
  - Evaluation of wound healing, ROM, and strength
  - New physical therapy orders to begin active-assisted ROM, active motion, and gentle early rotator cuff strengthening exercises
  - Removal of sling
  - Light duty work continued for a minimum of 6 additional weeks
- 12-week postoperative visit
  - Evaluate the progression of ROM and strength.
  - Determine the need for additional physical therapy.
  - Discuss the return to work plan.

Suggested Readings
Miller MD, Hart JA, MacKnight JM, editors: *Essential orthopaedics,* Philadelphia, 2010, Saunders.

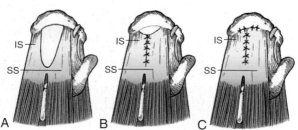

Figure 2-15. A to C, Margin convergence technique. IS, infraspinatus; SS, supraspinatus. *(From Miller MD, Cole BJ: Textbook of arthroscopy, Philadelphia, 2004, Saunders.)*

Morse K, Davis AD, Afra R, et al: Arthroscopic versus mini-open rotator cuff repair: a comprehensive review and meta-analysis, *Am J Sports Med* 36:1824–1828, 2008.

Willenborg MD, Miller MD, Safran MR: Shoulder arthroscopy. In Miller MD, Chhabra AB, Safran MR, editors: *Primer of arthroscopy,* Philadelphia, 2010, Saunders.

Wolf BR, Dunn WR, Wright RW: Clinical sports medicine update: indications for repair of full-thickness rotator cuff tears, *Am J Sports Med* 35:1007–1016, 2007.

SHOULDER INSTABILITY

History

- Shoulder instability may be traumatic or atraumatic.
- Traumatic shoulder dislocations most commonly occur with the shoulder in an abducted and externally rotated position causing immediate pain, shoulder deformity, and loss of motion.
- Patients may report a "dead" arm syndrome resulting from transient traction on the brachial plexus or the axillary nerve.
- Atraumatic shoulder instability may be more vague, with pain or subluxation events during activity such as overhead throwing or swimming.
- It is important to differentiate dislocation from subluxation during the history, as well as the number of episodes (acute, recurrent).
- Other causes of shoulder dislocation include seizure disorders and electric shock (posterior dislocation).
- Hyperligamentous laxity can predispose to instability, as can a history of such conditions as Ehlers-Danlos syndrome or Marfan syndrome.

Physical Examination

- Acute dislocations produce deformity and loss of motion.
- Decreased sensation occurs over the "deltoid patch" initially and resolves with time.
- Apprehension and relocation tests are positive.
- A positive sulcus sign with inferior instability, often bilateral, indicates multidirectional instability.
- A positive supraspinatus stress test may indicate an associated rotator cuff tear in patients who are more than 40 years old.

Imaging: Figures 2-16 and 2-17

- AP and axillary views are indicated at a minimum (the **axillary view** is important to confirm reduction).
- Stryker notch and West Point views can be helpful for chronic, recurrent instability:
  - Stryker notch: Hill Sachs lesion
  - West Point view: bony Bankart lesion
- MRI arthrogram is used to evaluate labral tear (patients <40 years old) or rotator cuff tear (patient >40 years old) with shoulder dislocation or instability.
- CT scan may be helpful in recurrent shoulder instability to evaluate the glenoid for bone loss (important to determine the need for a concomitant bony procedure).

Classification System

- Direction of instability (anterior, posterior, multidirectional)

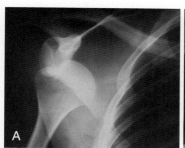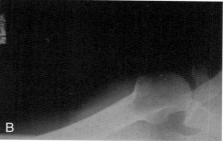

Figure 2-16. A, Anteroposterior view of anterior shoulder dislocation. **B,** Axillary view; note the large Hill Sachs lesion.

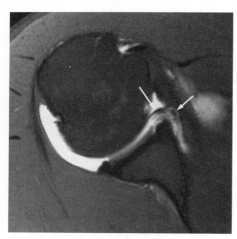

Figure 2-17. Magnetic resonance imaging appearance of anterior labral tear (cartilaginous Bankart lesion; arrows). *(From Miller MD, Sanders TG, editors:* Presentation, imaging, and treatment of common musculoskeletal conditions: MRI-arthroscopy correlation, *Philadelphia, 2012, Saunders, p 56.)*

- Chronicity (acute or chronic, first-time dislocation, recurrent)
- By anatomic description of disease:
  - Glenoid labrum articular disruption (GLAD)
  - Anterior labral periosteal sleeve avulsion (ALPSA)
  - Humeral avulsion of the glenoid labrum (HAGL)

Initial Treatment
Patient Education
Shoulder dislocations should be reduced as soon as possible, usually in an emergency department. Pain improves rapidly after the shoulder is reduced and can usually be controlled with antiinflammatory medications and ice. Typically, the shoulder remains sore for several weeks after an acute dislocation. Shoulder strengthening with physical therapy is helpful after acute shoulder dislocation. The rate of recurrence is highest in younger patients.

First Treatment Steps
- Acute dislocation should be treated with reduction, although this may need to be done in the emergency department because sedation may be required.
- A sling is useful for patient comfort initially.
- Antiinflammatory medication and/or narcotic pain medication should be provided for early postinjury pain.
- Follow up in the clinic 1 to 2 weeks after acute dislocation should be set up to reevaluate motion and strength.

Treatment Options
Nonoperative Management
- Nonoperative management is indicated for most first-time shoulder dislocations and cases of multidirectional instability.
- Narcotic pain medications should be used only for initial postinjury pain and discontinued as soon as the patient is comfortable. NSAIDs may be used at that point if necessary.
- A sling can be used and discontinued based on patient comfort.
- Physical therapy can be helpful to decrease pain, restore normal ROM, and improve rotator cuff and scapula stabilizer strength.
- Recurrent episodes of instability or failure to improve with this nonoperative treatment plan may necessitate MRI with arthrogram to evaluate the labrum.
- Clinicians should have a high index of suspicion for rotator cuff tear in patients more than 40 years old who have shoulder dislocation.

Operative Management: Arthroscopic Bankart Repair and Capsulorrhaphy
Codes
ICD-9 codes: 718.81 Shoulder instability
    718.31 Shoulder instability, recurrent
    831.00 Shoulder dislocation
CPT codes: 29806 Arthroscopy, shoulder, surgical; capsulorrhaphy

Operative Indications
- Recurrent shoulder dislocation
- Symptomatic shoulder instability
- Multidirectional instability with failure of appropriate course of conservative treatment

Informed Consent and Counseling
- Routine surgical risks should be discussed with the patient (infection, bleeding, bruising, surgical pain, continued symptoms, and anesthesia complications).
- If your institution routinely uses nerve blocks as part of the postoperative pain management, the expected duration of action of these blocks should be discussed.
- Generally, the patient is expected to be in a sling for approximately 6 weeks postoperatively.
- Physical therapy is generally started after the first postoperative appointment and continued for 12 weeks.
- Return to sport should be restricted until 6 months postoperatively.

Anesthesia
- General with or without nerve block

Patient Positioning
- Beach chair or lateral decubitus (surgeon preference)

Surgical Procedures
- Arthroscopic Bankart repair (with or without capsulorrhaphy)
- Open Bankart repair (with or without capsulorrhaphy)
- Latarjet procedure
- Open glenoid bone grafting

Arthroscopic Bankart Repair
- Routine diagnostic arthroscopy is performed.
- Examination under anesthesia with arthroscopic visualization can identify engaging Hill Sachs lesions.
- Labral tears should be identified and may require mobilization and elevation up onto the face of the glenoid if the tissue has scarred down medially.
- The "bumper pad" effect of the labrum is restored by passing suture secured to anchors placed on the glenoid rim.

Estimated Postoperative Course
- Initial postoperative visit (7 to 14 days)
  - Suture removal
  - Physical therapy orders given to focus on passive ROM, with

avoidance of extreme abduction and external rotation
  - Pain medication refill, if necessary
  - Continued use of the sling, removed only for pendulum exercises and elbow motion
  - Review of work or sports status; light duty desk work begun as tolerated by the patient, with no use of surgical arm or athletics
- 6-week postoperative visit
  - Evaluation of wound healing, ROM, and strength
  - New physical therapy orders to advance ROM and begin strengthening exercises
  - Removal of sling
- 12-week postoperative visit
  - Evaluate the progression of ROM and strength.
  - Determine the need for additional physical therapy.
  - Discuss the return to work and sports plan (usually no collision or throwing sports until 6 months postoperatively).

Suggested Readings
McCarty ED, Ritchie P, Gill HS, et al: Shoulder instability: return to play, *Clin Sports Medi,* 23:335–351, 2004.

Provencher MT, Bhatia S, Ghodadra NS, et al: Recurrent shoulder instability: current concepts for evaluation and management of glenoid bone loss, *J Bone Joint Surg Am* 92(Suppl 2):133–151, 2010.

Shah AS, Karadsheh MS, Sekiya JK: Failure of operative treatment for glenohumeral instability: etiology and management, *Arthroscopy* 27(5):681–694, 2011.

Young AA, Maia R, Berhouet J, et al: Open Latarjet procedure for management of bone loss in anterior instability of the glenohumeral joint, *J Shoulder Elbow Surg* 20(2):S61–S69, 2011.

SUPERIOR LABRAL TEARS AND BICEPS TENDON DISORDERS
History
- These injuries are common in overhead throwing athletes from repetitive stress on the biceps anchor.
- They may be traumatic, mostly commonly from a fall on the outstretched hand or a traction injury (e.g., catching oneself

from a fall by grabbing something overhead).

- Patients typically report pain anterior and deep in the shoulder that is worse with overhead reaching and the throwing motion.
- They can be associated with mechanical catching.

Physical Examination

- Several special tests have been described to identify SLAP tears such as the O'Brien (active compression) test.
- Glenohumeral internal rotation deficit (GIRD) should be documented because this is a common finding with internal impingement in throwing athletes.
- Otherwise, ROM and strength are generally normal.

Imaging

- Standard AP, outlet, and axillary radiographs (usually normal)
- MRI with arthrogram (the preferred imaging modality)

Magnetic Resonance Imaging: Figure 2-18

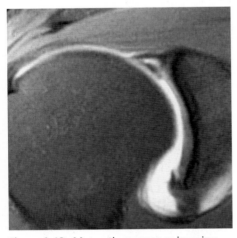

Figure 2-18. Magnetic resonance imaging appearance of superior labrum anterior to posterior (SLAP) tear. *(From Miller MD, Sanders TG, editors:* Presentation, imaging, and treatment of common musculoskeletal conditions: MRI-arthroscopy correlation, *Philadelphia, 2012, Saunders, p 69.)*

Classification System: Figure 2-19

- The original Snyder classification system of SLAP tears included types I to IV, but types V to VII were added later:
  - Type I: degenerative tearing of the superior labrum with intact biceps anchor
  - Type II: detachment of the superior labrum and biceps anchor (most common)
  - Type III: bucket handle tear of the superior labrum but intact biceps anchor
  - Type IV: tearing of the superior labrum that extends up into the biceps tendon
  - Type V: superior labral tear in addition to anterior or posterior labral tear
  - Type VI: flap tear of the superior labrum
  - Type VII: superior labral tear with extension to the capsule
- Classification of proximal biceps disease is typically descriptive (tendinopathy, partial tear, complete rupture).

Initial Treatment
Patient Education

Although tears of the biceps tendon attachment in the shoulder can result from an injury, they more commonly occur from repetitive activity that stresses this area. Injections may provide some temporary relief, but these conditions often require surgery for correction.

First Treatment Steps

- Any loss of motion should first be corrected with physical therapy (sleeper stretch may be necessary for GIRD to stretch the posterior capsule).
- NSAIDs may be helpful if the patient is in pain and has pain-related difficulty doing exercises.
- Glenohumeral injections may temporarily relieve pain and can be diagnostic if the patient has other symptoms that confuse the clinical picture.

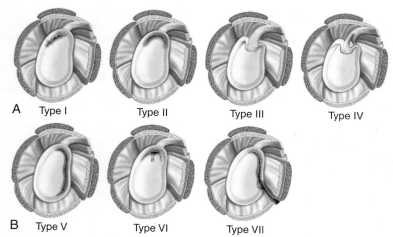

A Type I   Type II   Type III   Type IV

B Type V   Type VI   Type VII

Figure 2-19. Classification of superior labrum anterior to posterior (SLAP) tears. *(From Miller MD, Thompson S, Hart JA, editors:* Review of orthopaedics, *ed 6, Philadelphia, 2012, Saunders. Adapted from Kepler CL, Nho SJ, Sherman SL, et al: Superior labral tear. In Reider B, Terry M, Provencher MT, editors:* Operative techniques: sports medicine surgery, *Philadelphia, 2009, Saunders.)*

Treatment Options
Nonoperative Management
- Nonoperative management can be initiated early with NSAIDs, activity modification, glenohumeral injection, and/or physical therapy.
- MRI with arthrogram should be performed when conservative treatment fails or in high-level athletes who are unable to perform at their normal level of activity.
- If surgery is considered, tenotomy versus tenodesis should be discussed because the best procedure is still debated in the literature.
- Complete ruptures of the proximal biceps tendon are treated conservatively with reassurance, ice, NSAIDs, and rest.

Operative Management
Codes
ICD-9 codes: 840.7 Superior glenoid labrum lesion (SLAP tear)
   840.8 Biceps rupture, proximal
   726.12 Biceps tendinitis
CPT codes: 29807 Arthroscopy, shoulder, surgical; repair of SLAP lesion
   29822 Arthroscopy, shoulder, débridement, limited (biceps tenotomy)
   29828 Arthroscopy, shoulder, biceps tenodesis
   23430 Tenodesis of long tendon of biceps, open

Operative Indications
- Symptomatic SLAP tears
- Biceps tendinopathy that has failed to improve with conservative treatment
- Symptomatic biceps tendon subluxation

Informed Consent and Counseling
- Routine surgical risks (infection, bleeding, bruising, surgical pain, continued symptoms, and anesthesia complications) should be discussed, as well as expectations of nerve blocks if these blocks are used at your institution.
- For patients considered for biceps tenotomy or tenodesis, the difference between these two procedures should be discussed (e.g., "popeye" deformity for tenotomy, longer sling for tenodesis).
- Generally, the patient is expected to be in a sling for approximately 6 weeks postoperatively for SLAP repairs and biceps tenodesis and only

to comfort (about 2 weeks) for tenotomy.
- Physical therapy is generally started after the first postoperative appointment and is continued for 12 weeks.
- Return to sport should be restricted until 6 months postoperatively.

Anesthesia
- General, with or without a nerve block

Patient Positioning
- Beach chair or lateral decubitus (surgeon preference)

Surgical Procedures
- Arthroscopic débridement
- Arthroscopic superior labral repair
- Biceps tenotomy
- Biceps tenodesis

Arthroscopic Labral Débridement or Repair
- Diagnostic arthroscopy is initially performed according to routine protocol.
- Classification of the superior labral tear is performed to determine appropriate treatment:
  - Type I: débridement
  - Type II: SLAP repair
  - Type III: débridement, repair if unstable
  - Type IV: SLAP repair or tenodesis
  - Type V: labral repair
  - Type VI: débridement
  - Type VII: repair or stabilization
- Repair of the superior labrum is performed by placing anchors on either side of the biceps tendon and passing or tying sutures.

Arthroscopic Biceps Tenotomy or Tenodesis
- Diagnostic arthroscopy is initially performed according to routine protocol.
- The biceps tendon should be visually inspected by using a probe to pull the proximal tendon into the joint.
- Biceps tenotomy is performed by simply releasing the proximal biceps and débriding the stump.
- Biceps tenodesis is performed by first releasing the tendon and then reattaching it by suturing it to the rotator

cuff or securing it to the proximal humerus through a bone tunnel.
- The tenodesis is secured by anchors or a screw.

Estimated Postoperative Course
- Initial postoperative visit (7-14 days)
  - Suture removal
  - Physical therapy orders given to focus on passive ROM, with avoidance of resisted elbow flexion (biceps tenotomy can progress strengthening immediately)
  - Pain medication refill, if necessary
  - Continued use of sling, with removal only for pendulum exercises and elbow motion (biceps tenotomy, can remove as comfortable)
  - Review of work or sports status, light duty desk work begun as tolerated by the patient, with no use of surgical arm or athletics
- 6-week postoperative visit
  - Evaluation of wound healing, ROM, and strength
  - New physical therapy orders to advance ROM and begin strengthening exercises
  - Removal of sling
- 12-week postoperative visit
  - Evaluate the progression of ROM and strength.
  - Determine the need for additional physical therapy.
  - Discuss the return to work and sports plan (usually no collision or throwing sports until 6 months postoperatively).

Suggested Readings
Abrams GD, Safran MR: Diagnosis and management of superior labrum anterior to posterior lesions in overhead athletes, *Br J Sports Med* 44(5):311–318, 2010.
Keener JD, Brophy RH: Superior labral tears of the shoulder: pathogenesis, evaluation, and treatment, *Am Acad Orthop Surg* 17(10): 627–637, 2009.
Longo UG, Loppini M, Marineo G, et al: Tendinopathy of the tendon of the long head of the biceps, *Sports Med Arthrosc* 19(4):321–332, 2011.
Milewski M, Hart JA, Miller MD: Sports medicine. In Miller MD, Thompson S, Hart JA, editors: *Review of Orthopaedics,* ed 6, Philadelphia, 2012, Saunders.
Rainey R, Miller MD, Anderson M, et al: Superior labral injuries. In Miller MD, Sanders TG,

editors: *Presentation, imaging, and treatment of common musculoskeletal conditions: MRI-arthroscopy correlation,* Philadelphia, 2012, Saunders, 65–69.

GLENOHUMERAL OSTEOARTHRITIS

History

- Most commonly a progressive degenerative condition
- May be posttraumatic
- Often seen in patients with a history of shoulder instability and a remote history of surgical treatment of that instability (e.g., Putti-Platt or Magnuson procedure)
- Complaints of pain, crepitus, and progressive loss of motion

Physical Examination

- Active and passive ROM is often limited.
- Crepitus is frequently noted during motion testing.
- Strength is typically not affected, except in cases of associated rotator cuff disease (e.g., rotator cuff arthropathy).

Imaging

- AP and axillary radiographs are usually sufficient to make the diagnosis.
- The most common findings are an inferior humeral osteophyte and glenohumeral joint space narrowing.

Radiographic Image: Figure 2-20

Classification

- Mild, moderate, or severe, based on the amount of glenohumeral joint space narrowing

Initial Treatment

Patient Education

Glenohumeral osteoarthritis refers to progressive "wear and tear" changes to the ball and socket joint in the shoulder. Although this can occur from an old injury, it more commonly develops with increasing age from use. Arthritis has no definitive cure, so treatment is based on modifying activities and trying various treatments to control the pain that range from antiinflammatory drugs to injections to shoulder replacement.

First Treatment Steps

- Ice, NSAIDs, rest, activity modification
- Glenohumeral steroid injections, usually done under fluoroscopic guidance for improved accuracy
- Physical therapy to improve ROM and rotator cuff strengthening

Treatment Options

Nonoperative Management

- Ice, NSAIDs, rest, activity modification
- Glenohumeral steroid injections, usually done under fluoroscopic guidance for improved accuracy
- Physical therapy to improve ROM and rotator cuff strengthening

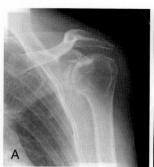
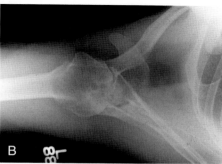

Figure 2-20. A and **B,** Radiographic appearance of glenohumeral osteoarthritis. Note inferior humeral osteophyte and joint space narrowing.

Operative Management
Codes
ICD-9 codes: 715.1 Osteoarthritis shoulder
CPT codes: 29823 Shoulder arthroscopy, débridement, extensive
23472 Total shoulder replacement

Operative Indications
- Shoulder osteoarthritis that has failed to respond to nonoperative treatment
- Pain secondary to shoulder osteoarthritis that affects activities of daily living

Informed Consent and Counseling
- Standard surgical risks should be discussed in detail (e.g., bleeding, infection, failure, anesthesia risks).
- Shoulder arthroscopy can be useful in relieving some mechanical catching and locking related to osteoarthritis, but it rarely relieves all the symptoms.
- Total shoulder replacements are effective at treating pain from osteoarthritis but they do not usually restore normal function and ROM (some stiffness should be expected postoperatively).

Anesthesia
- General, likely with nerve block

Patient Positioning
- Beach chair or lateral decubitus (arthroscopy)
- Modified beach chair (total shoulder replacement)

Surgical Procedures
- Arthroscopic débridement
- Total shoulder arthroplasty

Total Shoulder Arthroplasty
- A standard deltopectoral approach is used to access the glenohumeral joint.
- The biceps tendon is released within the bicipital groove.
- Osteotomy of the lesser tuberosity is performed, and the subscapularis is taken down to allow dislocation of the joint for access.
- The humeral canal is reamed, and a humeral head cutting jig is used for the humeral head osteotomy.
- The glenoid is exposed, the labral tissue is excised, and the glenoid bone is reamed in preparation for the implant.
- The appropriately sized implants are cemented into place, and the shoulder is reduced; the final position is confirmed with imaging.
- After copious irrigation, the wound is closed in layers according to routine protocol.

Estimated Postoperative Course
- Initial postoperative visit (7 to 14 days)
  - Suture or staple removal
  - Physical therapy orders given to focus on ROM in the early period
  - Pain medication refill, if necessary
  - Sling used for comfort and discontinued as tolerated by the patient
- 6-week postoperative visit
  - Evaluation of wound healing, ROM, and strength
  - New physical therapy orders to advance ROM and begin strengthening exercises
- 12-week postoperative visit
  - Evaluate the progression of ROM and strength.
  - Determine the need for additional physical therapy.
  - Counsel the patient that ROM and strength improvements continue over upcoming months.

Suggested Readings
Boileau R, Sinnerton R, Chuinard C, et al: Arthroplasty of the shoulder, *J Bone Joint Surg Br* 88:562–575, 2006.
Denard PJ, Wirth MA, Orfaly RM: Management of glenohumeral arthritis in the young adult, *J Bone Joint Surg Am* 93(9):885–892, 2011.
Miller MD: Shoulder and arm. In Miller MD, Chhabra AB, Hurwitz SR, et al, editors: *Orthopaedic surgical approaches,* Philadelphia, 2008, Saunders.

ADHESIVE CAPSULITIS
History
- The patient has progressive loss of motion.
- Pain is worse at the end ROMs.
- The origin of adhesive capsulitis not well understood, but the condition is believed to be an inflammatory process and is often seen in patients with

a history of an autoimmune disorder, especially diabetes mellitus.

- Other related factors may include history of trauma, thyroid disease, period of immobilization, associated cervical disease, and multiple medical comorbidities, but often occurs in the absence of all these conditions.

Physical Examination
- Both passive ROM and active ROM are restricted.
- The patient exhibits increased pain at the end ROM during the examination.
- Often supine ROM measurements are more accurate with this condition.
- Careful documentation is important to assess improvement after treatment.

Imaging
- Standard AP, axillary, and outlet radiographs are usually normal but are important to evaluate for other conditions that can affect ROM, such as shoulder osteoarthritis.

Initial Treatment
Patient Education
Adhesive capsulitis is better known as "frozen shoulder." It is caused by scarring of the joint capsule that causes pain and stiffness in the shoulder joint. It is more common in diabetic patients but can also be seen in completely healthy patients with no history of shoulder problems. Generally, frozen shoulder is self-limiting, but the process can be long and can take more than a year or two to resolve without appropriate treatment steps.

First Treatment Steps
- Ice and antiinflammatory medications are generally used to help control pain.
- The use of a sling should be avoided because this can increase joint stiffness.
- Glenohumeral joint steroid injections, generally done under fluoroscopic guidance for improved accuracy, are extremely helpful initially.
- Physical therapy is the key to the nonoperative management, with the focus on both passive and active ROM.

- Patients should be encouraged to work on passive ROM exercises on their own at home in addition to formal physical therapy sessions.

Treatment Options
Nonoperative Management
- Ice and antiinflammatory medications are generally used to help control pain.
- The use of a sling should be avoided because this can increase joint stiffness
- Glenohumeral joint steroid injections, generally done under fluoroscopic guidance for improved accuracy, are extremely helpful initially.
- Physical therapy is the key to the nonoperative management, with the focus on both passive and active ROM.
- Patients should be encouraged to work on passive ROM exercises on their own at home in addition to formal physical therapy sessions.

Operative Management: Arthroscopic Lysis of Adhesion and Manipulation under Anesthesia
Codes
ICD-9 codes: 726.0 Adhesive capsulitis, shoulder
CPT codes: 29825 Arthroscopic lysis of adhesions and manipulation under anesthesia

Operative Indications
- Adhesive capsulitis that has been refractory to conservative treatment (often two glenohumeral injections and a minimum of 12 weeks of physical therapy)

Informed Consent and Counseling
- Standard surgical risks should be discussed in detail (e.g., bleeding, infection, failure, anesthesia risks).
- Physical therapy should be set up before surgery to begin in the immediate postoperative period (postoperative day 1 or 2).
- Recurrence of this condition is common even with surgical treatment.

Anesthesia
- General, with or without a block
- Consideration of leaving a catheter in place for continuous block infusion for severe refractory cases, to allow early aggressive physical therapy

Patient Positioning
- Beach chair or lateral decubitus (surgeon preference)

Surgical Procedures
Arthroscopic Lysis of Adhesions and Manipulation under Anesthesia
- Examination under anesthesia should be done before beginning the surgical procedure and preoperative ROM recorded.
- Standard arthroscopic portals are made, and diagnostic arthroscopy is performed as described earlier.
- A shaver is used to débride the rotator interval, and the middle glenohumeral ligament is released along with the capsular tissue, with caution used to avoid the rotator cuff tendon.
- After changing portals, the posterior joint is similarly débrided, and tight posterior capsular tissue is released.
- Postoperative ROM should be measured and recorded to ensure that adequate release was performed before portal closure.

Estimated Postoperative Course
- Early postoperative period (days 0 to 6)
  - Physical therapy to emphasize ROM should start as early as 1 to 2 days after surgery.
  - Use of a sling should be avoided, and home ROM exercises should be encouraged immediately.
- Initial postoperative visit (7 to 14 days)
  - Suture or staple removal
  - Physical therapy orders given to focus on ROM in the early period
  - Pain medication refill, if necessary
  - Sling used for comfort and discontinued as tolerated by the patient
- 6-week postoperative visit
  - Evaluation of wound healing, ROM, and strength.
  - New physical therapy orders to advance ROM and begin strengthening exercises
- 12-week postoperative visit
  - Evaluate the progression of ROM and strength.
  - Determine the need for additional physical therapy.
  - Counsel the patient that ROM and strength improvements continue over upcoming months.
  - Additional fluoroscopically guided glenohumeral injections may be necessary for patients with persistent symptoms postoperatively, but these injections are typically delayed for at least 6 weeks after surgery.

Suggested Readings
Hannafin JA, Chiaia TA: Adhesive capsulitis: a treatment approach, *Clin Orthop Relat Res* 372:95–109, 2000.

MacKnight JM: Adhesive capsulitis (frozen shoulder). In Miller MD, Hart JA, MacKnight JM, editors: *Essential orthopaedics,* Philadelphia, 2010, Saunders, pp 172–174.

Neviaser AS, Neviaser RJ: Adhesive capsulitis of the shoulder, *Am Acad Orthop Surg* 19(9): 536–542, 2011.

Shaffer B. Tibone JE, Kerlan RK: Frozen shoulder: a long-term follow-up, *J Bone Joint Surg Am* 72:738–746, 1992.

ACROMIOCLAVICULAR JOINT INJURIES AND DISORDERS
History
- AC separations
  - Trauma with most likely reported mechanism a fall onto the lateral point of the shoulder
  - Common in collision sports (e.g., football) from a direct hit to the shoulder
  - Pain localized over the AC joint
  - Often a "lump" or deformity reported over the AC joint
- AC joint osteolysis and osteoarthritis
  - Usually more insidious onset of pain, although old trauma possibly reported
  - Pain again localized over the AC joint
  - Pain worse when reaching across the body (adduction)

- Possible history of weight lifting or other repetitive activity

Physical Examination

- Possible deformity over the AC joint in acute or chronic separations
- Focal tenderness over the AC joint
- Palpation of the entire clavicle and also the sternoclavicular joint in cases of trauma
- Cross-body adduction pain

Imaging

- Plain radiographs of the shoulder include a bilateral AP view of the AC joint (comparison), as well as an axillary view of the affected shoulder (type IV AC separation; see later).
- The Zanca view may be helpful to visualize the AC joint for osteolysis or osteoarthritis.

Radiographic Image: Figure 2-21

Classification System

- AC separation (Fig. 2-22)
  - Type I: AC sprain only, possible widening of the AC joint but no elevation of the distal clavicle
  - Type II: Complete tear of the AC ligament but intact coracoclavicular (CC) ligament
  - Type III: AC and CC ligament rupture, elevation of distal clavicle up to 100% of the contralateral side
  - Type IV: *Posterior* displacement of the distal clavicle through the trapezius (need axillary view to diagnose)

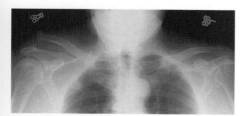

Figure 2-21. Radiographic appearance of acromioclavicular separation. Note bilateral radiographs for comparison of coracoclavicular distance.

- Type V: AC and CC ligament injury with elevation greater than 100% of the contralateral side (twice the other CC distance)
- Type VI: inferior displacement of the distal clavicle below the coracoid (rare)
- AC osteolysis and osteoarthritis
  - Mild, moderate, severe

Initial Treatment

Patient Education

- AC separation
  - AC separations are very painful in the first few weeks of injury, and treatment is based on the degree of separation. More minor separations begin to improve rapidly after that time, and symptoms generally resolve within 6 to 8 weeks. More severe separations may require surgery to repair the damaged structures.
- AC osteolysis and osteoarthritis
  - These conditions occur secondary to repetitive stresses across this small joint and can affect people of all ages. Generally, treatment is conservative with antiinflammatory medications (pills or injections) and avoidance of activities that aggravate the pain. If symptoms persist, surgery to remove the affected bone end surfaces is an option.

First Treatment Steps

- Treatment of AC separations begins with identifying the severity of the injury (radiographs)
  - Types I and II AC separations are treated conservatively with rest, activity modification, and antiinflammatory medications.
  - Type III separations are most commonly treated conservatively initially, and surgery is considered only for patients with persistent symptoms.
  - Types IV, V, and VI separations require surgery to restore the AC joint.
- Treatment of AC joint osteolysis and osteoarthritis should begin with ice, rest, activity modification, and antiinflammatory medications.

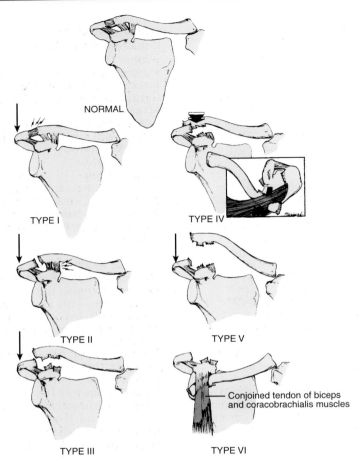

Figure 2-22. Classification of acromioclavicular (AC) separations. Type I: AC sprain. Type II: Complete AC tear, intact coracoacromial (CC) ligament. Type III: AC and CC ligament tear, displacement up to 100% of contralateral side. Type IV: Posterior displacement of clavicle through trapezius muscle; requires axillary view for diagnosis. Type V: Displacement of more than 100% of the contralateral side. Type VI: (Rare) inferior displacement of clavicle below coracoids. *(From Rockwood CA Jr, Young DC: Disorders of the acromioclavicular joint. In Rockwood CA Jr, Matsen FA III, editors: The shoulder, ed 2, Philadelphia, 1998, Saunders.)*

Treatment Options
Nonoperative Management

- Conservative treatment for AC joint injuries (types I, II, and most type III), as well as osteolysis or osteoarthritis, should begin with resting the shoulder and avoiding activities that aggravate the pain.
- Antiinflammatory medications are useful.

- AC joint injections are very effective in controlling pain and are also useful to localize symptoms in cases of more generalized pain.
- Activities can progress as pain improves.
- AC joint padding should be used for collision athletes (e.g., football players) as they return to play.

Operative Management: Acromioclavicular Joint Reconstruction and Distal Clavicle Excision

Codes
ICD-9 codes: 716.91 AC joint arthritis (unspecified arthropathy of the shoulder)
840.0 Sprain, acromioclavicular joint/ligament
CPT codes: 29824 Shoulder arthroscopic distal claviculectomy
23120 Open distal claviculectomy
23550 Open treatment of acromioclavicular dislocation
23552 Open treatment of acromioclavicular dislocation, with graft

Operative Indications
- Types IV, V, and VI AC separations
- Type III AC separations that are persistently symptomatic despite adequate conservative treatment
- AC joint osteolysis, AC joint degenerative disease, very distal clavicle fractures (distal clavicle excision)

Informed Consent and Counseling
- Standard surgical risks should be discussed in detail (e.g., bleeding, infection, failure, anesthesia risks).
- The use of a sling will be necessary for a minimum of 6 weeks postoperative (AC joint reconstruction).
- No heavy lifting, reaching, or repetitive activity with this shoulder is permitted for 3 to 6 months.
- Recurrence is a relatively common complication of AC joint reconstruction procedures.

Anesthesia
- General anesthesia, with or without nerve block

Patient Positioning
- Beach chair or lateral decubitus (arthroscopic distal clavicle excision)
- Beach chair or modified beach chair (AC reconstruction)

Surgical Procedures

Arthroscopic Distal Clavicle Excision
- Standard arthroscopic portals are made, and diagnostic arthroscopy performed as previously described.
- The coracoacromial ligament is incised, with care taken to limit the dissection medially to avoid vascular injury.
- An arthroscopic bur is used to remove 1 to 1.5 cm of bone from the distal clavicle, with careful evaluation to ensure that adequate bony resection is performed before closure.

Acromioclavicular Joint Reconstruction (Modified Weaver-Dunn Procedure)
- An incision is made starting approximately 2 to 3 cm posterior to the AC joint and extending to the tip of the coracoid.
- The approach is carried down to expose the lateral clavicle and the AC joint.
- The distal clavicle (1 to 1.5 cm) is resected, and then the coracoid is exposed.
- Reconstruction is performed using surgical tape, braided suture, or tendon graft (allograft or autograft) according to the preference of the surgeon.
- This tape, suture, or graft is passed either through drill holes through the coracoid and distal clavicle or looped around the bone and secured after appropriate reduction of the AC joint is obtained.
- Reduction should be confirmed and maintained through passive ROM of the shoulder before irrigating and closing the wound in layers according to routine protocol.

Estimated Postoperative Course
- Early postoperative period (days 0 to 6)
  - Sling at all times, with removal only for elbow motion (AC joint reconstruction)

- Sling for comfort only (AC joint resection)
- Initial postoperative visit (7 to 14 days)
  - Suture or staple removal
  - Physical therapy generally delayed until the 2- to 6-week point (surgeon's preference) for reconstructions but may begin immediately for distal clavicle excision
  - Pain medication refill, if necessary
  - Sling continued for AC joint reconstruction but weaned as tolerated by the patient after simple AC joint resection
- 6-week postoperative visit
  - Evaluate wound healing and distal clavicle deformity.
  - Radiographs of AC joint should be obtained.
  - Begin physical therapy to start gentle ROM exercises.
- 12-week postoperative visit
  - Evaluate the progression of ROM and strength.
  - Obtain new radiographs of the AC joint.
  - Assess job status and consider continued light duty for next 2 to 3 months.

Suggested Readings

Emberg LA, Potter HG: Radiographic evaluation of the acromioclavicular and sternoclavicular joints, *Clin Sports Med* 22:255–275, 2003.

Rabalais RD, McCarty E: Surgical treatment of symptomatic acromioclavicular joint problems: a systematic review, *Clinical Orthop Relat Res* 455:30–37, 2007.

Rokito AS, Oh, YH, Zuckerman JD: Modified Weaver-Dunn procedure for acromioclavicular joint dislocations, *Orthopedics* 27(1):21, 2004.

Simpson M, Howard MS: Acromioclavicular degenerative joint disease. In Miller MD, Hart JA, MacKnight JM, editors: *Essential orthopaedics,* Philadelphia, 2010, Saunders, pp 178–181.

FRACTURES OF THE SHOULDER
History
- The patient usually has a history of a fall or other trauma.
- Pain is the most common symptom.

- Deformity may be present at the site of injury.
- Numbness or tingling into the hand or discoloration distal to the shoulder should prompt neurovascular evaluation.

Physical Examination
- Inspect for laceration or skin defects (possible open fracture), ecchymosis, and deformity.
- Skin tenting is common with displaced clavicle fractures, and the integrity of skin overlying fracture fragment is important in determining possible surgical treatment.
- ROM should be evaluated, with acute loss concerning for fracture-dislocation.
- Tenderness and crepitus are noted over the fracture site.
- A thorough neurovascular examination of the extremity should be performed.

Imaging
- Radiographs
  - AP and axillary radiographs are indicated at a minimum.
  - AP and tangential views of the clavicle should be added for suspected clavicle fracture.
  - Scapula views are useful for posterior pain and suspicion of scapula fracture.
- CT scan may be necessary for displaced proximal humerus fractures and scapula fractures.

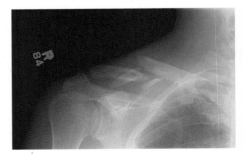

Figure 2-23. Radiographic appearance of midshaft clavicle fracture.

Radiographic Image: Figures 2-23
and 2-24

Classification System
Clavicle Fractures
- Described by displacement and location (middle third, medial third, lateral third)
- Distal clavicle fractures are further classified based on involvement of the CC ligaments:
  - Type I: intact CC ligaments, nondisplaced fracture
  - Type II: displaced fracture, medial to CC ligaments
    - Type IIA: CC ligaments attached to fracture fragment (Fig. 2-25)
    - Type IIB: fracture between the CC ligaments
  - Type III: intra-articular fracture (involves AC joint)

Proximal Humerus Fractures
- Neer classification (Fig. 2-26)

Initial Treatment
Patient Education
Fractures around the shoulder joint commonly occur from falls and motor vehicle accidents. These injuries can be very painful, and a sling is helpful to limit shoulder motion and reduce pain. Many shoulder fractures can be treated without surgery, but others may require a surgical procedure to align the bone ends more accurately for improved outcome. Radiographs and/or CT scan will be necessary to make the best treatment decision.

First Treatment Steps
- Treatment depends on the degree of displacement of the fracture.
- Minimally displaced fractures may be treated with the application of a sling or shoulder immobilizer.
- Adequate pain control may require narcotic pain medications; the use of antiinflammatory medications in fracture care is controversial.

Treatment Options
Nonoperative Management
- Treatment depends on the degree of displacement of the fracture.
- Minimally displaced fractures may be treated with the application of a sling or shoulder immobilizer.
- Adequate pain control may require narcotic pain medications; the use of antiinflammatory medications in fracture care is controversial.

Operative Management: Open Reduction and Internal Fixation of Clavicle Fractures
Codes
ICD-9 code: 810.0 Fracture of clavicle
CPT code: 23515 Clavicle open reduction, internal fixation

Operative Indications
- Still controversial: traditionally, most clavicle fractures treated nonoperatively, but more of these fractures currently managed surgically for improved shoulder mechanics

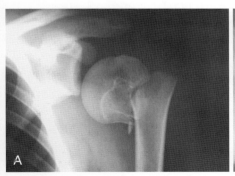
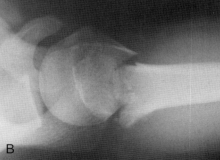

Figure 2-24. Radiographic appearance of proximal humerus fracture. **A,** Anteroposterior view. **B,** Axillary view.

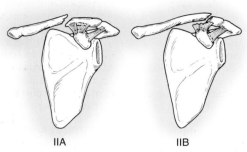

IIA   IIB

Figure 2-25. Neer type II clavicle fractures. *(From Canale ST, Beaty JH, editors:* Campbell's operative orthopaedics, *ed 11, Philadelphia, 2008, Mosby, p 3372.)*

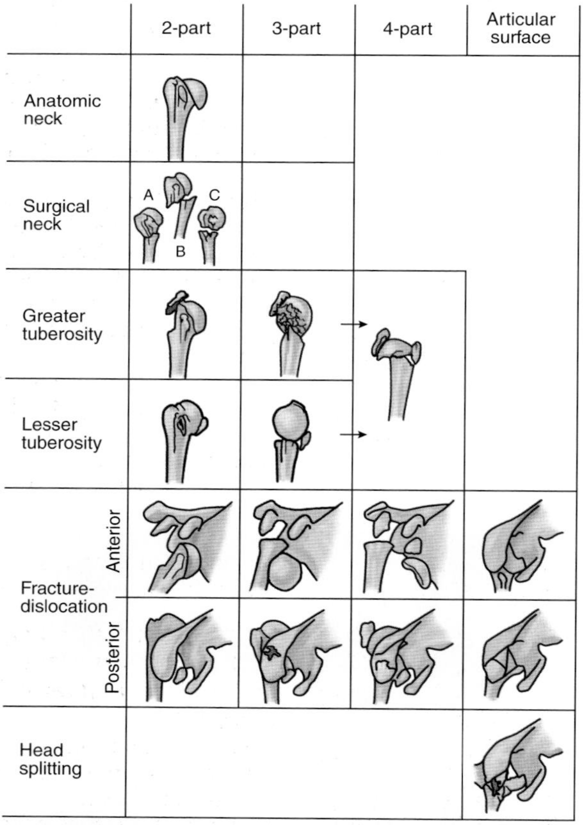

	2-part	3-part	4-part	Articular surface
Anatomic neck				
Surgical neck	A B C			
Greater tuberosity				
Lesser tuberosity				
Fracture-dislocation (Anterior / Posterior)				
Head splitting				

Figure 2-26. Neer classification of proximal humerus fractures. *(From Miller MD, Hart JA, MacKnight JM, editors:* Essential orthopaedics, *Philadelphia, 2010, Saunders, p 201.)*

- Open fracture or skin compromise (severe skin tenting from fracture fragment)
- More than 2 cm of clavicle shortening, 100% displacement, or severe comminution

Informed Consent and Counseling
- Standard surgical risks should be discussed in detail (e.g., bleeding, infection, failure, anesthesia risks).
- Hardware failure and nonunion are known complications of fracture treatment.
- A minimum of 6 to 8 weeks in a sling is usually required following surgery.

Anesthesia
- General anesthesia, with or without nerve block

Patient Positioning
- Beach chair or modified beach chair

Surgical Procedure: Clavicle Open Reduction, Internal Fixation: Figure 2-27
- A 5- to 8-cm longitudinal incision is made in line with the clavicle.
- The deltotrapezius fascia is stripped off the clavicle.
- The fracture fragments may be reduced by Steinmann pins and the reduction verified with fluoroscopy.
- A four- to five-hole low-profile clavicle plate should be fitted to the contour of the clavicle.
- Screws are placed carefully with an instrument placed along the inferior

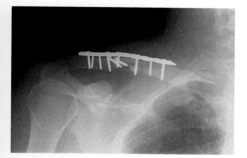

Figure 2-27. Open reduction, internal fixation of a clavicle fracture.

clavicle border to protect the subclavian vessels.
- Closure is in layers according to routine protocol.

Operative Management: Proximal Humerus Fractures
Codes
ICD-9 code: 812.0 Fracture of humerus, upper end
CPT codes: 23615 Open treatment of proximal humerus fracture, with internal fixation
23470 Arthroplasty glenohumeral joint, hemiarthroplasty

Operative Indications
- Displaced two-part surgical neck fractures
- Displaced three- and four-part fractures in relatively young, healthy patients
- Greater tuberosity fractures with more than 5 mm displacement (also require surgical open reduction, internal fixation [ORIF])

Informed Consent and Counseling
- Standard surgical risks should be discussed in detail (e.g., bleeding, infection, failure, anesthesia risks).
- Hardware failure and nonunion are known complications of fracture treatment.
- A minimum of 6 to 8 weeks in a sling is usually required following surgery.

Anesthesia
- General anesthesia, with or without nerve block

Patient Positioning
- Beach chair or modified beach chair

Surgical Procedure: Open Reduction, Internal Fixation of Proximal Humerus Fracture: Figure 2-28
- An anterior shoulder incision is made for a standard deltopectoral approach to the shoulder.
- The fracture is exposed by releasing the deltoid, and the fracture fragments are reduced using a Cobb elevator or threaded pin.

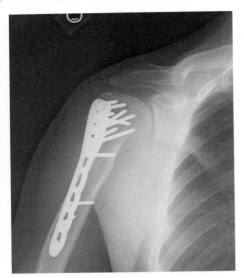

Figure 2-28. Open reduction, internal fixation of a proximal humerus fracture.

- Kirschner wires (K-wires) are used to hold the reduction in place, as confirmed with fluoroscopy.
- A proximal humerus plate is placed on the lateral aspect of the bone posterior to the biceps tendon and is secured with locking screws in the humeral head and nonlocking screws in the shaft.
- The rotator cuff is sutured to the proximal plate, and the wound is closed in layers according to routine protocol.

Estimated Postoperative Course
- Early postoperative period (days 0 to 6)
  - A sling should be used at all times, except for elbow motion.
- Initial postoperative visit (7 to 14 days)
  - Sutures should be removed, and the wound should be inspected.
  - Refill pain medications.
  - Address the patient's work status.
  - Check AP and tangential views of the clavicle or AP and axillary views of the shoulder for proximal humerus fracture.
- 6-week postoperative visit
  - Repeat radiographs.
  - Consider physical therapy for early gentle passive ROM.

- Continue light duty work status with limited to no use of the affected arm.
- 12-week postoperative visit
  - Repeat radiographs (last time if united).
  - Advance physical therapy to include active ROM and strengthening.
  - Determine the need for additional follow-up visits.

Suggested Readings
Crenshaw AH Jr, Perez EA: Fractures of the shoulder, arm, and forearm. In Canale ST, Beaty JH, editors: *Campbell's operative orthopaedics*, vol 3, ed 11, Philadelphia, 2008, Mosby, pp 3371–3460.
Johnston PS, Bushnell BD, Taft TN: Proximal humerus fractures. In Miller MD, Hart JA, MacKnight JM, editors: *Essential orthopaedics*, Philadelphia, 2010, Saunders, pp 199–203.
Rubright JH, Bushnell BD, Taft TN: Clavicle fractures. In Miller MD, Hart JA, MacKnight JM, editors: *Essential orthopaedics*, Philadelphia, 2010, Saunders, pp 212–216.

ORTHOPAEDIC PROCEDURES (SHOULDER)
Subacromial Injection
CPT code: 20610

Indications
- Shoulder impingement
- Partial rotator cuff tear
- Rotator cuff arthropathy
- Shoulder pain (diagnostic)

Contraindications
- Shoulder infection
- Local skin rash or active skin lesion over the injection site
- Allergy to injection material

Equipment Needed
- Ethyl chloride
- Topical cleansing agent (e.g., povidone-iodine [Betadine])
- Sterile gloves
- Syringe with a 21-gauge 1½-inch or longer needle
- Steroid (e.g., triamcinolone [Kenalog], 40 mg/mL)
- Anesthetic (e.g., lidocaine, 1% without epinephrine)
- Sterile dressing and tape or self-adhesive bandage

Procedure

1) Palpate and locate the injection site (Fig. 2-29).
2) Apply ethyl chloride to the area before injection (not sterile).
3) Prepare the area with a cleaning agent such as povidone-iodine (Betadine) and include the skin well beyond the injection site.
4) Insert the needle just below the inferior border of the acromion.
5) As you insert the needle past the acromion, angle the need tip up into the subacromial space.
6) Inject the steroid or anesthesia medication.
7) Withdraw the needle, remove any residual cleansing agent from the skin, and apply a dressing.

Aftercare Instructions

1) Apply ice to the area if local pain is present that day.
2) Expect the anesthetic to wear off later that same day, but know that the steroid does not take effect for an average of 3 to 5 days.
3) Call the office with any local erythema, increased pain, fever, or chills.
4) Call the office if symptoms fail to improve or if pain returns within 2 to 3 weeks of injection because this may indicate the need for additional imaging to evaluate the rotator cuff.

Acromioclavicular Joint Injection

CPT code: 20605

Indications
- AC joint osteoarthritis
- AC joint osteolysis
- AC joint pain

Contraindications

- Shoulder infection
- Local skin rash or active skin lesion over the injection site
- Allergy to injection material

Equipment Needed

- Ethyl chloride
- Topical cleansing agent (e.g., povidone-iodine [Betadine])
- Sterile gloves
- Syringe with a 21-gauge 1½-inch or longer needle
- Steroid (e.g., triamcinolone [Kenalog], 40 mg/mL)
- Anesthetic (e.g., lidocaine, 1% without epinephrine)
- Sterile dressing and tape or self-adhesive bandage

Procedure

- Palpate and locate the injection site at the lateral tip of the clavicle (Fig. 2-30).
- Apply ethyl chloride to the area before injection (not sterile).
- Prepare the area with cleaning agent such as povidone-iodine (Betadine) and include the skin well beyond the injection site.
- Hold the syringe vertically, and insert the needle with a slight medial angle until it passes between the acromion and clavicle and a small "pop" is felt when the joint capsule is penetrated (Fig. 2-31).
- Inject the steroid or anesthesia medication.
- Withdraw the needle, remove any residual cleansing agent from skin, and apply a dressing.

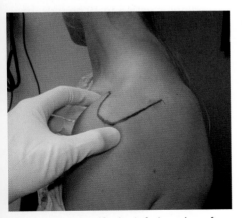

Figure 2-29. Identify the inferior edge of the acromion as the site for the injection. *(From Miller MD, Hart JA, MacKnight JM, editors:* Essential orthopaedics, *Philadelphia, 2010, Saunders, p 226.)*

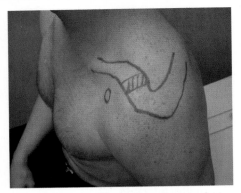

Figure 2-30. Identify the bony landmarks to visualize the area of the injection just lateral to the end of the clavicle *(hashed line)*. *(From Miller MD, Hart JA, MacKnight JM, editors:* Essential orthopaedics, *Philadelphia, 2010, Saunders, p 229.)*

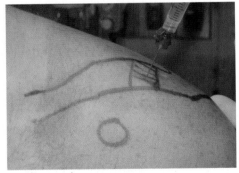

Figure 2-31. Injection just lateral to the end of the clavicle *(hashed line)*. *(From Miller MD, Hart JA, MacKnight JM, editors:* Essential orthopaedics, *Philadelphia, 2010, Saunders, p 230.)*

Aftercare Instructions
1) Apply ice to the area if local pain is present that day.
2) Expect the anesthetic to wear off later that same day, but know that the steroid does not take effect for an average of 3 to 5 days.
3) Call the office with any local erythema, increased pain, fever, or chills.

Shoulder Reduction
CPT code: 23650 Closed treatment with manipulation of shoulder dislocation not requiring anesthesia
23655 Closed treatment with manipulation of shoulder dislocation requiring anesthesia

Indications
- Shoulder dislocation, anterior

Contraindications
- Multitrauma in which medical status is unstable
- Displaced, unstable fracture

Anesthesia
- Intra-articular lidocaine or
- Conscious sedation

Equipment Needed
- Minimal equipment necessary; traction/countertraction method requiring the use of weights or intravenous bags

Procedure
Traction/Countertraction Technique (Stimson Method)
1) The patient is placed prone on the table, with his or her arm hanging down vertically off the side.
2) Weights are added to the arm, beginning with 5 to 10 pounds, or manual pressure is applied to the arm to provide gentle traction (the table provides countertraction).
3) This may take time (15 to 20 minutes typically) as the muscles fatigue.
4) Scapula manipulation may be helpful to facilitate reduction.

Kocher Method: Figure 2-32
1) With the patient's arm adducted and the elbow flexed to 90 degrees, externally rotate the arm.
2) At the point of resistance, maximally forward flex the shoulder then internally rotate it until reduction is felt.

Milch Method: Figure 2-33
1) The patient is placed either supine or prone, and the patient's arm is placed in an abducted position with the elbow flexed to 90 degrees.

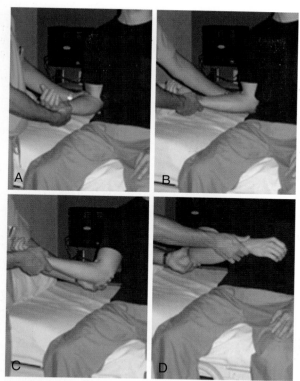

Figure 2-32. Kocher method of shoulder reduction. **A,** Start with adduction at the shoulder and elbow flexion. **B,** Externally rotate the arm at the shoulder. **C,** Flex the arm forward at the shoulder until resistance is felt. **D,** Internally rotate the arm at the shoulder. *(From Miller MD, Hart JA, MacKnight JM, editors:* Essential orthopaedics, *Philadelphia, 2010, Saunders, p 218.)*

2) The arm is passively abducted and externally rotated while the examiner's other hand gently pushes the humeral head back into proper position.

Aftercare Instructions

1) The arm is placed in a sling for patient comfort, with instructions to remove the sling for pendulum exercises and elbow motion, to prevent stiffness.

2) External rotation slings are increasingly popular after shoulder reduction because some literature suggests improved healing in this position.

3) Follow-up evaluation should be set for 1 to 2 weeks after to assess motion and rotator cuff strength.

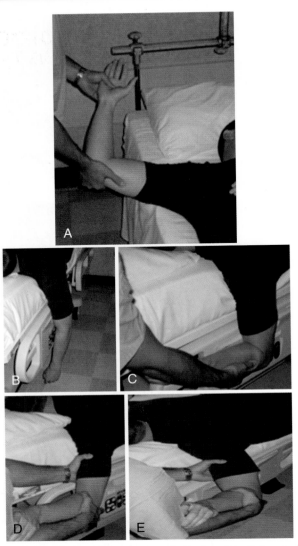

Figure 2-33. Milch method of shoulder reduction. **A,** Supine. **B** to **E,** Prone. *(From Miller MD, Hart JA, MacKnight JM, editors:* Essential orthopaedics, *Philadelphia, 2010, Saunders, pp 218–219.)*

Elbow and Forearm 3
Sara D. Rynders

ANATOMY
Bones: Figure 3-1

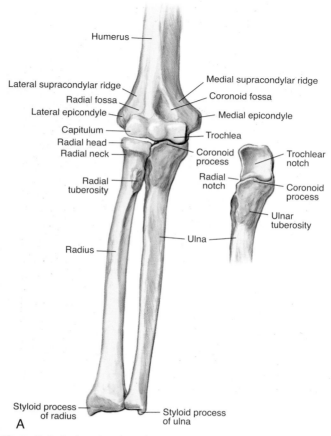

Figure 3-1. A, Anterior view of the elbow and forearm bony anatomy.

Continued

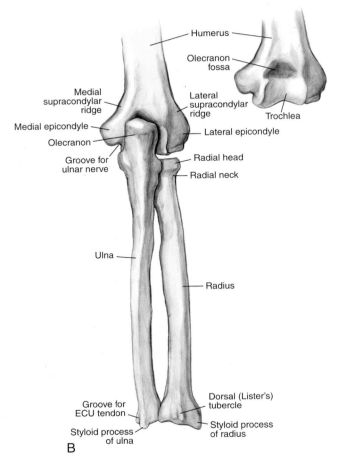

Figure 3-1, cont'd. B, Posterior view of the elbow and forearm bony anatomy. ECU, extensor carpi ulnaris. *(From Chhabra AB: Elbow and forearm. In Miller MD, Chhabra AB, Hurwitz S, et al, editors: Orthopaedic surgical approaches, Philadelphia, 2008, Saunders, pp 63, 64.)*

Ligaments: Figure 3-2

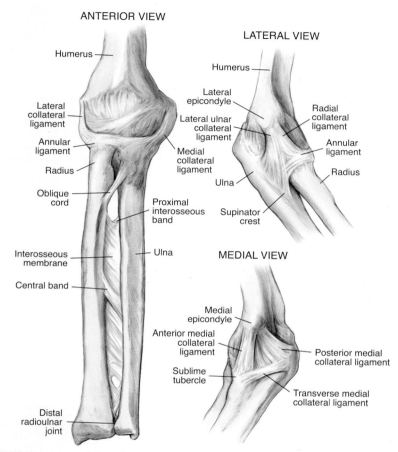

Figure 3-2. Ligaments of the elbow and forearm. Components of the elbow ligaments—ulnar collateral ligament: anterior band, posterior band, and transverse band; lateral collateral ligament: annular ligament, radial collateral ligament, accessory collateral ligament, and lateral ulnar collateral ligament. *(From Chhabra AB: Elbow and forearm. In Miller MD, Chhabra AB, Hurwitz S, et al, editors: Orthopaedic surgical approaches, Philadelphia, 2008, Saunders, p 67.)*

Muscles and Tendons:
Figure 3-3

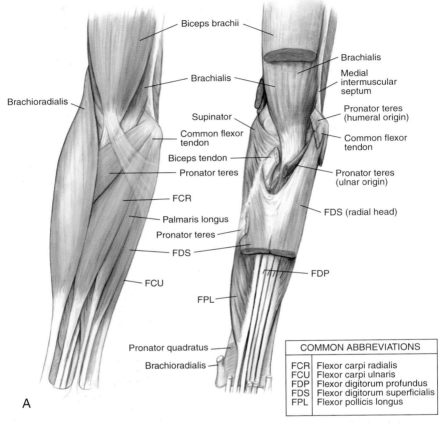

Figure 3-3. A, Muscles and tendons of the anterior elbow and forearm: superficial and deep compartments.

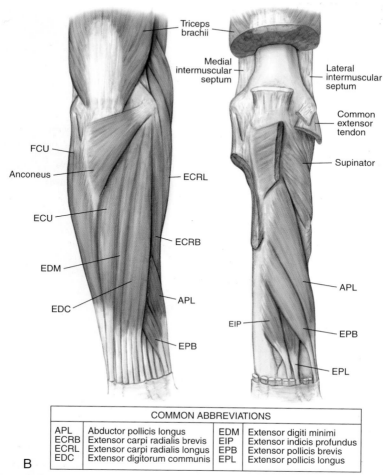

COMMON ABBREVIATIONS			
APL	Abductor pollicis longus	EDM	Extensor digiti minimi
ECRB	Extensor carpi radialis brevis	EIP	Extensor indicis profundus
ECRL	Extensor carpi radialis longus	EPB	Extensor pollicis brevis
EDC	Extensor digitorum communis	EPL	Extensor pollicis longus

Figure 3-3, cont'd. B, Muscles and tendons of the posterior elbow and forearm: superficial and deep compartments. *(From Chhabra AB: Elbow and forearm. In Miller MD, Chhabra AB, Hurwitz S, et al, editors:* Orthopaedic surgical approaches, *Philadelphia, 2008, Saunders, pp 68, 69.)*

Nerves and Arteries:
Figure 3-4 and Table 3-1

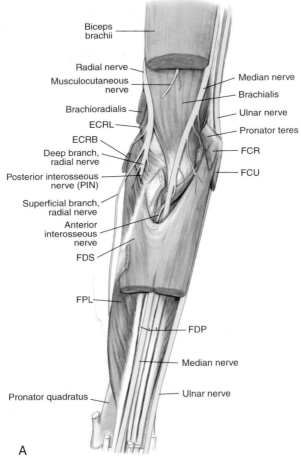

Figure 3-4. A, Anterior view of the nerves of the elbow and forearm.

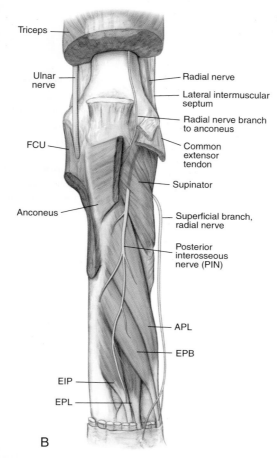

Triceps

Ulnar nerve

FCU

Anconeus

Radial nerve

Lateral intermuscular septum

Radial nerve branch to anconeus

Common extensor tendon

Supinator

Superficial branch, radial nerve

Posterior interosseous nerve (PIN)

APL

EPB

EIP

EPL

B

Figure 3-4, cont'd. B, Posterior view of the nerves of the elbow and forearm.

Continued

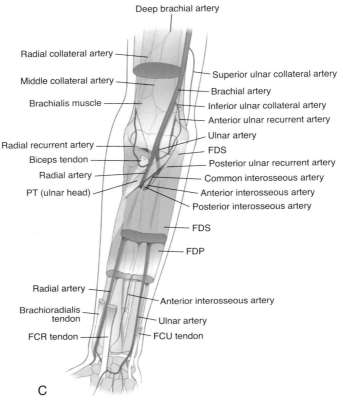

C

Figure 3-4, cont'd. C, Arteries of the elbow and forearm. APL, abductor pollicis longus; ECRB, extensor carpi radialis brevis; ECRL, extensor carpi radialis longus; EIP, extensor indicis profundus; EPB, extensor pollicis brevis; EPL, extensor pollicis longus; FCR, flexor carpi radialis; FCU, flexor carpi ulnaris; FDP, flexor digitorum profundus; FDS, flexor digitorum superficialis; FPL, flexor pollicis longus; PT, pronator teres. *(From Chhabra AB: Elbow and forearm. In Miller MD, Chhabra AB, Hurwitz S, et al, editors:* Orthopaedic surgical approaches, *Philadelphia, 2008, Saunders, pp 74, 75, 81.)*

Table 3-1. Muscle Innervation and Testing

NERVE	BRANCH	MOTOR	TEST	SENSORY
Musculocutaneous	Proper	Biceps brachii, brachialis	Elbow flexion, forearm supination	
	Lateral antebrachial cutaneous			To lateral elbow and forearm
Medial cord	Medial antebrachial cutaneous			To anterior antebrachium and medial forearm
Radial	Proper	Triceps, anconeus, brachioradialis	Elbow extension, elbow flexion	

Table 3-1. Muscle Innervation and Testing—cont'd

NERVE	BRANCH	MOTOR	TEST	SENSORY
	Superficial sensory radial nerve (SSRN)			To dorsal aspect of radial wrist and thumb, dorsal hand
	Posterior interosseous nerve (PIN)	ECRB, EDM, ECRL, APL, ECU, EPB, supinator, EPL, EIP	Wrist extension, thumb extension, finger extension	
Median	Proper	Pronator teres, FCR, FDS, palmaris longus, index and middle finger lumbricals	Radial wrist flexion, finger flexion, pronation	Thumb, index finger, middle finger, and radial half of ring finger
	Recurrent motor branch	Thenar muscles: APB	Thumb abduction	
	Anterior Interosseous nerve (AIN)	FDP to index finger, FPL, pronator quadratus	Index finger DIP joint flexion, thumb IP joint flexion, pronation	
	Superficial sensory palmar branch			Sensation to palm
Ulnar	Proper	FDP to ring and small fingers, FCU	Flexion of ring and small fingers, ulnar wrist flexion	
	Superficial sensory branch			Sensation to volar fifth finger and ulnar half of ring finger
	Deep motor branch	Adductor pollicis, hypothenar muscle, interosseous muscle, ring and small finger lumbricals, deep branch of FPB	Finger abduction and adduction, thumb adduction	
	Dorsal sensory branch			Dorsal sensation to small finger and ulnar half of ring finger

APB, abductor pollicis brevis; APL, abductor pollicis longus; DIP, distal interphalangeal; ECRB, extensor carpi radialis brevis; ECRL, extensor carpi radialis longus; ECU, extensor carpi ulnaris; EDM, extensor digiti minimi; EIP, extensor indicis proprius; EPB, extensor pollicis brevis; EPL, extensor pollicis longus; FCR, flexor carpi radialis; FCU, flexor carpi ulnaris; FDP, flexor digitorum profundus; FDS, flexor digitorum superficialis; FPB, flexor pollicis brevis; FPL, flexor pollicis longus; IP interphalangeal.

Surface Anatomy: Figure 3-5

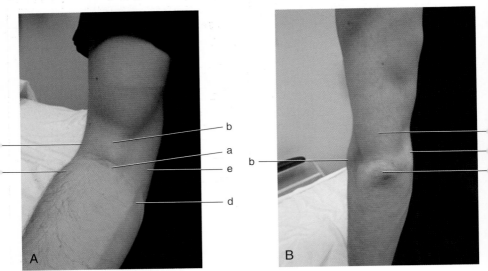

Figure 3-5. Surface anatomy of the anterior and posterior elbow and forearm. **A,** Anterior labels: **a)** antebrachial fossa, **b)** biceps tendon, **c)** common extensor tendons, **d)** common flexor tendons, **e)** medial epicondyle, **f)** lateral epicondyle. **B,** Posterior labels: **a)** medial epicondyle, **b)** lateral epicondyle, **c)** olecranon process, **d)** triceps tendon.

Normal Radiographic Appearance: Figures 3-6 and 3-7

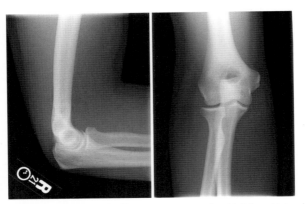

Figure 3-6. Normal radiographs of the elbow. Anteroposterior *(right)* and lateral *(left)* views. *(From Hart JA: Overview of the elbow. In Miller MD, Hart JA, MacKnight JM, editors: Essential orthopaedics, Philadelphia, 2010, Saunders, 2010, p 239.)*

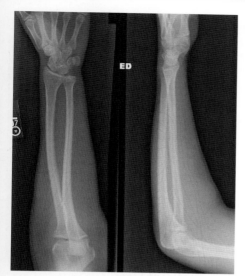

Figure 3-7. Normal radiographs of the forearm. Anteroposterior *(left)* and lateral *(right)* views.

PHYSICAL EXAMINATION
(Table 3-2, 3-3, 3-4)

Inspect for edema, deformity, ecchymosis, biceps muscle.

Palpate:

- Medial epicondyle
- Ulnar nerve in cubital tunnel
- Lateral epicondyle
- Radial head
- Distal biceps tendon
- Brachial artery
- Common extensor muscles (also known as "mobile wad")
- Olecranon and olecranon bursa

Table 3-2. Normal Elbow and Forearm Range of Motion

Extension	0 degrees
Flexion	135 degrees
Supination	90 degrees
Pronation	90 degrees

Table 3-3. Neurovascular Examination

NERVE	LOCATION OF TEST	TESTS
Ulnar nerve	Cubital tunnel at elbow	Tinel sign, look for subluxation over medial epicondyle; distally, check Froment and Wartenburg sign (see cubital tunnel syndrome on p. 84)
Median nerve	Wrist and hand	Radial-sided wrist flexion and finger flexion checked distally
Radial nerve	Triceps	Resisted elbow extension
Posterior interosseous nerve	Test strength distally at wrist and hand	Resisted wrist extension, finger extension, thumb extension
Brachial artery; radial and ulnar artery	At medial brachium; at volar wrist	

Table 3-4. Differential Diagnosis of Elbow Pain

Medial-sided elbow pain	Medial epicondylitis Ulnar collateral ligament injury Arthritis Cubital tunnel syndrome
Lateral-sided elbow pain	Lateral epicondylitis Radial head fracture Lateral collateral ligament injury
Anterior elbow pain	Biceps tendinitis or biceps tendon rupture
Posterior elbow pain	Olecranon bursitis Triceps tendinitis
Forearm pain	Radial tunnel syndrome Muscle strain

LATERAL EPICONDYLITIS
History
- Definition: tendinitis of the common extensor tendon origin, also known as tennis elbow
- Lateral-sided elbow pain
- Possible reported history of injury or repetitive trauma
- Pain worse with lifting and gripping
- Pain also possible at night when the elbow is moved from a resting position

Physical Examination
- Possible mild edema over lateral epicondyle
- Point tenderness to palpation over lateral epicondyle
- Pain with resisted wrist extension
- Pain at the lateral epicondyle caused by grip strength testing with a dynamometer; pain worse when test performed with the elbow extended rather than flexed

Imaging: Figure 3-8
- Not always necessary for diagnosis; considered if history of injury
- Elbow: anteroposterior (AP), lateral, oblique views
- Diagnosis confirmed by magnetic resonance imaging (MRI)

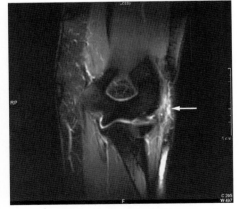

Figure 3-8. Magnetic resonance image of lateral epicondylitis. Edema and high-grade partial tearing of the common extensor tendon origin are visible (*arrow*).

Differential Diagnosis
- Lateral collateral ligament (LCL) sprain
- Radial tunnel syndrome (compression of the posterior interosseous nerve [PIN] in the supinator)
- Distal humerus fracture

Initial Treatment
Patient Education
Lateral epicondylitis is also known as tennis elbow and is a form of tendinitis. It is an inflammatory condition. Treatment revolves around decreasing the inflammation, using proper lifting techniques, and strengthening the musculature. Because the tendons that are inflamed are responsible for wrist extension, the pain is worse with grip and lifting.

First Treatment Steps
- Patient education and activity modification are paramount to successful treatment.
- Good results are reported in the literature after 12 months of conservative management.
- Measures include avoidance of aggravating activities and repetitive lifting and gripping, correction of improper lifting or gripping techniques, a nonsteroidal antiinflammatory drug (NSAID) regimen if tolerated, possible use of transdermal anesthetic patches, heat and ice modalities with stretching, and occupational therapy referral.
- Some advocate use of a wrist brace to limit wrist extension during activities.

Treatment Options
Nonoperative Management
- Conservative management is reserved for patients with no previous treatment or whose previous treatment was successful but the problem recurred after several months or years.
- In addition to initial treatments listed earlier, a cortisone injection may be performed (see p. 107 for lateral epicondyle injection).
- Avoid multiple repeat injections over a short time because they can result in local tissue destruction and possible tendon or ligament rupture.

- Advise the patient on a period of rest and activity modification after injection.
- If referring patient to occupational therapy, the referral should include instructions to provide elbow stretching, gradual protected strengthening, counseling on lifting techniques, and use of local modalities for inflammation.
- If the patient notes no improvement or diminishing improvement in symptoms with injections, consider an MRI scan to evaluate for any other causes of lateral elbow pain such as an LCL injury. Lateral epicondylitis may be described on an MRI as "high-grade partial tearing of the common extensor tendon origin."
- Interest in the use of platelet-rich plasma (PRP) injections is increasing, but no definitive data on its efficacy are available, and this treatment is still considered experimental.

Operative Management
Codes
ICD-9 code: 726.32 Lateral epicondylitis
CPT code: 24359 Débridement of soft tissue and/or bone at lateral epicondyle

Operative Indications
- Conservative management for at least 1 year has failed.
- Indications and techniques vary, and more studies are necessary for an evidence-based approach.

Informed Consent and Counseling
- Surgical débridement has shown good results in the literature, but the risk of partial or no relief of symptoms is approximately 15%.
- The surgical procedure is not likely to be successful if the patient fails to modify activities or cease repetitive trauma postoperatively.
- The patient will require a 2- to 3-month recovery period with monitored progressive occupational therapy.

Anesthesia
- Regional block with sedation, or general anesthesia

Patient Positioning
- Supine with the arm on an arm board, with the shoulder internally rotated and the elbow flexed
- Nonsterile tourniquet high on the brachium

Surgical Procedures
- Lateral approach for tendon débridement
- Arthroscopy with débridement

Lateral Epicondyle Débridement
- An oblique incision is made just anterior to the lateral epicondyle and common extensor tendon origin. Care is taken to avoid injury to the **lateral antebrachial cutaneous nerve.**
- The lateral epicondyle is identified, and a split is made in the common extensor tendon origin parallel to the fibers. The tissue is divided in layers until the underlying joint capsule is identified.
- A rongeur or curette is used to débride the dysvascular tissue and to stimulate bleeding. Avoid injury to the underlying LCL. Sometimes, a Kirschner wire (K-wire) is used to puncture the lateral epicondyle several times and stimulate bleeding at the origin of the tendon.
- Once débridement has concluded, the common extensor tendon is repaired in layers using a suture. The fascia is also closed followed by the subcutaneous tissues and the skin. Most surgeons immobilize the patient in a **long-arm posterior splint** for 10 to 14 days.

Estimated Postoperative Course
- Postoperative days 10 to 14
  - Perform a wound check and suture removal.
  - *Therapy:* Start therapy for gentle elbow ROM. The patient should avoid lifting with the operative extremity.
- Postoperative 6 weeks
  - Perform a motion check. Evaluate and document whether the patient has tenderness to palpation at the lateral epicondyle.
  - *Therapy:* Start a graduated strengthening program.

- Postoperative 3 months
  - Perform a motion and strength check. Evaluate and document whether the patient has tenderness at the lateral epicondyle, and test for pain with resisted wrist extension.
  - If the patient is asymptomatic, release him or her to regular activities.

Suggested Readings

Buchbinder R, Johnston RV, Barnsley L, et al: Surgery for lateral elbow pain, *Cochrane Data-Base Syst Rev* 16(3):CD003525, 2011.

Dorf ER, Chhabra AB, Golish SR, et al: Effect of elbow position on grip strength in the evaluation of lateral epicondylitis, *J Hand Surg Am* 32:882–886, 2007.

Faro F, Wolf JM: Lateral epicondylitis: review and current concepts, *J Hand Surg Am* 32:1271–1279, 2007.

Hall MP, Band PA, Meislin RJ, et al: Platelet-rich plasma: current concepts and application in sports medicine, *J Am Acad Orthop Surg* 17:602–608, 2009.

Jobe FW, Ciccotti MG: Lateral and medial epicondylitis of the elbow, *J Am Acad Orthop Surg* 2: 1–8, 1994.

Nirschl RP, Ashman ES: Elbow tendinopathy: tennis elbow, *Clin Sports Med* 22:813–836, 2003.

MEDIAL EPICONDYLITIS
History
- Definition: tendinitis of the common flexor tendon origin, also known as golfer's elbow
- Medial-sided elbow pain
- Possible reported history of injury or repetitive trauma
- Possible patient-reported associated paresthesias in the fourth and fifth fingers (possible simultaneous cubital tunnel syndrome resulting from inflammation)

Physical Examination
- Possible mild edema over medial epicondyle
- Point tenderness to palpation over medial epicondyle
- Pain with resisted wrist flexion
- Elbow stable to stress testing of the ulnar collateral ligament (UCL)
- Evaluation of the ulnar nerve at the cubital tunnel for subluxation or neuritis (see p. 84 for cubital tunnel syndrome)

Imaging: Figure 3-9
- Not necessary for diagnosis but possibly warranted if history of recent trauma or examiner suspects arthritis
- Elbow AP, lateral, and oblique views
- MRI of the elbow can aid in diagnosis and evaluation for other causes of medial-sided elbow pain

Differential Diagnosis
- UCL sprain
- Cubital tunnel syndrome
- Distal humerus fracture

Initial Treatment
Patient Education
Medial epicondylitis is also known as golfer's elbow and is a form of tendinitis. It is an inflammatory condition, and treatment revolves around decreasing the inflammation and strengthening the musculature. Because the tendons that are inflamed are responsible for wrist flexion and pronation, the pain is occasionally worse with gripping, lifting, and twisting.

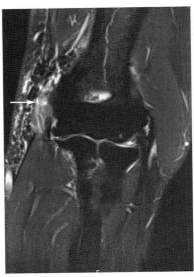

Figure 3-9. Magnetic resonance image of medial epicondylitis. Edema and high-grade partial tearing of the common flexor tendon origin are visible (*arrow*).

First Treatment Steps
- Patient education and activity modification are paramount to successful treatment.
- Measures include avoidance of aggravating activities and repetitive activities, correction of improper techniques, NSAID regimen if tolerated, heat and ice modalities with stretching, and occupational therapy referral.
- Some advocate use of a wrist brace to limit wrist flexion during activities.
- If fourth and fifth finger paresthesias are present, consider obtaining an electromyography and nerve conduction study (EMG/NCS) to evaluate for concomitant cubital tunnel syndrome.

Treatment Options
Nonoperative Management
- Conservative management is reserved for patients with no previous treatment or whose previous treatment was successful but the problem recurred after several months or years.
- In addition to initial treatments listed earlier, a cortisone injection may be performed (see p. 108 for medial epicondyle injection).
- Avoid multiple repeat injections over a short time because this can result in local tissue destruction and possible tendon or ligament rupture.
- A relative contraindication to injection is a subluxating ulnar nerve.
- Advise the patient on a period of rest and activity modification after injection.
- If referring the patient to occupational therapy, the referral should include instructions to provide elbow stretching, gradual protected flexor-pronator strengthening, and use of local modalities for inflammation.
- If the patient notes no improvement or diminishing improvement in symptoms with injections, consider an MRI scan to evaluate for any other causes of medial elbow pain such as a UCL injury.

Operative Management
Codes
ICD-9 code: 726.31 Medial epicondylitis
CPT code: 24359 Débridement of soft tissue and/or bone at medial epicondyle

Operative Indications
- Conservative management for at least 1 year has failed.
- Indications and techniques vary, and more studies are necessary for an evidence-based approach.

Informed Consent and Counseling
- The surgical procedure is not likely to be successful if the patient fails to modify activities or cease repetitive trauma postoperatively.
- The patient will require a 2- to 3-month recovery period with monitored progressive occupational therapy.

Anesthesia
- Regional block with sedation, or general anesthesia

Patient Positioning
- Supine with the arm on an arm board, with the shoulder externally rotated and the elbow flexed
- Nonsterile tourniquet placed high on the brachium

Surgical Procedures
- The medial approach is used for tendon débridement.
- If cubital tunnel syndrome is present, an ulnar nerve transposition can be performed simultaneously with this procedure (see p. 84 for cubital tunnel syndrome).

Medial Epicondyle Débridement
- An oblique incision is made just anterior to the medial epicondyle. Care is taken to avoid injury to the **medial antebrachial cutaneous nerve and ulnar nerve in the cubital tunnel.**
- The medial epicondyle is identified, and a split is made in the common flexor tendon origin parallel to the fibers. The tissue is divided in layers until the underlying joint capsule is identified.
- A rongeur or curette is used to débride the dysvascular tissue and to stimulate bleeding. Avoid injury to the underlying **UCL.** Sometimes, a K-wire is used to puncture the medial epicondyle several times to stimulate bleeding at the origin of the tendon.

- The common flexor tendon is then repaired in layers using a suture. The fascia is also closed followed by the subcutaneous tissues and the skin. Most surgeons immobilize the patient in a **long-arm posterior splint** for 10 to 14 days.

Estimated Postoperative Course
- Postoperative days 10 to 14
  - Perform a wound check and suture removal.
  - *Therapy:* Start gentle elbow ROM. The patient is to avoid lifting with the operative extremity.
- Postoperative 6 weeks
  - Perform a motion check. Evaluate and document whether the patient has tenderness to palpation at the medial epicondyle.
  - *Therapy:* Start a graduated strengthening program.
- Postoperative 3 months
  - Perform a motion and strength check. Evaluate and document whether the patient has tenderness to palpation at the medial epicondyle, and test for pain with resisted wrist flexion.
  - If the patient is asymptomatic, release him or her to regular activities.

Suggested Readings
Ciccotti MG, Ramani MN: Medial epicondylitis, *Tech Hand Up Extrem Surg* 7:190–196, 2003.

Jobe FW, Ciccotti MG: Lateral and medial epicondylitis of the elbow, *J Am Acad Orthop Surg* 2:18, 1994.

Mierisch C: Golfer's elbow (medial epicondylitis). In Miller MD, Hart JA, MacKnight JM, editors: *Essential orthopaedics*, Philadelphia, 2010, Saunders, pp 247–248.

CUBITAL TUNNEL SYNDROME
History
- Definition: Ulnar nerve compression at the elbow
- Medial-sided elbow pain
- Numbness and tingling in the fourth and fifth fingers
- Achy pain radiating down the ulnar side of the forearm to the wrist and hand
- Worse when the elbow is flexed or while leaning on the elbow; possibly while sleeping
- Hand weakness (late finding)

Physical Examination
- Tenderness over the ulnar nerve at the cubital tunnel
- Positive Tinel sign over the ulnar nerve at the cubital tunnel, with symptoms radiating to the fourth and fifth fingers
- Placement of the elbow into flexion and palpation for subluxation of the ulnar nerve over the medial epicondyle
- Altered or decreased sensation to touch (or two-point discrimination) of the ulnar border of the fourth finger and the entire fifth finger
- Inspection for intrinsic muscle atrophy in the hand, or claw deformity (late finding)

Wartenburg Test: *Figure 3-10*
- This test evaluates for weakness of the adductor digiti minimi, which is the earliest sign of muscle weakness.
- Ask the patient to adduct all fingers together.
- A positive test result is when the fifth finger remains in an abducted position.

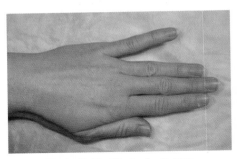

Figure 3-10. Wartenburg test.

Froment Sign: *Figure 3-11*
- This test evaluates for weakness of the adductor pollicis muscle caused by ulnar nerve injury.
- Ask the patient to hold a piece of paper between the thumb and index finger while the fingers are extended. The examiner then tries to remove paper from the patient's grip.
- A positive sign is when the patient flexes the thumb interphalangeal joint and thereby activates the flexor pollicis longus (a median nerve innervated muscle) to hold the paper, instead of using the adductor pollicis.

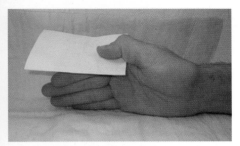

Figure 3-11. Froment sign.

Imaging
- Not necessary for diagnosis; considered only if symptoms are trauma-related

Additional Tests
Electromyography and Nerve Conduction Study
EMG/NCS can identify ulnar nerve compression at the cubital tunnel and can determine severity of compression. Ask the electromyographer to evaluate for the differential diagnosis, which includes carpal tunnel syndrome, cervical radiculopathy, and peripheral neuropathy. Sometimes an "inching study" is performed across the elbow to identify an area of compression.

Differential Diagnosis
- Medial epicondylitis
- Cervical radiculopathy
- Ulnar tunnel syndrome: compression of the ulnar nerve at the hand
- Carpal tunnel syndrome

Initial Treatment
Patient Education
Cubital tunnel syndrome is compression of the ulnar nerve or "funny bone" as it crosses behind the elbow. If left untreated, this condition can result in permanent loss of sensation to the fourth and fifth fingers and permanent weakness of the hand with a claw deformity. Sometimes, simply avoiding flexing the elbow and leaning on the elbow can eliminate the problem.

First Treatment Steps
- Provide the patient with education about how to avoid leaning on the

elbow and flexing it for long periods of time.
- Discuss activity modifications.
- Suggest that the patient obtain an elbow pad to protect the nerve and possibly refer the patient to an occupational therapist to have a night-time splint made. Wrapping a towel around the elbow at night can also work to prevent flexion and protect the nerve from compression.

Treatment Options
Nonoperative Management
- Conservative management is reserved for patients with no evidence of muscle wasting on EMG/NCS or physical examination and for those without any previous treatment.
- Patient education is key. Discuss in detail how the patient should avoid leaning on the elbow and flexing the elbow repetitively or for long periods of time. Discuss sleep posture.
- NSAIDs can help with pain.
- Attempt nonoperative management for at least 6 weeks.

Rehabilitation
- Refer the patient to an occupational therapist for ulnar nerve gliding exercises, night splinting with the elbow in 45 degrees of flexion, and discussion of activity modifications.

Operative Management
Codes
ICD-9 code: 354.2 Lesion of ulnar nerve
CPT code: 64718 Ulnar nerve neuroplasty and/or transposition at elbow

Operative Indications
- Nonoperative management has failed.
- Patient has evidence of severe ulnar nerve compression and/or muscle denervation on EMG/NCS.
- Surgical treatment may be appropriate for patients with evidence of intrinsic wasting on physical examination, to prevent further progression.

Informed Consent and Counseling
- Care will be taken to avoid injury to the cutaneous nerves at the elbow, but some residual numbness

occasionally occurs near the incision site at the elbow.

- The purpose of the surgical procedure is to relieve the sites of compression, and the goal is to prevent progression of nerve damage; if the patient has advanced disease, the operation may not restore normal sensation to the fingers, and strength may never return.
- The patient can expect to have limited use of the arm for about 6 to 8 weeks.

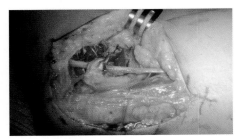

Figure 3-12. Intraoperative photograph of a transposed ulnar nerve. The nerve now lies anterior to the medial epicondyle and is held in place by lengthened flexor-pronator fascia.

Anesthesia
- Regional upper extremity block, with sedation or general anesthesia

Patient Positioning
- Supine, with the shoulder abducted and externally rotated and the arm on the hand table
- Nonsterile tourniquet high on the brachium

Surgical Procedures
- Medial approach over the ulnar nerve at the elbow
- Ulnar nerve decompression or decompression and transposition of the ulnar nerve
- Nerve transposed subcutaneously (best reserved for those with adequate subcutaneous fat) or submuscularly
- Endoscopic ulnar nerve decompression gaining popularity

Ulnar Nerve Transposition (Subcutaneous or Submuscular): Figure 3-12
- Instruments: Vessel loops are used to hold the nerve gently during dissection.
- A longitudinal incision is made over the medial elbow. Take care to identify and protect the **medial antebrachial cutaneous nerve**. Elevate the subcutaneous flaps off the fascia overlying the flexor-pronator mass. Identify the medial epicondyle. Just posteriorly, identify the **ulnar nerve** within the cubital tunnel. With tenotomy scissors and smooth forceps, the ulnar nerve is carefully decompressed. Minimal traction and manipulation of the nerve are ideal, and a vessel loop can be used to retract and control the nerve gently while operating.

- All sites of ulnar nerve compression at the elbow are addressed: arcade of Struthers, medial intramuscular septum of the triceps, Osborne ligament, the flexor carpi ulnaris (FCU) fascia, and the heads of the FCU.
- If transposing subcutaneously, a sling is created within the medial subcutaneous flap. The nerve is transposed, and then a suture is used to tack the subcutaneous tissue back down to the flexor pronator fascia, thus securing the nerve anterior to the medial epicondyle.
- If transposing submuscularly, the flexor-pronator fascia may be lengthened using a steplike incision. A trough may also be created in the musculature and the nerve transposed anterior to the medial epicondyle. The fascia is then sutured back together over the nerve but in a lengthened position.
- Once the nerve has been transposed, the elbow is placed through ROM to ensure that the nerve no longer subluxes with flexion, has no areas of compression, and is not under tension. The wound is then irrigated and the skin closed. **A Jackson-Pratt (JP) drain or similar drain may be placed into the wound to be removed before discharge home or on postoperative day 1.** Most surgeons place the patient in a postoperative long-arm posterior splint with the elbow at 90 degrees and the forearm in neutral.

Estimated Postoperative Course

- Postoperative days 3 to 5
  - Some clinicians advocate for an early therapy session for gentle elbow ROM and edema control to prevent stiffness. A removable thermoplastic long-arm posterior splint may be fabricated to support the arm between therapy sessions.
- Postoperative days 10 to 14
  - Sutures are removed, and ROM is assessed.
  - Inquire about and document changes in preoperative paresthesias.
  - Check and document Froment and Wartenburg signs.
- Postoperative 6 weeks
  - Reassess ROM.
  - Perform a wound check, and evaluate for hypersensitivity.
  - Inquire about and document changes in preoperative paresthesias.
  - Check and document Froment and Wartenburg signs.
  - The patient can start strengthening exercises between 6 and 8 weeks and gradually return to everyday activities without restrictions.

Suggested Readings

Cobb TK: Endoscopic cubital tunnel release, *J Hand Surg* 35:1690–1697, 2010.

Palmer BA, Hughes TB: Cubital tunnel syndrome, *J Hand Surg Am* 35:153–163, 2010.

Szabo RM, Kwak C: Natural history and conservative management of cubital tunnel syndrome, *Hand Clin* 23:311–318, 2007.

Zlowodzki M, Chan S, Bhandari M, et al: Anterior transposition compared with simple decompression for treatment of cubital tunnel syndrome: a meta-analysis of randomized, controlled trials, *J Bone Joint Surg Am* 89:2591–2598, 2007.

OLECRANON BURSITIS

History

- Definition: inflammation or infection of the olecranon bursa
- Possible history of elbow trauma, repetitive activity, or abrasion
- Patient-reported edema and sometimes pain over the posterior elbow
- Possible erythema and warmth
- Possible pain with ROM

Physical Examination

- Evaluation of the posterior elbow reveals an inflamed olecranon bursa.
- Note the presence of any erythema and whether it is localized to the bursa or extends to the surrounding tissues in a cellulitic pattern.
- Palpation of the bursa reveals bogginess and mild tenderness. Severe tenderness could indicate infection.
- Evaluate ROM and assess whether it is painful. Painful ROM could suggest deeper joint infection.

Imaging

- This is generally not necessary for diagnosis and is indicated only to evaluate for any underlying elbow joint injury or if a septic joint is suspected. Elbow, AP, and lateral views are used.

Classification System: Inflammatory versus Infectious

- Sometimes the difference can be subtle.
- Infectious olecranon bursitis generally appears as beefy red, taut skin and looks very aggressive. It is generally more painful with palpation and ROM and is more likely to have associated surrounding cellulitis.
- Inflammatory olecranon bursitis generally has localized erythema, and edema is isolated to the bursa itself. Usually, this type of bursitis is less tender to palpation.
- Both conditions can have warmth.

Differential Diagnosis

- Rheumatoid nodules
- Elbow joint effusion
- Cellulitis
- Gouty arthritis or gouty tophi
- Pigmented villonodular synovitis

Initial Treatment

Patient Education

Olecranon bursitis is a condition of inflammation or infection of the olecranon bursa. It can occur from repetitive leaning on the elbow or from mild trauma. The bursa can be filled with sterile serous fluid or infection. Recurrences are possible and may require repeat aspiration, but nonoperative treatment is successful most of the time. If the bursitis is mild and clinically deemed to be aseptic, avoid aspiration, to reduce the risk of iatrogenic infection.

First Treatment Steps
- Determine whether bursitis is inflammatory or infectious.
- This distinction may be made by physical examination and history, or an aspirate may be necessary to identify a pathogen.
- If possible, avoid aspiration and treat conservatively.

Treatment Options
Nonoperative Management
- **For mild inflammatory bursitis:** Suggest ice, NSAIDs, an elbow pad or elastic (Ace) wrap for compression, and avoidance of leaning on the elbow. These treatments may take several weeks to be successful.
- **For symptomatic inflammatory bursitis:** Suggest aspiration in addition to the foregoing treatments. Use of a compression wrap over the decompressed bursa is key to prevent recurrence. The patient may need to apply constant compression for 7 to 10 days. Repeat aspirations may be necessary, but treatment is usually successful (70% of cases resolve at 1 month and 90% at 6 months, according to one retrospective study). If the aspirated fluid is cloudy or purulent, suspect infection, and send cultures as described next.
- **For questionable or suspected infectious bursitis:** Aspirate bursa and send fluid for **Gram stain, aerobic and anaerobic culture with sensitivities, white blood cell (WBC) count, crystals, and fluid glucose**. A WBC count greater than 10,000 is considered diagnostic for septic bursitis. A fluid glucose level less than half of the blood glucose level is also indicative of septic bursitis. Consider empiric oral antibiotic treatment in addition to ice, rest, and a compression wrap because most infections are caused by *Staphylococcus aureus* or other gram-positive bacteria. Intravenous antibiotics can also be used. Once the susceptibility of the pathogen is known, a 2-week course of oral antibiotics is indicated (see Olecranon Bursa Aspiration, p. 109).

- Incision and drainage with wound packing are reserved for cases of infectious olecranon bursitis that does not resolve after treatment with antibiotics. An incision is made just lateral to the olecranon process (an incision directly over the process can lead to delayed wound healing, a chronic open wound, and pain over the posterior elbow). A wick can be placed into the bursa and changed frequently. Avoid overpacking the wound, and use less packing with each dressing change, to encourage healing and wound closure.
- Intrabursal steroid injections are not indicated because of the risk of infection, residual pain, and skin atrophy.

Operative Management
Codes
ICD-9 code: 726.33 Olecranon Bursitis
CPT code: 24105 Excision of olecranon bursa

Operative Indications
- Surgery should be reserved for chronic or severe infections and for failure of multiple aspirations.

Informed Consent and Counseling
- The risk of wound breakdown over the olecranon is high. The skin over the olecranon may become painful or hypersensitive.

Anesthesia
- General anesthesia or a regional anesthetic with sedation

Patient Positioning
- Supine, with the operative arm extended on the arm table, the shoulder internally rotated, and the elbow flexed so that the lateral aspect of the elbow is easily exposed
- Nonsterile tourniquet placed high on the brachium

Surgical Procedures
Olecranon Bursectomy
- An oblique incision is made just lateral to the olecranon. Take care to avoid injury to the **lateral antebrachial cutaneous nerve**. The inflamed or infected bursa is usually easily identified and

completely excised. Consider sending the bursa for pathologic examination and for cultures. Care should be taken to avoid injury to the insertion of the triceps tendon. The wound is then copiously irrigated, and the skin is closed using suture. Most surgeons advocate for a 2-week period of postoperative splinting in a long-arm posterior elbow splint with the elbow at 90 degrees and neutral forearm rotation, to reduce the risk of hematoma formation.

Estimated Postoperative Course
- Postoperative days 10 to 14
  - Return to the clinic for a wound check and for splint and suture removal.
  - A therapy referral may be necessary to encourage elbow ROM and strengthening.
- Postoperative 6 weeks
  - A wound and motion check is performed.
  - If the injury is healed, return to all activities as tolerated.

Suggested Readings
Aaron DL, Patel A, Kayiaros S, et al: Four common types of bursitis: diagnosis and management, *J Am Acad Orthop Surg* 19:359–367, 2011.
McAfee JH, Smith DL: Olecranon and prepatellar bursitis: diagnosis and treatment, *West J Med* 149:607–610, 1988.
Weinstein PS, Canosos JJ, Wohlgethan JR: Long-term follow-up of corticosteroid injection for traumatic olecranon bursitis, *Ann Rheum Dis* 43:44–46, 1984.

DISTAL BICEPS TENDON RUPTURE
History
- Generally, patients are men 30 to 50 years old.
- Patients may have prior history of some biceps tendinitis.
- Patients report a "pop" while lifting or using the arm with an extension load.
- Patients may report pain and a "pop-eye deformity" of the biceps muscle.
- A chronic tear may manifest with arm weakness as the primary complaint.

Physical Examination
- Observe for prominence of the biceps muscle belly ("pop-eye deformity"),

and compare it with the contralateral side.
- The distal biceps tendon in the antecubital fossa is nonpalpable.

Hook Test
- The examiner attempts to hook the distal biceps tendon in the antecubital fossa with the index finger while the patient's elbow is flexed and the forearm is supinated.
- Sensitivity and specificity for complete rupture are reported to be nearly 100% for this test.
- The distal biceps tendon insertion site is tender to palpation just distal to the antecubital fossa.
- Pain or weakness is noted with resisted forearm supination and flexion. (Remember: The brachialis muscle is the primary elbow flexor; the biceps brachii is a primary forearm supinator when the elbow is flexed.)

Imaging
- Radiographs of the elbow should be obtained: AP, lateral, and oblique views. The images are usually normal, however.

Additional Imaging
Magnetic Resonance Imaging
- Usually, this diagnosis is made clinically. MRI may be indicated if the diagnosis is unclear, if a partial tear is suspected, or if the surgeon requires additional studies for operative planning.

Classification
- Complete or partial
- Acute (<4 weeks old)
- Chronic (>4 weeks old)

Initial Treatment
Patient Education
- It is important to repair the tendon within 2 to 3 weeks of injury.
- Repair is usually recommended to limit weakness of elbow flexion and supination, but in some situations (patient is low demand, is of advanced age, or has significant medical comorbidities), an argument can be made against repair.
- If the injury is left unrepaired, the patient can expect a loss of about 25%

of flexion strength and up to 40% of supination strength.

- After tendon repair, a significant amount of rehabilitation is necessary, and full strength is not usually recovered until 6 months postoperatively.

First Treatment Steps
- Splint the elbow in a posterior splint with the elbow at 90 degrees, and provide a sling for comfort.
- The patient should be seen by orthopaedic surgeon as soon as possible and within 2 weeks of injury so that surgery can be performed within the first 21 days.

Treatment Options
Nonoperative Management
- Conservative management is indicated for partial ruptures of less than 50% of the tendon insertion, or if patient is low demand, is older, or has significant medical comorbidities.
- If nonoperative management is indicated, splint the elbow for no more than 3 weeks to allow pain and edema to subside.
- Use a hinged elbow brace with low-grade partial tears, and gradually increase the arc of motion over several weeks. Strengthening can begin at 3 months.
- For nonoperative complete tears, start early elbow ROM with a skilled occupational therapist. Later, the patient can start strengthening ancillary elbow muscles to minimize loss of strength.

Operative Management
Codes
ICD-9 code: 840.8 Rupture of the distal biceps tendon
CPT code: 24342 Reinsertion of distal biceps tendon

Operative Indications
- Acute rupture of the distal biceps tendon
- Partial ruptures of more than 50% of the tendinous insertion

Informed Consent and Counseling
- Recovery time is 6 months until return to full strength.

- Success of surgery depends on the patient's compliance with the postoperative therapy program.
- There is a risk of development of heterotopic ossification (HO), which could limit motion and result in the need for additional procedures. Compliance with therapy is crucial.
- A small (5%) risk of injury to the PIN exists, but usually this injury is transient neurapraxia.

Anesthesia
- Regional upper extremity block, with general anesthesia

Patient Positioning
- The patient is supine, with the arm extended on the arm table.
- A nonsterile tourniquet is placed high on the brachium.
- A sterile towel roll or upside-down basin may be used under the forearm to place the elbow in flexion once the repair is complete; this limits tension on the repair.

Surgical Procedures
- The most common repair is with suture anchors or a bone tunnel at the radial tuberosity.
- Multiple approaches and techniques for repair have been described. These include:
  - Single incision extended Henry Approach (S-type or horizontal incision at the antecubital fossa)
  - Dual incision technique incorporating the S-type antecubital incision with a dorsal forearm incision that splits the extensor carpi ulnaris (ECU)
  - Tendon repair using a bone tunnel, suture anchor technique, intraosseous screw fixation, or suspensory cortical button

Distal Biceps Tendon Repair:
Figure 3-13
- Instruments include suture anchors if applicable, as well as a burr if using a bone tunnel.
- A lazy-S incision is made over the antecubital fossa with the proximal aspect of the incision medially. Avoid

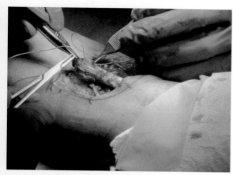

Figure 3-13. Repair of the distal biceps tendon.

injury to the **lateral antebrachial cutaneous nerve**, which lies just lateral to the biceps tendon in the antecubital fossa. The radial artery and the basilic vein and its tributaries are also protected during this procedure. The proximal stump of the biceps tendon is identified, and a hematoma is frequently encountered. The lacertus fibrosis (also known as the bicipital aponeurosis) often prevents the tendon from retracting. The stump of the tendon is mobilized and freed of adhesions. An interval is developed between the brachioradialis and the pronator teres. The forearm is placed in supination to avoid injury to the PIN, and blunt dissection is used to identify the radial tuberosity.

- The radial tuberosity is identified and prepared by débridement with a rongeur. If suture anchors are used for repair, these are then placed at the radial tuberosity. If a bone tunnel is used, a second incision is made posteriorly through the ECU tendon. The forearm is maintained in pronation during this portion of the surgical procedure. The radius is identified posteriorly, and a burr is used to create the tunnel at the radial tuberosity. A 2-mm drill bit is used to create two or three holes about 1 cm apart on the lateral side of the radius.
- The biceps tendon is then prepared with a double-limbed running locking suture, also known as a Krackow suture technique. The suture limbs are then pulled down into the bone tunnel

or to the suture anchor and are tied in place. The elbow must be flexed during this procedure.
- After irrigation and closure of the wound, a posterior elbow splint is applied with the elbow flexed to 90 degrees and the forearm in neutral.

Estimated Postoperative Course
- Postoperative days 10 to 14
  - A wound check and suture removal are performed.
  - The elbow is continuously maintained in 90 degrees of flexion during examination.
  - Occupational therapy is initiated for edema control, wrist and finger ROM, and shoulder pendulum exercises with the elbow in a splint. A splint is fabricated, or a hinged elbow brace is provided and locked at 90 degrees.
- Postoperative 3 weeks
  - Therapy starts to increase dynamic elbow flexion. Elbow extension is incrementally increased from weeks 3 to 6 while in the hinged brace. The patient can perform active extension in the brace, but no active flexion. The patient also begins gentle active forearm pronation with the elbow at 90 degrees.
- Postoperative 6 weeks
  - The patient returns for a clinic visit for a wound and motion check.
  - The patient continues with therapy for progressive extension.
- Postoperative 8 weeks
  - The patient can start gentle active elbow flexion.
- Postoperative 12 weeks through 6 months
  - The patient returns for a clinic visit at 3 months and 6 months postoperatively for a motion check.
  - The patient continues with therapy for ROM and can start strengthening.

Suggested Readings
Bain GI, Johnson LJ, Turner PC: Treatment of partial distal biceps tendon tears, *Sports Med Arthrosc Rev* 16:154–161, 2008.

Cohen MS: Complications of distal biceps tendon repairs, *Sports Med Arthrosc Rev* 16:148–153, 2008.

Morrey BF, Askew NL, An KN, et al: Rupture of the distal tendon of the biceps brachii, *J Bone Joint Surg Am* 67:418–421, 1985.

Sutton KM, Dodds SD, Ahmad CS, et al: Surgical treatment of distal biceps rupture, *J Am Acad Orthop Surg* 18:139–148, 2010.

ELBOW SPRAIN

History

- Fall onto an outstretched hand
- Possible report of a "pop" at the time of injury
- Elbow pain, stiffness, and edema after a fall
- Overhead throwing athletes prone to UCL sprains or chronic instability
- Overhead throwing athlete with report of medial-sided elbow pain worse during late cocking and acceleration phases of throwing, decreased velocity, and loss of control.

Physical Examination

- Observe edema, ecchymosis, and position of the elbow.
- Observe active elbow ROM including supination and pronation.
- Palpate for tenderness to palpation at the following areas:
  - Medial epicondyle and the UCL complex just anterior to the medial epicondyle
  - Lateral epicondyle and the LCL complex just anterior to the lateral epicondyle
  - Radial head
- Palpate the ulnar nerve in the cubital tunnel, and document a thorough neurovascular examination.

Evaluation of the Ulnar Collateral Ligament Complex

Valgus Stress Test: Figure 3-14
The examiner places one hand on the lateral aspect of the patient's brachium and the other hand on the patient's forearm. The examiner stabilizes the brachium and places the elbow in about 30 degrees of flexion to "unlock" the olecranon and then applies valgus stress on the UCL. A positive test result is characterized by pain, apprehension, or instability of the ligament.

Milking Maneuver: Figure 3-15
The patient lies supine on the examining table. The shoulder is abducted to

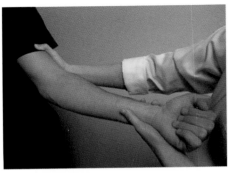

Figure 3-14. Valgus stress test.

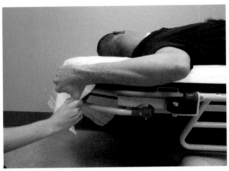

Figure 3-15. Milking maneuver.

90 degrees, and the elbow is flexed to 90 degrees, with the thumb pointing toward the floor. The examiner grabs the patient's thumb and pulls downward toward the floor (hence, "milking maneuver"). This maneuver places stress over the UCL. A positive test result is characterized by pain, apprehension, or frank instability.

Evaluation of the Lateral Collateral Ligament Complex

Varus Stress Test
This test is similar to the valgus stress test. The examiner places one hand on the medial side of the patient's elbow and holds the medial and lateral epicondyles. With the other hand, the examiner places the patient's elbow in about 30 degrees of flexion to "unlock" the olecranon and then applies varus stress across the LCL complex. A positive test result is characterized by pain, apprehension, or instability.

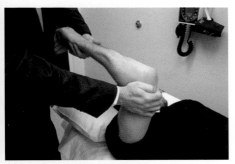

Figure 3-16. Lateral pivot shift test.

Lateral Pivot Shift Test: Figure 3-16

This tests the lateral-UCL (LUCL) for posterolateral rotatory instability. The patient lies supine on the examining table. The shoulder is extended over the patient's head. The examiner stands at the head of the bed. The examiner places a hand on the posterolateral aspect of the patient's elbow and grasps the medial and lateral epicondyles. The maneuver starts with the elbow in an extended position. The examiner applies axial force to the elbow joint and simultaneously flexes and supinates the forearm. A positive test result is characterized by pain, apprehension, a "clunk," or frank dislocation.

Imaging

- Elbow AP, lateral, and oblique views
- Varus or valgus stress views

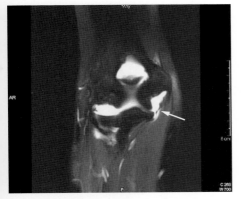

Figure 3-17. Elbow magnetic resonance imaging with arthrogram with a partial ulnar collateral ligament tear. A small strand of ligament is still attached to the ulna.

- Observation for unilateral widening of the joint or avulsion fractures
- Radiographs often normal in simple dislocations
- MRI with arthrogram helpful in the diagnosis of a partial or complete tear (Fig. 3-17).

Initial Treatment

Patient Education
- Most simple elbow sprains heal with nonoperative treatment.
- The patient may experience elbow stiffness as a result of this injury.

First Treatment Steps
- Confirm that the elbow joint is reduced on a radiograph.
- Place the elbow in a long-arm posterior splint.
- Refer the patient to be seen in follow-up in 10 to 14 days.

Treatment Options

Nonoperative Management
- Reserved for sprained but intact ligaments and/or stable reduced joints.
- Remove the initial splint, and assess ROM.
- Place the patient in a hinged elbow brace, and allow gentle elbow ROM in the brace.
- Refer the patient to an occupational therapist to help guide protected elbow ROM.
- The patient is to be non–weight bearing for 6 to 8 weeks.
- Retest elbow ROM, and assess stability after about 2 months of treatment. If the joint is stable and there is no pain, the patient can return to all regular activities (overhead throwing athletes can return to a graduated throwing program at about 3 months).
- If the patient has continued pain or instability, obtain an MRI with an arthrogram of the elbow to evaluate the location and degree of tear.

Operative Management
Codes
ICD-9 codes:
  841.0 Sprain of elbow radial (lateral) collateral ligament

841.1 Sprain of elbow ulnar (medial) collateral ligament

841.9 Sprain of elbow or forearm unspecified site

CPT codes:

24344 Reconstruction of radial (lateral) collateral ligament with tendon graft

24346 Reconstruction of ulnar (medial) collateral ligament with tendon graft

Operative Indications
- UCL injury
  - Complete tear with significant elbow instability
  - A partial tear with no improvement after 2 to 3 months of conservative management
  - High-level overhead throwing athlete in whom 6 weeks of splinting and rehabilitation fail
- LCL injury
  - The presence of posterolateral rotatory instability

Informed Consent and Counseling
- A significant amount of postoperative therapy is required for a successful outcome.
- The medial antebrachial cutaneous nerve and the ulnar nerve are at risk for injury during UCL surgery.
- This procedure carries a risk of elbow stiffness.
- Overhead throwing athletes will not be back to baseline for at least 1 year and may not be able to achieve preinjury level of performance.

Anesthesia
- Regional block with general anesthesia

Patient Positioning
- The patient is supine, with the arm extended on an arm table. The elbow is flexed.
- A nonsterile tourniquet is placed high on the brachium.

Surgical Procedures
Ulnar Collateral Ligament Reconstruction or Lateral Collateral Ligament Reconstruction
- Direct ligament repair is performed on acute injuries usually associated with

elbow dislocation or an acute avulsion from the humerus (see p. 95 for elbow dislocation).

Ulnar Collateral Ligament Reconstruction (also known as Tommy John Surgery): Figure 3-18
- An incision is made just anterior to the medial epicondyle. Blunt dissection is used in the subcutaneous tissue so that the **medial antebrachial cutaneous nerve** can be identified and protected. The underlying medial epicondyle and common flexor tendon origin are identified. Note whether the tendon origin has been injured because this is a secondary stabilizer of the elbow.
- A longitudinal incision is made through the common flexor tendon origin running parallel to the muscle fibers. A plane is developed between the tendon origin and the underlying joint capsule and UCL. At this point, it may be pertinent to dissect, identify, and protect the ulnar nerve in the cubital tunnel for the remainder of the procedure. The UCL is identified, and injuries are noted, most of which occur in the midsubstance of the anterior bundle.
- Bone tunnels are created next with a 3.5-mm or similar drill bit. **Extreme care should be taken to protect the ulnar nerve while drilling.** Two converging holes are made in the humerus at the origination point of the UCL.

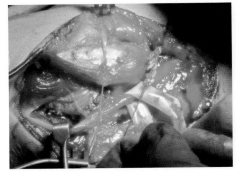

Figure 3-18. Reconstruction of the ulnar collateral ligament with a palmaris longus tendon graft (also known as Tommy John surgery).

- Next, a single tunnel is created in the ulna at the insertion point of the UCL. An autologous tendon graft is harvested (usually the palmaris longus tendon, or a strip of the Achilles or hamstring). With the elbow in 45 degrees of flexion, the graft is woven through the bone tunnels in a figure-8 fashion and is sutured together.
- The elbow is placed through ROM, and the graft is stressed to ensure stability and appropriate tightening. At this point, the surgeon may choose to transpose the ulnar nerve. The joint capsule is then closed, and the common flexor tendon origin is repaired as indicated. Some surgeons use a temporary drain. The patient is placed in a long-arm posterior splint with the elbow in 90 degrees of flexion and the forearm in neutral.

Lateral Collateral Ligament Reconstruction

- A posterior midline approach or Kocher approach is used. The common extensor tendon origin is identified, and an interval is created through the ECU and anconeus to expose the underlying LCL and joint capsule. The elbow is placed under varus stress, and the ligamentous injury is identified.
- Anteriorly converging bone tunnels are then created on the posterior surface of the lateral epicondyle with a 3.5-mm or similar drill bit. A single tunnel is created on the ulna from the supinator tubercle to the ulnar attachment of the annular ligament.
- An autologous tendon graft is harvested (usually the Palmaris longus, or a strip of the Achilles or hamstring). The graft is then woven through the bone tunnels in a figure of 8 or similar fashion.
- The elbow is placed through ROM and varus stress to ensure proper stability and graft tension.
- The joint capsule is closed, and the common extensor tendon origin is repaired as needed. The wound is closed in layers. A long-arm posterior splint is applied with the elbow in 90 degrees of flexion and the forearm in neutral.

Estimated Postoperative Course

Ulnar Collateral and Lateral Collateral Ligament Reconstruction

- Postoperative day 7
  - Remove the postoperative dressing for a wound check.
  - UCL: Start gentle elbow ROM under the guidance of an occupational therapist or athletic trainer. For protection, a hinged elbow brace may be prescribed with full ROM.
  - LCL: Provide a hinged elbow brace locked at 30 degrees of extension and gradually extend the elbow at 10-degree increments over a 6-week period. Initiate gentle elbow ROM in the brace as guided by an occupational therapist.
  - The patient is non–weight bearing for 6 to 8 weeks.
- Postoperative 2 weeks
  - Return for suture removal.
- Postoperative 4 weeks
  - Start strengthening of the wrist and forearm.
- Postoperative 6 weeks
  - Start gradual strengthening of the elbow.
- Postoperative 3 months
  - Most patients return to activities as tolerated.
  - A graduated throwing program may be initiated for the overhead throwing athlete.
- Postoperative 9 to 18 months
  - Overhead throwing athletes can usually return to play at preinjury level.

Suggested Readings

Cain EL Jr, Dugas JR, Wolf RS, et al: Elbow injuries in throwing athletes: a current concepts review, *Am J Sports Med* 31:621–35, 2003.

Chen FS, Rokito AS, Jobe FW: Medial elbow problems in the overhead throwing athlete, *J Am Acad Orthop Surg* 9:99–113, 2001.

Mehta JA, Bain GI: Posterolateral rotatory instability of the elbow, *J Am Acad Orthop Surg* 12:405–415, 2004.

ACUTE ELBOW DISLOCATIONS
History

- Fall onto an outstretched arm
- High-energy trauma or fall from a height

Physical Examination
- Inspect for evidence of elbow deformity, and identify open injuries.
- Inspect skin integrity, and identify abrasions.
- Palpate known landmarks: lateral epicondyle, medial epicondyle, olecranon process, and radial head.
- Assess neurovascular function and, in particular, the distal motor and sensory function of the median, ulnar, and radial nerves, the brachial artery, and the radial and ulnar arteries distally. Document findings before and after reduction.
- Neurovascular injury is rare and usually transient. The brachial and radial pulse may be diminished initially but should return to normal once the joint is reduced. The ulnar or median nerve may incur stretch neurapraxia while the joint is dislocated, and this should resolve once the injury is reduced.

Imaging: Figure 3-19
- Radiographs of the elbow: AP, lateral, and oblique views

Ligaments: see Figure 3-2
Classification
- Of dislocations, 90% are posterior or posterolateral (radius and ulna dislocate posterior to humerus).

Simple Instability
- Injury to the UCL or the LCL (specifically the LUCL)

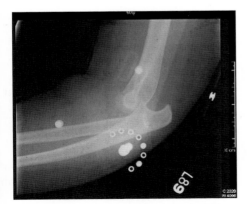

Figure 3-19. Radiograph of a posterior elbow dislocation.

- General pattern of simple dislocation (described by O'Driscoll et al): stage 1, disruption of the LUCL; stage 2, disruption of the remainder of the LCL in addition to the anterior and posterior capsules; stage 3, partial (posterior band only) or complete UCL disruption

Complex Instability: Ligamentous and Osseous Injury
- Radial head fracture with dislocation
- Coronoid fracture with dislocation
- Monteggia fracture-dislocation
- Transolecranon fracture-dislocation
- Terrible triad: a constellation of elbow dislocation, radial head fracture, and coronoid fracture

Primary Stabilizers of the Elbow
- LCL complex
- UCL complex
- Ulnohumeral joint

Secondary Stabilizers of the Elbow
- Radial head
- Common flexor and extensor tendon origins
- Elbow joint capsule

Initial Treatment
Patient Education
- Most acute simple injuries can be treated with reduction followed by a period of immobilization and do not require surgery. If the elbow remains unstable or a complex injury pattern exists, surgical treatment is necessary.
- Chronic elbow instability after a simple dislocation is unusual and occurs in less than 1% to 2%.
- Some loss of elbow ROM, especially in terminal extension, can result after an elbow dislocation.
- HO can occur after a dislocation but rarely limits function.
- Recovery and rehabilitation can take 6 to 8 weeks.

First Treatment Step
Elbow Joint Closed Reduction: Figure 3-20
Code
CPT code: 24605 Closed reduction with anesthesia

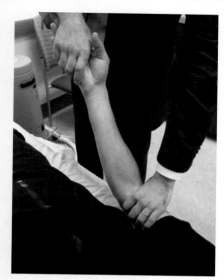

Figure 3-20. Closed reduction of a dislocated elbow.

Procedure
- Obtain adequate pain control, and use conscious sedation to provide muscle relaxation and to ease reduction.
- Perform and document prereduction and postreduction neurovascular examinations.
- For posterior dislocations, the patient is supine on a stretcher. An assistant is used to apply traction at the brachium. Apply traction at the forearm with one hand. With the other hand, apply pressure to the posterior aspect of the olecranon by pushing it anteriorly into the trochlea. Varus or valgus stress may also be applied to reduce the joint. The elbow can be flexed during this maneuver to aid in reducing the ulnohumeral joint. An audible "clunk" usually accompanies successful reduction.
- Once reduced, the elbow is placed through passive ROM to ensure reduction and stability. Occasionally, the elbow redislocates in extension. When this occurs, the elbow should be reduced again, and an extension blocking splint should be applied to maintain the reduction.
- Postreduction radiographs are taken: AP and true lateral views of the elbow.

Evaluate for adequate reduction and a congruent joint.

Postreduction Procedures and Therapy
- After the elbow joint is reduced, document a neurovascular examination of the median, ulnar, and radial nerves, as well as the radial and ulnar arteries.
- Place the patient in a sugar tong splint with the elbow flexed to 90 degrees and the forearm in neutral rotation, and advise the patient not to remove the splint.
- The patient should return to the clinic in 10 to 14 days for repeat radiographs to ensure that the joint has stayed reduced. The splint can be removed and replaced with a hinged elbow brace or sling.
- Gentle ROM is initiated; the extremity is non–weight bearing; the patient may require supervised therapy visits for ROM.
- If the elbow feels unstable in extension, an extension block should be applied to the hinged elbow brace and gradually increased over 3 to 6 weeks.
- The patient should return to the clinic in 6 to 8 weeks. If the elbow is stable on repeat examination, the patient can be released to gradual weight bearing at 6 to 8 weeks.

Treatment Options
Nonoperative Management
Indications
- Simple dislocations
- Stable and congruent elbow joint after reduction or a stable joint through 50 to 60 degrees of flexion

Operative Management
Codes
ICD-9 codes: 832.0 Closed dislocation of the elbow
CPT codes: 24615 Open treatment of acute or chronic elbow dislocation
    24586 Open treatment of elbow periarticular fracture and/or dislocation
    24343 Repair of radial (lateral) collateral ligament
    24345 Repair of ulnar (medial) collateral ligament

Operative Indications
- An unreducible joint
- Acute dislocations that require more than 50 to 60 degrees of flexion to maintain reduction
- Elbow dislocation with an associated unstable periarticular fracture

Informed Consent and Counseling
- Significant stiffness may occur after an elbow fracture-dislocation; therefore, extensive therapy is needed postoperatively.
- Posttraumatic stiffness may need to be addressed later with anterior or posterior capsulotomies. Functional ROM of the elbow is 30 to 130 degrees.

Anesthesia
- Regional upper extremity block with general anesthesia

Patient Positioning
- Supine on the operating table, with the arm extended on an arm board
- Sterile or nonsterile tourniquet applied high on the brachium

Surgical Procedures
- Repair of collateral ligaments
- External fixation (rigid or dynamic): for persistent instability after ligament repair
- Other:
  - Open reduction, internal fixation (ORIF) is indicated for fractures (radial head, coronoid) with repair of collateral ligaments as needed. External fixators can be applied during this procedure.
  - Occasionally, implants such as a radial head implant are used.

Collateral Ligament Repair
- Hardware includes suture anchors and intraoperative fluoroscopy equipment.
- The medial collateral ligament and LCL are approached through two separate incisions. On the medial side of the elbow, an incision is made over the medial epicondyle. Care is taken to avoid injury to the **ulnar nerve**, which is identified in the cubital tunnel and is protected. The flexor-pronator mass is identified, as is the injured UCL. Often, the entire flexor pronator mass is disrupted from the medial epicondyle in addition to the UCL. The ligament and flexor pronator mass can be repaired back to their origins either with suture through bone tunnels or with suture anchors.
- Next, an incision is made over the lateral aspect of the elbow by using a posterior midline or Kocher approach. The lateral epicondyle and the common extensor tendon origin are identified. Often, the common extensor tendon insertion is disrupted, and the underlying ruptured LCL is easily identified. The ligament and common extensor tendon origin can be repaired back to their origins either with suture through bone tunnels or with suture anchors. The elbow is then placed through ROM, and intraoperative fluoroscopy is used to confirm joint reduction through ROM.
- It may be necessary to apply an external fixator if the joint is unstable. The fixator is applied with two pins in the humerus and two pins in the ulna. Care should be taken when placing the humeral pins to avoid injury to the **axillary nerve**, which lies 4 to 7 cm distal to the acromion, and the radial nerve in the spiral groove, which is found 9 cm from the acromion and 10 cm from the lateral epicondyle. Pins are placed through small incisions under direct visualization. A drill guide firmly seated on bone is used to avoid soft tissue injury. The fixator is usually left in place for 3 to 4 weeks to allow the ligaments to heal.

Estimated Postoperative Course
- Postoperative days 10 to 14
  - Remove sutures, and perform a wound check.
  - Document a neurovascular examination.
  - Obtain radiographs of the elbow: AP and lateral.
  - Therapy for stable elbows after ligament repair: Some clinicians advocate for early protected motion. The patient is taken out of the postoperative splint and placed into a hinged

elbow brace, and protected motion is started.
- For elbows in external fixators: Provide pin site care education.
■ Postoperative 4 weeks
- For stable elbows after ligament repair: Obtain radiographs to check joint reduction after initiation of therapy.
- For elbows in an external fixator: The fixator can be removed in the clinic. Provide a hinged elbow brace, and start gentle protected motion now or in 2 more weeks, depending on strength of repair and the severity of injury.
■ Postoperative 8 weeks
- Perform a motion check.
- Obtain radiographs to confirm joint reduction.
- Therapy: Progress ROM and start a gradual strengthening program.
■ Postoperative 3 months
- Perform a final check for ROM and strengthening.
- Continue to follow the patient if ROM is not yet functional (30 to 130 degrees).

Suggested Readings

Chen NC, Julka A: Hinged external fixation of the elbow, *Hand Clin* 26:423–433, 2010.
Cohen MS, Hastings H 2nd: Acute elbow dislocation: evaluation and management, *J Am Acad Orthop Surg* 6:15–23, 1998.
Ebrahimzadeh MH, Amadzadeh-Chabock H, Ring D: Traumatic elbow instability, *J Hand Surg* 35:1220–225, 2010.
Morrey BF: Current concepts in the management of complex elbow trauma, *Surgeon* 7:151–161, 2009.

FOREARM (RADIUS AND ULNA) FRACTURES AND DISLOCATIONS

■ Ulnar shaft fracture (night-stick fracture)
■ Radial shaft fracture
■ Both bone forearm fracture (Figure 3-21)
■ Galeazzi fracture-dislocation: distal third radius fracture with dislocation of the distal ulna (Figure 3-22)
■ Monteggia fracture-dislocation: proximal third ulna fracture with dislocation of the proximal radius (Figure 3-23)

History

■ Usually high-energy trauma such as motor vehicle crash (MVC) or a fall from a height
■ Pain and deformity in the forearm and/or elbow

Physical Examination

■ Look for evidence of open injury, inspect skin integrity, and identify abrasions.
■ Edema and deformity may be present.
■ Palpate for instability of the forearm bones and crepitus, and palpate for concomitant wrist injury.
■ Assess compartments for compartment syndrome.
■ Assess distal motor function for finger and wrist flexor and extensors.
■ Assess the neurovascular examination, especially function of the PIN, and document it.

Imaging: Figures 3-21 through 3-23

■ Obtain routine elbow, forearm, and wrist films as indicated

Classification System: Monteggia Fractures

Type I (most common): Anterior dislocation of the radial head and ulnar diaphysis fracture
Type II: Posterior or posterolateral dislocation of the radial head and ulnar diaphysis fracture
Type III: Lateral or anterolateral dislocation of the radial head and fracture through the ulnar metaphysis
Type IV (rare): Anterior dislocation of radial head and fracture of both forearm bones

Initial Treatment

Patient Education

■ Bone forearm fractures, Monteggia fractures, and Galeazzi fractures should be treated with ORIF unless medical status prohibits.
■ The recovery period is 6 to 8 weeks, depending on bone healing.

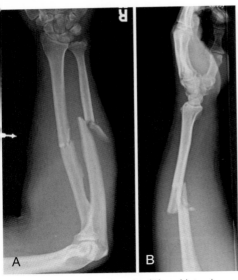

Figure 3-21. Anteroposterior (**A**) and lateral (**B**) radiographs of a comminuted displaced both bone forearm fracture.

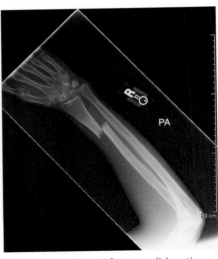

Figure 3-22. Galeazzi fracture-dislocation: distal third radius fracture with dislocation of the ulna at the distal radioulnar joint. PA, posteroanterior. *(From Dacus AR: Radial and ulnar shaft fractures. In Miller MD, Hart JA, MacKnight JM, editors: Essential orthopaedics, Philadelphia, 2010, Saunders, 2010, p 280.)*

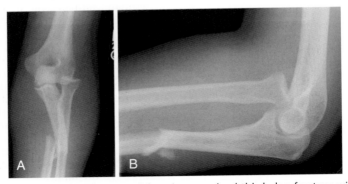

Figure 3-23. Type I Monteggia fracture-dislocation: proximal third ulna fracture with dislocation of the radial head. **A,** Anteroposterior view; **B,** lateral view.

First Treatment Steps
- All patients with open injuries should be taken to the operating room urgently.
- Reduce closed fractures by using traction and manipulation, if necessary.
- Splint the forearm in a sugar tong splint or a long-arm posterior splint with the elbow at 90 degrees and the forearm in neutral pronation.

Treatment Options
Nonoperative Management
Both Bone Forearm Fractures
- Nonoperative treatment generally not recommended

Ulnar Shaft Fractures and Radial Shaft Fractures

- Nonoperative management is indicated if the patient has less than 10 degrees of angulation and at least 50% cortical contact.
- A sugar tong splint is used for 1 to 2 weeks.
- Apply a short arm cast or a Muenster cast for an additional 4 weeks.
- Place a functional splint for 2 weeks, and start elbow and therapy referral for forearm ROM.
- Monitor fractures with radiographs at each visit to evaluate for displacement.

Galeazzi Fracture-Dislocation

- Nonoperative treatment generally not recommended

Monteggia Fracture-Dislocation

- Nonoperative treatment generally not recommended

Operative Management
Codes
ICD-9 codes: Radial shaft fracture, closed 813.21, open 813.31
Ulnar shaft fracture: closed 813.22, open 813.32
Radius and ulna shaft fractures: closed 813.23, open 813.33
- CPT codes: 25515 ORIF radial shaft fracture
  25525 ORIF radial shaft fracture and closed treatment of DRUJ dislocation
  25526 ORIF radial shaft fracture and open treatment DRUJ dislocation
  24635 ORIF Monteggia fracture
  25545 ORIF ulnar shaft fracture
  25575 ORIF radius and ulna shaft fractures
  +20690 Application of uniplanar external fixator

Operative Indications
- All open injuries
- Both bone forearm fractures
- Galeazzi fractures
- Monteggia fractures
- Radial or ulnar shaft fractures with more than 10 degrees of angulation or a more than 50% loss of cortical contact

Informed Consent and Counseling
- Treatment of open injuries has a higher risk of infection and nonunion.
- Significant elbow stiffness can result from these injuries, and aggressive postoperative therapy is the key to a good functional outcome.
- A risk of PIN injury or palsy related to exposure of the proximal and middle radius exists.

Anesthesia
- Regional upper extremity block with sedation or general anesthesia

Patient Positioning
- The patient is supine on the operating table, with the arm extended on an arm board.
- A nonsterile tourniquet is placed high on the brachium.
- Intraoperative fluoroscopy is used.

Surgical Procedures
Open Reduction, Internal Fixation of the Radius and Ulna Shaft:
Figure 3-24
- Two approaches are needed: the approach to the ulnar shaft and the Thompson approach to the dorsal forearm.

Open Reduction, Internal Fixation of Both Bone Forearm Fractures
- Equipment: 3.5-mm dynamic compression plate, intraoperative fluoroscopy, and mini–C-arm

Approach to the Ulna Shaft
Make a longitudinal incision directly over the midulnar shaft at the interval between the ECU and FCU muscle bellies. Use a periosteal elevator to lift the ECU and FCU from their attachments on the ulna. Identify the fracture site, and débride any hematoma. Reduce the fracture with the aid of retractors or towel clips. Apply an appropriate plate, and use lag screws across the fracture site as necessary. Use intraoperative fluoroscopy to confirm the placement of hardware and fracture reduction. Once fixation is in place, the wound is irrigated, and the fascia is closed using suture. The skin is closed in layers.

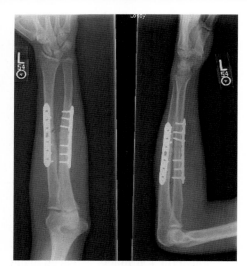

Figure 3-24. Radiographs of a both bone forearm fracture treated with open reduction, internal fixation. *Left,* Anteroposterior view; *right,* lateral view.

Thompson (Dorsal) Approach to the Radius

The forearm is pronated, and a longitudinal incision is made between the extensor carpi radialis brevis (ECRB) and extensor digitorum communis (EDC) muscle bellies. The interval lies just anterior to the lateral epicondyle and travels distally toward the Lister tubercle on the dorsal radius. The ECRB and EDC muscles are retracted at this interval to expose the underlying supinator and abductor pollicis longus (APL). Extreme care should be taken to identify the **PIN** as it runs through and exits the supinator. The radius is identified between the supinator and the APL, and a periosteal incision is made down its shaft. The periosteum can be elevated down the length of the radius as needed. The APL and extensor pollicis brevis are retracted to expose more distal fractures. An appropriate plate is selected, and lag screws are used as indicated. Intraoperative fluoroscopy is used to confirm hardware placement and fracture reduction. Once the fracture is fixed, the wound is irrigated,

and the fascia is closed. The skin is closed in layers.

Henry Approach (Volar Approach) to the Forearm (for Galeazzi Fractures)

A longitudinal incision is made directly over the FCR tendon. Sharp dissection is carried down through the skin and subcutaneous tissues, the FCR tendon sheath is divided, and the tendon is mobilized. The interval of this approach is between the FCR and the brachioradialis. The FCR and the underlying flexor pollicis longus are retracted. The flexor compartment with the **median nerve** is retracted ulnarly as a unit and is protected. Care is taken to protect the **radial artery** and the **superficial sensory radial nerve** on the radial aspect of the surgical field. If operating on the distal aspect of the radius, the pronator quadratus is visible once the tendons have been retracted. If operating on the radial shaft, the interval of exposure lies between the flexor digitorum superficialis and the pronator teres. The periosteum of the radius is sharply incised and elevated from the bone at the fracture site. Usually, the distal radioulnar joint (DRUJ) will reduce once the radius fracture has been stabilized.

A sugar tong or long-arm posterior splint is applied. It is important to assess the patient's PIN postoperatively during exposures of the proximal forearm if a nerve block was not used.

Estimated Postoperative Course

- Postoperative days 10 to 14
  - Wound check and suture removal
  - Radiographs are obtained as follows: for shaft fractures, forearm posteroanterior (PA) and lateral views; for Monteggia fracture, elbow AP and lateral views; for Galeazzi fracture, wrist PA and lateral views.
  - If fixation is stable, the patient can wear a removable custom forearm splint and start therapy for gentle hand, wrist, forearm, and elbow ROM. The patient is non–weight bearing on the extremity.
  - For severely comminuted fractures, a long-arm or Muenster cast may

be necessary for several weeks. In addition, consider casting in patients who need to bear weight on the forearm such as with a platform attachment on a walker.
- Postoperative 6 weeks
  - Radiographs are obtained as described earlier.
  - If healing is evident, start strengthening and gradual weight bearing.
  - If no healing is present, continue the current program.
- Postoperative 3 months
  - Radiographs are obtained as described earlier.
  - If healing is evident, release the patient to all regular activities.
  - If no healing is present, consider supplying the patient with a bone stimulator. Consider reasons for nonunion including infection. It may be beneficial to order appropriate laboratory tests.

Suggested Readings

Chhabra AB: Elbow and forearm. In Miller MD, Chhabra AB, Hurwitz S, et al, editors: *Orthopaedic surgical approaches*, Philadelphia, 2008, Saunders, pp 61–144.

Eathiraju S, Mudgal CS, Jupiter JB: Monteggia fracture-dislocations, *Hand Clin* 23:165–177, 2007.

Giannoulis FS, Sotereanos DG: Galeazzi fractures and dislocations, *Hand Clin* 23:153–163, 2007.

Moss JP, Bynum DK: Diaphyseal fractures of the radius and ulna in adults, *Hand Clin* 23:143–151, 2007.

Sauder DJ, Athwal GS: Management of isolated ulnar shaft fractures, *Hand Clin* 23:179–184, 2007.

Sebastin SJ, Chung KC: A historical report on Riccardo Galeazzi and the management of Galeazzi fractures, *J Hand Surg* 35:1870–1877, 2010.

RADIAL HEAD FRACTURES
History
- Fall on an outstretched hand
- Lateral elbow pain, edema, and stiffness

Physical Examination
- Possible elbow edema
- Possible limited and/or painful ROM
- Tenderness to palpation at the radial head and pain and possible crepitus with forearm rotation

Imaging: Figures 3-25 and Figure 3-26
- AP, lateral, and oblique radiographic views, and possibly a "radial head view," of the elbow are obtained.
- A radial head view or Greenspan view is a modified lateral view with the beam angled 45 degrees toward the radial head.
- Look for the "sail sign" on the radiograph. This is a shadow created by the anterior fat pad when elbow effusion is present. This sign may indicate intra-articular injury even if radiographic findings are negative.

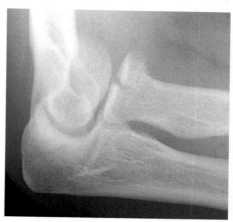

Figure 3-25. Radial head view or Greenspan view of a type I radial head fracture.

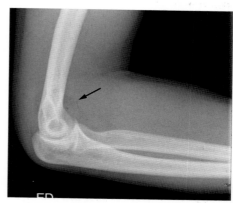

Figure 3-26. Radiograph of an occult radial head fracture with a "sail sign" (*arrow*).

- A computed tomography (CT) scan may be helpful to characterize comminuted fracture fragments further.

Mason Classification System (as Modified by Hotchkiss):
Figure 3-27 **and** Table 3-5

Initial Treatment
Patient Education
- Type I nondisplaced radial head fractures do not require prolonged immobilization.
- Elbow stiffness can develop after this fracture; the patient may require occupational therapy during healing.
- Intra-articular fractures are associated with an increased risk of posttraumatic arthritis.

First Treatment Steps
- Evaluate ROM. If a significant block to supination or pronation is noted,

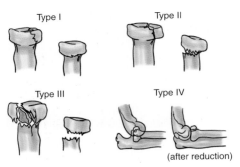

Type I   Type II   Type III   Type IV

(after reduction)

Figure 3-27. Classification of radial head fractures. *(From Dacus AR: Radial head or neck fractures. In Miller MD, Hart JA, MacKnight JM, editors:* Essential orthopaedics, *Philadelphia, 2010, Saunders, 2010, p 274.)*

Table 3-5. Mason Classification System (as Modified by Hotchkiss)	
Type I	Minimally displaced radial head fracture (<2 mm intra-articular step-off) with no block to motion
Type II	Radial head fracture displaced >2 mm or angulated
Type III	Comminuted fracture of the radial head with block to motion
Type IV	Radial head fracture with elbow dislocation

attempt hematoma aspiration and/or intra-articular injection of 1% plain lidocaine. If block remains, a CT scan may be necessary to evaluate for displaced, intra-articular fracture.
- Splint the elbow in a long-arm posterior splint.

Treatment Options
Nonoperative Management
- Nonoperative management is indicated for a nondisplaced or minimally displaced (1-mm intra-articular step-off or less) fracture without block to motion.
- Maintain in a posterior splint for 7 to 14 days, and no longer than 21 days, to prevent permanent elbow stiffness.
- Obtain a repeat radiograph of the elbow at the first follow-up visit to evaluate for displacement.
- If reduction is maintained, transition the patient to a hinged elbow brace, and start gentle elbow ROM. Based on the patient's level of discomfort, the brace may need to have a limited arc of motion initially, with graduated progression to full ROM.
- Monitor more severe fractures with weekly radiographs to ensure maintenance of reduction.
- The patient will require 6 to 8 weeks of protected ROM and is non–weight bearing during this time.
- If the patient is asymptomatic and radiographs show evidence of healing at 6 to 8 weeks, release the patient to regular activities.

Operative Management
Codes
ICD-9 code: 813.05 Closed fracture of head of radius
CPT codes: 24665 ORIF radial head or neck fracture (includes radial head excision)
24666 With radial head prosthetic replacement

Operative Indications
- Displaced and or comminuted fracture or evidence of bony block to motion

Informed Consent and Counseling
- A risk of permanent elbow stiffness exists.

- The patient will require weeks of therapy to regain elbow ROM.
- A risk of injury or neurapraxia of the PIN exists.
- A risk of the development of HO exists.
- If the fracture is severe, the patient should be counseled on the possibility of converting an ORIF procedure to a radial head replacement.

Anesthesia
- Regional block with sedation or general anesthesia

Patient Positioning
- The patient is supine, with the arm on a hand table, the elbow flexed, and the forearm pronated.
- A sterile or nonsterile tourniquet is used high on the brachium.
- Intraoperative fluoroscopy is used.

Surgical Procedures
- ORIF with screws is used for most fractures.
- Radial head prosthetic replacement is used for severely comminuted fractures.
- ORIF with radial head plate is used for fractures that extend into the radial neck.
- Radial head excision is falling out of favor with more advanced technology. It is associated with proximal migration of the radius resulting in an Essex-Lopresti lesion and wrist pain.

Open Reduction, Internal Fixation of a Radial Head Fracture
- A Kocher approach to the elbow is used to gain access to the radial head. A lateral incision is made from the lateral epicondyle to the ECU. The muscle fascia over the common extensor tendon and ECU insertions is identified and divided at the interval between the ECU and anconeus. A plane is developed between the muscles and the underlying joint capsule and LCL.
- It is important to keep the forearm in pronation during the procedure to protect the **PIN** in the supinator.
- The joint capsule is incised anterior to the LUCL from the lateral epicondyle

to the annular ligament. The annular ligament can be incised and later repaired to gain access to the radial neck. With the radiocapitellar joint now exposed, the fracture is débrided, and individual pieces are aligned. K-wires are used for provisional fixation of the fracture fragments.
- Then, mini-fragment screws are used for definitive fixation. Alternatively, a plating system can also be used, especially if there is involvement of the radial neck or a radial head replacement in an older patient with a severely comminuted fracture.
- Once fracture reduction and hardware placement are confirmed by intraoperative fluoroscopy, the wound is irrigated and closed in layers to avoid development of a synovial sinus tract. A long-arm posterior splint is applied with the elbow in 90 degrees of flexion and the forearm in neutral rotation.

Estimated Postoperative Course
- Postoperative days 10 to 14
  - Return to the clinic for a wound check and suture removal.
  - Some clinicians advocate for early protected elbow ROM if fixation is good and comminution is minimal.
  - Radiography: Obtain routine postoperative radiographs: AP, lateral, and oblique views of the elbow.
  - Therapy: Provide a hinged elbow brace and start gentle, protected ROM with no weight bearing. The brace may need to be placed in an extension block, depending on the patient's motion, elbow stability, or fracture severity.
- Postoperative 4 weeks
  - Return to the clinic for a wound and motion check.
  - Radiography: Obtain routine radiographs to evaluate for healing.
  - Therapy: Progress ROM.
- Postoperative 6 to 8 weeks
  - Return to the clinic for a motion check.
  - Radiography: Obtain routine radiographs to evaluate for healing.
  - Therapy: Start aggressive ROM and weight bearing.

- Postoperative 3 months
  - Return for a motion check.
  - Obtain radiographs if concerned for healing.
  - Release to regular activities without restrictions.

Suggested Readings

Dacus AR: Radial head or neck fractures. In Miller MD, Hart JA, MacKnight JM, editors: *Essential orthopaedics*, Philadelphia, 2010, Saunders, pp 273–275.

Pike JM, Athwal GS, Faber KJ, et al: Radial head fractures: an update, *J Hand Surg* 34:557–565, 2009.

Tejwani NC, Mehta H: Fractures of the radial head and neck: current concepts in management, *J Am Acad Orthop Surg* 15:380–387, 2007.

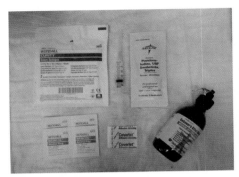

Figure 3-28. Equipment needed for intra-articular elbow injection and aspiration. Manufacturers and supplies may vary.

ORTHOPAEDIC PROCEDURES
Intra-articular Elbow Injection and Aspiration
Code
CPT code: 20605

Indications
- Elbow arthritis
- Intra-articular block for fracture reduction
- Diagnostic injection
- Elbow aspiration

Contraindications
- Steroid injections contraindicated if infection suspected
- Skin abrasions over lateral elbow

Equipment Needed: Figure 3-28
- Gloves
- Iodine and alcohol swabs or another antiseptic of choice
- Injection: 5-mL syringe and 25-gauge needle
- Injectate: 3 mL of 1% plain lidocaine mixed with 1 mL of 40 mg/mL triamcinolone (Kenalog) or other corticosteroid
- Aspiration: 20-mL empty syringe and 18-gauge needle
- Adhesive bandage

Procedure: Figure 3-29
1) Position the patient's elbow in 90 degrees of flexion with the arm internally rotated so that the lateral aspect of the elbow is exposed.

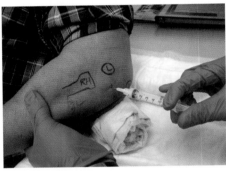

Figure 3-29. Intra-articular elbow injection and aspiration.

2) Identify the lateral epicondyle, radial head, and olecranon process. Triangulate the area among these three structures, and identify the "soft spot" that is the location for the intra-articular injection. Mark the injection site.
3) Prepare the skin with iodine and alcohol swabs or antiseptic of choice.
4) Ethyl chloride spray may be used for patient comfort
5) Place the needle directly into the "soft spot," and inject the medication or aspirate synovial fluid.
6) Withdraw the needle, and apply an adhesive bandage.

Aftercare Instructions
1) The elbow joint may be sore and even mildly edematous for the 24-hour period following the injection.

2) A risk of subcutaneous fat atrophy, skin depigmentation, and damage to surrounding structures exists when cortisone is used as a treatment modality.
3) Apply ice and take acetaminophen (Tylenol) or NSAIDs if pain is intolerable
4) The injection may take several weeks to exert maximum effect.
5) The injection may provide temporary relief; return to the clinic if symptoms recur.

Lateral Epicondyle Injection
Code
CPT code: 20551

Indications
■ Lateral epicondylitis that has failed to respond to therapeutic exercise, rest, and NSAIDs.

Contraindications
■ Injection is contraindicated if the integrity of the skin over the lateral epicondyle has been compromised, such as from an abrasion or from subcutaneous fat atrophy from previous treatment.
■ Multiple repeated injections are a relative contraindication, and length between injections should be considered before administration.

Equipment Needed
■ Gloves
■ Iodine and alcohol swabs or topical antiseptic of choice
■ Ethyl chloride spray considered for patient comfort
■ 5-mL syringe and 25-gauge needle
■ Injectate: 3 mL of 1% plain lidocaine mixed with 1 mL of 40 mg/mL triamcinolone (Kenalog) or other corticosteroid
■ Adhesive bandage

Procedure: Figure 3-30
1) Position the patient's elbow in 90 degrees of flexion with the arm in internal rotation so that the lateral epicondyle is exposed.
2) Palpate the lateral epicondyle and mark the area for the injection directly over the bony prominence of the epicondyle. Administration of the

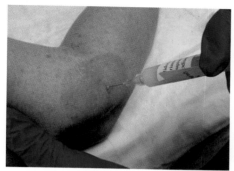

Figure 3-30. Injection for lateral epicondylitis.

injection too far distal, posterior, and anterior could result in damage to surrounding structures such as the LCL or the PIN.
3) Prepare the skin directly over the lateral epicondyle with the iodine and alcohol swabs or antiseptic of choice.
4) Ethyl chloride may be used before injection for patient comfort.
5) Administer the injection directly over the lateral epicondyle into the common extensor tendon origin. Manipulate the needle during the injection so that the injectate is distributed evenly over the fanlike insertion of the tendons. However, do not administer the injection distal to the epicondyle.
6) Withdraw the needle, and place an adhesive bandage over the injection site.

Aftercare Instructions
1) The injection site may be sore and even mildly edematous for the 24-hour period following the injection.
2) A risk of subcutaneous fat atrophy, skin depigmentation, and damage to surrounding structures is present when cortisone is used as a treatment modality.
3) Apply ice and take acetaminophen (Tylenol) or NSAIDs if pain is intolerable.
4) The injection may take several weeks to exert maximum effect.
5) Avoid lifting heavy objects or returning to repetitive activity in the period following the injection, and ease back into such tasks gradually.

6) The injection may provide temporary relief; return to the clinic if symptoms recur.

Medial Epicondyle Injection

Code
CPT code: 20551

Indications
- Medial epicondylitis that has failed to respond to therapeutic exercise, rest, and NSAIDs.

Contraindications
- A subluxating ulnar nerve or previous ulnar nerve transposition is a relative contraindication, and the injection should be performed with extreme caution in this situation.
- Injection is contraindicated if the integrity of the skin over the medial epicondyle has been compromised such as from an abrasion or from subcutaneous fat trophy from previous treatment.
- Multiple repeated injections are a relative contraindication, and length between injections should be considered before administration

Equipment Needed
- Gloves
- Iodine and alcohol swabs or topical antiseptic of choice
- Ethyl chloride spray considered for patient comfort
- 5-mL syringe and 25-gauge needle
- Injectate: 3 mL of 1% plain lidocaine mixed with 1 mL of 40 mg/mL triamcinolone (Kenalog) or other corticosteroid
- Adhesive bandage

Procedure: Figure 3-31
1) Position the patient's elbow in **full extension**, and externally rotate the arm so that the medial epicondyle is exposed. The ulnar nerve should remain behind the medial epicondyle in the cubital tunnel when the elbow is extended.
2) Palpate the medial epicondyle and then ulnar nerve posteriorly to confirm its position. While palpating the medial epicondyle, ask the patient to confirm that he or she does **not** feel any distal paresthesias.

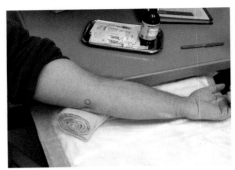

Figure 3-31. Elbow and arm positioning for medial epicondyle injection.

3) Mark the area for the injection directly over the medial epicondyle.
4) Prepare the skin directly over the medial epicondyle with the iodine and alcohol swabs or antiseptic of choice.
5) Ethyl chloride may be used before injection for patient comfort.
6) Administer the injection directly over the medial epicondyle and into the common flexor tendon origin with the elbow in extension. Discontinue injection if the patient reports paresthesias in the ulnar nerve. Minimal manipulation of the needle is ideal so that the injectate is distributed evenly over the tendon insertion but does not penetrate posteriorly into the cubital tunnel or anteriorly into the UCL (Fig. 3-32).
7) Withdraw the needle, and place an adhesive bandage over the injection site.

Aftercare Instructions
1) The injection site may be sore and even mildly edematous for the 24-hour period following the injection.
2) A risk of subcutaneous fat atrophy, skin depigmentation, and damage to surrounding structures exists when cortisone is used as a treatment modality.
3) Apply ice and take acetaminophen (Tylenol) or NSAIDs if pain is intolerable.
4) The injection may take several weeks to exert maximum effect.

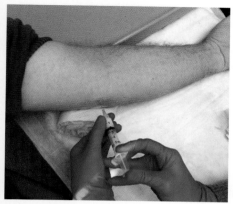

Figure 3-32. Injection for medial epicondylitis.

5) Avoid lifting heavy objects or return-ing to repetitive activity in the period following the injection, and ease back into such tasks gradually.
6) The injection may provide temporary relief; return to the clinic if symptoms recur.

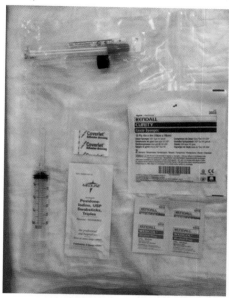

Figure 3-33. Equipment needed for olecranon bursa aspiration. Manufacturers and supplies may vary.

Olecranon Bursa Aspiration
Code
CPT code: 20605

Indications
- Symptomatic inflammatory bursitis
- Diagnostic aspiration of potential septic bursitis
- Treatment of septic bursitis

Contraindications
- Aspiration should be avoided in minimally symptomatic bursitis, to reduce the potential for iatrogenic infection.

Equipment Needed: *Figure 3-33*
- Gloves
- Iodine and alcohol swabs or other antiseptic of choice
- 30-mL syringe
- 21-gauge needle
- Adhesive bandage
- Compression wrap
- Culture swabs and specimen tube for aerobic or anaerobic culture with Gram stain

Procedure
1) Position the patient's elbow in 90 degrees of flexion with the lateral surface of the bursa exposed.
2) Identify area on the lateral side of bursa for aspiration site (avoid punc-tures directly posterior, because of sensitivity and increased risk for fistula formation, and in the ulnar direction, to avoid injury to the ulnar nerve).
3) Prepare the skin with antiseptic (Fig. 3-34).
4) Puncture the skin and bursa, and begin to aspirate fluid. Manual com-pression of the bursa may be neces-sary to extract all the fluid. No need exists to move the needle around in the bursa because it is one continu-ous space (Fig. 3-35).
5) Once the bursa is decompressed, apply an adhesive bandage.
6) Wrap the arm firmly with a compres-sion wrap (but avoid creating an arm tourniquet) (Fig. 3-36).
7) Send cultures if fluid looks cloudy or purulent or if infection is suspected (Fig. 3-37).

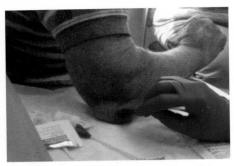

Figure 3-34. The elbow is positioned, and the skin is prepared.

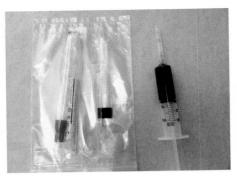

Figure 3-37. Cultures should be taken for suspected infection or if fluid looks cloudy or purulent.

8) Consider starting empiric antibiotics if infection is suspected.

Aftercare Instructions
1) Instruct the patient to leave the wrap on for at least 24 hours, then remove wrap only for bathing and replace it immediately. The wrap will be necessary for 7 to 10 days.
2) If the bursa recurs, the patient should return either for repeat aspiration or a discussion of surgical management.
3) If erythema, pain, or edema worsens, the patient is to return to the clinic.

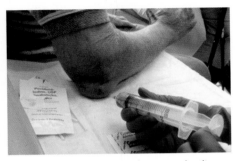

Figure 3-35. Olecranon bursa aspiration.

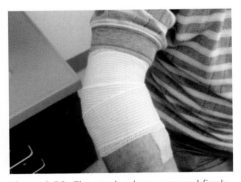

Figure 3-36. The arm has been wrapped firmly with a compression wrap. An arm tourniquet should not be created.

Wrist and Hand

Amy Radigan

4

ANATOMY
Bones: Figure 4-1

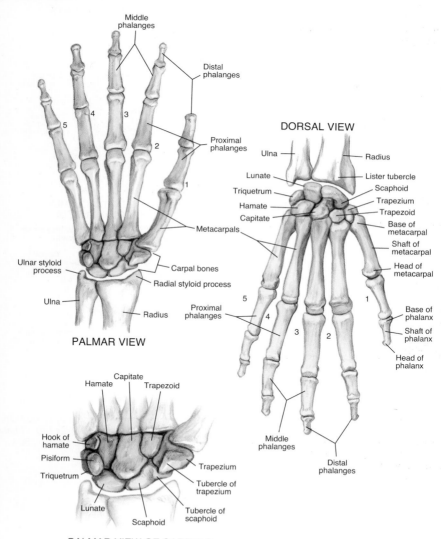

Figure 4-1. Bones of the hand and wrist. *(From Chhabra AB: Wrist and hand. In Miller MD, Chhabra AB, Hurwitz S, et al, editors:* Orthopaedic surgical approaches, *Philadelphia, 2008, Saunders, p 148.)*

Ligaments: Figure 4-2

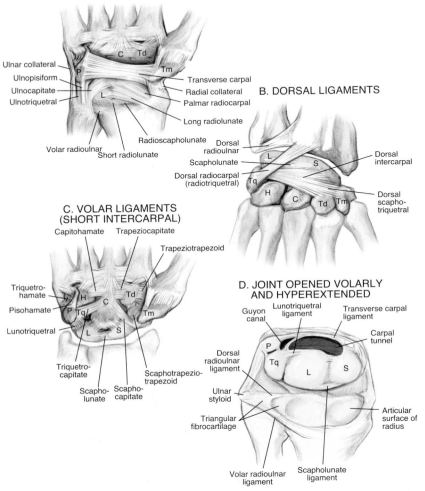

A. VOLAR LIGAMENTS (RADIOULNAR, RADIOCARPAL, ULNOCARPAL, AND TRANSVERSE CARPAL)

- Ulnar collateral
- Ulnopisiform
- Ulnocapitate
- Ulnotriquetral
- Transverse carpal
- Radial collateral
- Palmar radiocarpal
- Long radiolunate
- Radioscapholunate
- Volar radioulnar
- Short radiolunate

B. DORSAL LIGAMENTS

- Dorsal radioulnar
- Scapholunate
- Dorsal radiocarpal (radiotriquetral)
- Dorsal intercarpal
- Dorsal scapho-triquetral

C. VOLAR LIGAMENTS (SHORT INTERCARPAL)

- Capitohamate
- Trapeziocapitate
- Trapeziotrapezoid
- Triquetro-hamate
- Pisohamate
- Lunotriquetral
- Triquetro-capitate
- Scapho-lunate
- Scapho-capitate
- Scaphotrapezio-trapezoid

D. JOINT OPENED VOLARLY AND HYPEREXTENDED

- Guyon canal
- Lunotriquetral ligament
- Transverse carpal ligament
- Carpal tunnel
- Dorsal radioulnar ligament
- Ulnar styloid
- Triangular fibrocartilage
- Articular surface of radius
- Volar radioulnar ligament
- Scapholunate ligament

Figure 4-2. A to **D,** Ligaments of the wrist. Ca, capitate; H, hamate; L, lunate; P, pisiform; S, scaphoid; Td, trapezoid; Tm, trapezium; Tq, triquetrum. *(From Chhabra AB: Wrist and hand. In Miller MD, Chhabra AB, Hurwitz S, et al, editors:* Orthopaedic surgical approaches, *Philadelphia, 2008, Saunders, p 150.)*

Muscles and Tendons:
Figures 4-3 **through** 4-7

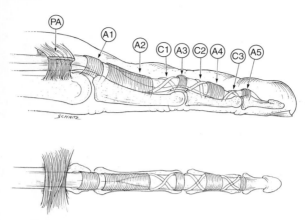

Figure 4-3. Flexor tendon pulley system. A1 to A5, annular pulleys; C1 to C3, cruciate pulleys; PA, palmar aponeurosis. *(From Strickland JW: Flexor tendons: acute injuries. In Green DP, editor: Operative hand surgery, ed 4, New York, 1999, Churchill Livingstone, p 1853.)*

VOLAR VIEW

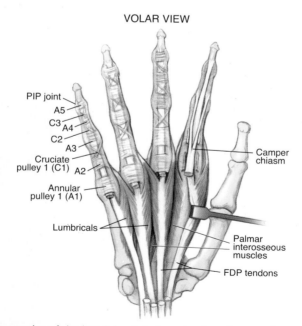

Figure 4-4. Volar muscles of the hand: lumbricals and palmar interossei. FDP, flexor digitorum profundus; PIP, proximal interphalangeal. *(From Chhabra AB: Wrist and hand. In Miller MD, Chhabra AB, Hurwitz S, et al, editors:* Orthopaedic surgical approaches, *Philadelphia, 2008, Saunders, p 154.)*

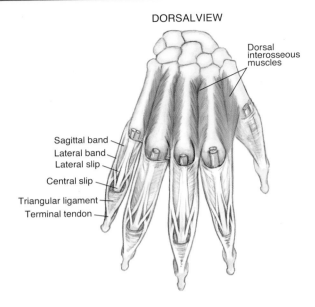

Figure 4-5. Dorsal muscles of the hand: dorsal interossei and extensor mechanism of the finger. *(From Chhabra AB: Wrist and hand. In Miller MD, Chhabra AB, Hurwitz S, et al, editors:* Orthopaedic surgical approaches, *Philadelphia, 2008, Saunders, p 155.)*

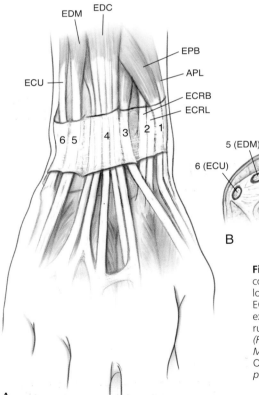

Figure 4-6. A and **B,** Extensor tendon compartments of wrist. APL, abductor pollicis longus; ECRB, extensor carpi radialis brevis; ECRL, extensor carpi radialis longus; ECU, extensor carpi ulnaris; EDC, extensor digitorum communis; EDM, extensor digiti minimi. *(From Chhabra AB: Wrist and hand. In Miller MD, Chhabra AB, Hurwitz S, et al, editors:* Orthopaedic surgical approaches, *Philadelphia, 2008, Saunders, p 157.)*

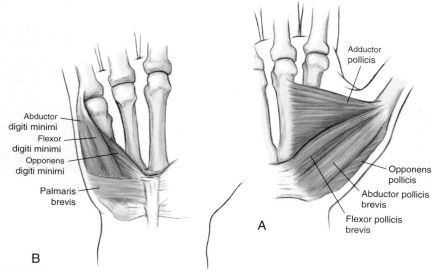

Figure 4-7. A and **B,** Thenar and hypothenar muscles of the hand. *(From Chhabra AB: Wrist and hand. In Miller MD, Chhabra AB, Hurwitz S, et al, editors:* Orthopaedic surgical approaches, *Philadelphia, 2008, Saunders, p 156.)*

Nerves and Arteries: Figures 4-8 through 4-10 and Table 4-1

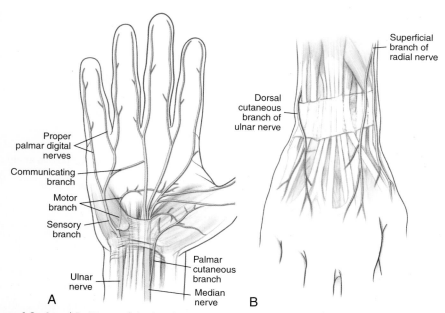

Figure 4-8. A and **B,** Nerves of the hand and wrist. *(From Chhabra AB: Wrist and hand. In Miller MD, Chhabra AB, Hurwitz S, et al, editors:* Orthopaedic surgical approaches, *Philadelphia, 2008, Saunders, p 159.)*

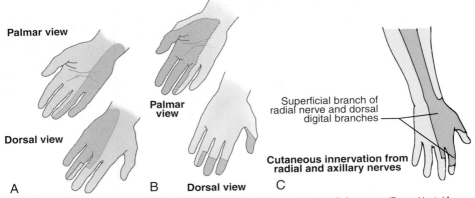

Palmar view

Dorsal view

A

Palmar view

Dorsal view

B

Superficial branch of radial nerve and dorsal digital branches

Cutaneous innervation from radial and axillary nerves

C

Figure 4-9. Sensory patterns of the (**A**), ulnar, (**B**), median, and (**C**), radial nerves. *(From Hart JA: Overview of the wrist and hand. In Miller MD, Hart JA, MacKnight JM, editors:* Essential orthopaedics, *Philadelphia, 2010, Saunders, p 297.)*

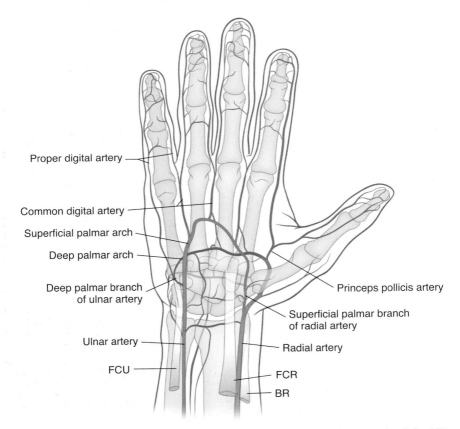

Proper digital artery

Common digital artery

Superficial palmar arch

Deep palmar arch

Deep palmar branch of ulnar artery

Ulnar artery

FCU

Princeps pollicis artery

Superficial palmar branch of radial artery

Radial artery

FCR

BR

Figure 4-10. Arteries of the hand and wrist. BR, brachioradialis; FCR, flexor carpi radialis; FCU, flexor carpi ulnaris. *(From Chhabra AB: Wrist and hand. In Miller MD, Chhabra AB, Hurwitz S, et al, editors:* Orthopaedic surgical approaches, *Philadelphia, 2008, Saunders, p 161.)*

Table 4-1. Nerves and Their Functional Testing

NERVE	BRANCH	MOTOR	TEST	SENSORY
Radial	Superficial sensory radial nerve			To dorsal aspect of radial wrist and thumb, dorsal hand
	PIN	ECRB EDM ECRL APL ECU EPB Supinator EPL EIP	Wrist extension Thumb extension Finger extension	
Median	Proper	Pronator teres FCR FDS Palmaris longus Index and middle finger lumbricals	Radial wrist flexion Finger flexion Pronation	Thumb, index finger, middle finger, and radial half of ring finger
	Recurrent motor branch	Thenar muscles: APB	Thumb abduction	
	AIN	FDP to index finger FPL Pronator quadratus	Index finger DIP joint flexion Thumb IP joint flexion Pronation	
	Superficial sensory palmar branch			Sensation to palm
Ulnar	Proper	FDP to 4 and 5 FCU	Flexion of ring and small fingers Ulnar wrist flexion	
	Deep motor branch	Adductor pollicis Hypothenar muscle Interosseous muscle Ring and small finger lumbricals Deep branch of FPB	Finger abduction and adduction Thumb adduction	
	Dorsal Sensory branch			Palmar and dorsal sensation to small finger and ulnar half of ring finger

APB, abductor pollicis brevis; APL, abductor pollicis longus; AIN, anterior interosseous nerve; DIP, distal interphalangeal; ECRB, extensor carpi radialis brevis; ECRL, extensor carpi radialis longus; ECU, extensor carpi ulnaris; EDM, extensor digiti minimi; EIP, extensor indicis proprius; EPB, extensor pollicis brevis; EPL, extensor pollicis longus; FCU, flexor carpi ulnaris; FCR, flexor carpi radialis; FDP; flexor digitorum profundus; FDS, flexor digitorum superficialis; FPB, flexor pollicis brevis; FPL, flexor pollicis longus; IP, interphalangeal; PIN, posterior interosseous nerve.

Surface Anatomy: Figure 4-11

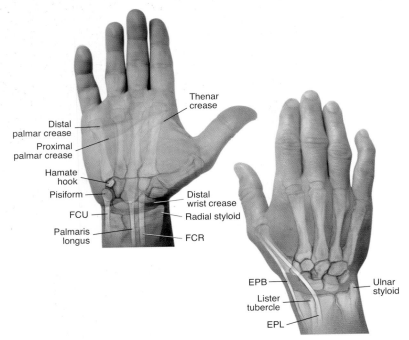

Figure 4-11. Surface anatomy of the hand and wrist. EPB, extensor pollicis brevis; EPL, extensor pollicis longus; FCR, flexor carpi radialis; FCU, flexor carpi ulnaris. *(From Chhabra AB: Wrist and hand. In Miller MD, Chhabra AB, Hurwitz S, et al, editors: Orthopaedic surgical approaches, Philadelphia, 2008, Saunders, p 163.)*

Normal Radiographic Appearance: Figures 4-12 **through** 4-14

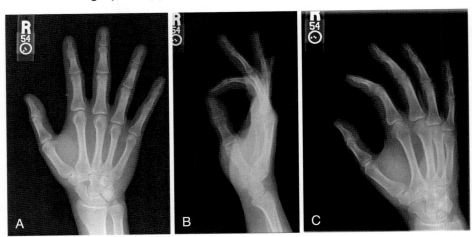

Figure 4-12. Normal radiographs of the hand. Anteroposterior (**A**), lateral (**B**), and oblique (**C**) views of the hand. *(From Hart JA: Overview of the wrist and hand. In Miller MD, Hart JA, MacKnight JM, editors: Essential orthopaedics, Philadelphia, 2010, Saunders, p 303.)*

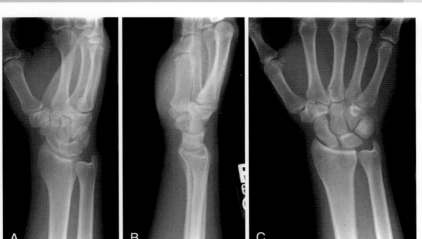

Figure 4-13. Normal radiographs of the wrist. *Anteroposterior (A) views of the wrist (B), and oblique (C), lateral.*

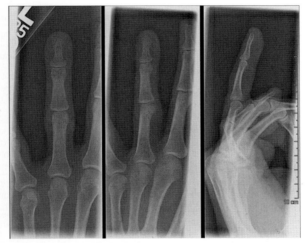

Figure 4-14. Normal radiographs of the finger. Anteroposterior (*left*), lateral (*middle*) views of the finger (*right*), and oblique.

HISTORY

1) Hand dominance
2) Occupation
3) Pain
4) Numbness
5) Tingling
6) Weakness
7) Discoloration
8) Edema
9) Clicking or snapping
10) Poor coordination

PHYSICAL EXAMINATION

Inspect for scars, muscle atrophy, edema, erythema or deformity.

Palpate specific structures to evaluate complaint:

• Distal radius
• Distal radioulnar joint (DRUJ)
• Distal ulna
• Anatomic snuffbox, scaphoid tubercle
• First extensor compartment, extensor carpi radialis ulnaris, extensor carpi

Table 4-2. Normal Wrist Range of Motion

Extension	80 degrees
Flexion	70 degrees
Supination	90 degrees
Pronation	90 degrees
Ulnar deviation	30 degrees
Radial deviation	20 degrees

Table 4-3. Neurovascular Examination of the Wrist and Hand

NERVE	LOCATION OF TEST	TESTS
Median nerve	Carpal tunnel	Tinel, Phalen, Durkan test (see page 140)
Ulnar nerve	Guyon canal/ medial epicondyle	Tinel test
Superficial sensory radial nerve	At radial styloid	Tinel test
Radial and ulnar artery	At volar wrist	Allen test for dominance or perfusion

radialis brevis, extensor carpi radialis longus
- Scapholunate (SL) interval (approximately 1 to 3 cm distal from Lister tubercle)
- First carpometacarpal (CMC) joint
- Flexor carpi ulnaris (FCU) tendon
- Extensor carpi ulnaris (ECU) tendon
- Pisotriquetral joint
- Triangular fibrocartilage complex (TFCC)
- Carpal tunnel
- Hook of the hamate
- A1 pulley

Normal wrist range of motion (ROM): Table 4-2

Neurovascular examination of the wrist and hand: Table 4-3

Differential Diagnosis of Wrist Pain: Table 4-4

Table 4-4. Differential Diagnosis of Wrist Pain

Radial-sided wrist pain	Distal radius fracture SLL tear Arthritis Scaphoid fracture Extensor tendinitis de Quervain tenosynovitis
Ulnar-sided wrist pain	TFCC tear FCU tendinitis Ulnar artery thrombosis Cubital tunnel syndrome Pisotriquetral arthritis ECU tendinitis Distal ulnar fracture Lunotriquetral tear Hook hamate fracture
Dorsal wrist pain	Extensor tendinitis Arthritis SLL tear Scaphoid fracture
Volar wrist pain	FCU or FCR tendinitis Carpal tunnel syndrome

ECU, extensor carpi ulnaris; FCU, flexor carpi ulnaris; FCR, flexor carpi radialis; SLL, scapholunate ligament; TFCC, triangular fibrocartilage complex.

Table 4-5. Differential Diagnosis of Finger Pain

Dorsal finger pain	Joint arthritis Extensor tendinitis Joint sprain Phalanx fracture
Volar finger pain	Trigger finger Joint arthritis Phalanx fracture

Differential Diagnosis of Finger Pain: Table 4-5

SCAPHOID FRACTURE
History
- Fall on an outstretched hand
- Patient-reported anatomic snuffbox pain, pain with motion and weight bearing

Physical Examination
- Radial-sided wrist edema and/or ecchymosis
- Tenderness to palpation at anatomic snuffbox and/or scaphoid tubercle
- Pain with all wrist motion

Imaging: Figure 4-15

- Order wrist radiographs: posteroanterior (PA), lateral, oblique, and scaphoid (also known as "navicular") views.

Classification

- Transverse, oblique, vertical oblique
- Proximal pole
- Waist fractures (70% to 80%)
- Distal pole

Differential Diagnosis

- SL ligament (SLL) injury (see page 129)
- First extensor compartment tendinitis
- First CMC joint arthritis
- Occult scaphoid fracture: If there is high level of suspicion for a scaphoid fracture but the initial radiographic findings are negative, place the patient into a thumb spica splint and obtain radiographs again at 3 weeks after injury. If follow-up radiographic findings are negative but patient is still symptomatic, order a magnetic resonance imaging (MRI) scan to evaluate for occult scaphoid fracture or SLL tear.

Initial Treatment
Patient Education

- The scaphoid is most commonly injured carpal bone (60% of carpal fractures). It has a tenuous blood supply, and if the injury is not treated appropriately, necrosis and subsequent wrist arthritis can develop.

First Treatment Steps

- A **short-arm thumb spica splint** is used until edema subsides (some clinicians argue for a long-arm splint or sugar tong splint).
- Refer the patient to an orthopaedic surgeon to be seen within 7 to 10 days from injury.

Treatment Options
Nonoperative Management

- Conservative management is reserved for nondisplaced fractures in which patient declines surgery or for patients too ill for surgery.
- Nondisplaced waist fractures have an 88% to 95% healing rate if treated within 3 weeks of injury.
- A short-arm thumb spica cast is used for a total of 8 to 12 weeks, depending on healing (some argue for long-arm cast).
- See the patient in follow-up at 4-week intervals to change the cast, obtain repeat radiographs of the fracture, and assess healing.
- A computed tomography (CT) scan may be necessary to confirm healing after 8 to 12 weeks.
- The fracture is considered healed if there is radiographic evidence of healing and patient is nontender to palpation at the anatomic snuffbox and scaphoid tubercle *or* if a CT scan confirms healing.

Rehabilitation

- Once the fracture is healed, the patient can start active wrist ROM. An off-the-shelf wrist brace may be used to transition from the cast.
- Restrictions: Non–weight bearing is indicated until the fracture is healed and patient is pain free.

Pearl

An MRI scan is a good way to diagnose an occult scaphoid fracture early. The scan is useful before 3 weeks in high-level athletes or in patients for whom remaining out of work for 3 weeks while in a splint would be financially detrimental.

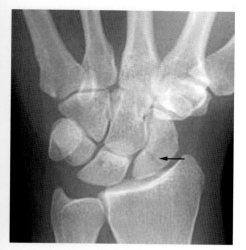

Figure 4-15. Nondisplaced scaphoid fracture.

ORTHOPAEDIC WARNING

If a scaphoid fracture is left undiagnosed or untreated, the patient will develop wrist arthritis within 10 to 15 years after the injury
- This pattern of arthritis is called scaphoid nonunion advanced collapse (SNAC) and is similar to the pattern of arthritis associated with an untreated scapholunate ligament tear (see page 129)
- If arthritis is present, proceed as if treating the underlying arthritis and not the scaphoid nonunion. Treatment would include a wrist support, activity modification, nonsteroidal antiinflammatory drugs, and possible intra-articular steroid injection.

Operative Management of Acute Scaphoid Fractures

Codes
ICD-9 code: 814.01 Scaphoid fracture
CPT code: 25628 Open reduction, internal fixation (ORIF) scaphoid fracture

Operative Indications
- Minimally displaced and displaced fractures of the scaphoid waist and proximal pole
- Nondisplaced fractures in patients who are athletes or who will benefit from early return to work

Informed Consent and Counseling
- Even with appropriate treatment and good surgical fixation, the rate of nonunion is 5% because of the scaphoid's tenuous blood supply. Proximal pole scaphoid fractures have the highest incidence of non-union.
- Smoking cessation is imperative for fracture healing.
- The patient can expect to be immobilized for approximately 6 weeks, although the type of immobilization depends on the surgeon's preference and on fracture fixation.
- The patient will require approximately 2 months of outpatient hand therapy to restore motion and strength.

Anesthesia
- Regional anesthetic such as a brachial plexus block, with sedation or general anesthesia

Patient Positioning
- Supine with the arm extended on a hand table
- Nonsterile tourniquet on the brachium

Surgical Procedures
- Dorsal approach for proximal pole fractures
- Volar approach for distal pole and waist fractures
- For either approach, placement of a forearm-based thumb spica splint

Open Reduction, Internal Fixation
- Hardware consists of a cannulated headless compression screw and multiple wires.
- Dorsal approach: A small longitudinal incision is made over the proximal pole of the scaphoid. Avoid the superficial sensory radial nerve.
- Volar approach: A small incision is made over the scaphoid tubercle. Avoid the radial artery during exposure.

Percutaneous Internal Fixation:
Figure 4-16
- This technique may be used preferentially for nondisplaced scaphoid fractures. The procedure is similar to the open technique, just performed percutaneously. With the patient's wrist flexed, a guidewire is placed down the central axis of the scaphoid. The guidewire is also used to measure the appropriate screw length. After fluoroscopic confirmation of adequate reduction, a screw is placed for fixation. Place the patient in a thumb spica splint following surgery.

Estimated Postoperative Course
- Postoperative days 10 to 14
  - Sutures are removed, and a wound check is performed.
  - Radiographs consist of wrist PA, lateral, oblique, and navicular views.
  - Immobilization: The patient is placed into a removable thumb spica splint.
  - *Therapy referral:* Start edema control and gentle finger and wrist ROM only.

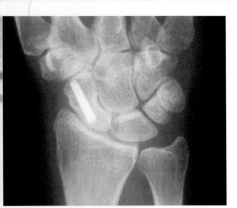

Figure 4-16. Percutaneous screw fixation of a scaphoid fracture. *(From Trumble T, Budoff J, Cornwall R, editors: Hand, elbow, and shoulder: core knowledge in orthopaedics. In Knoll, Victoria D and Tumble, Thomas E, editors:* Scaphoid Fractures and Nonunions, *Philadelphia, 2006, Mosby, p 123.)*

- Note: Some surgeons prefer cast immobilization in a thumb spica cast during the initial postoperative period, especially if the fracture was difficult to reduce or especially comminuted.
- Postoperative 6 weeks
  - The patient returns for a motion check.
  - Radiographs consist of wrist PA, lateral, and scaphoid views.
  - *Therapy:* If healing is present, progress therapy to more aggressive wrist ROM, wean from the splint, and start gradual weight bearing.
  - If no healing is noted, continue gentle ROM and have the patient wear the brace at all times until healing is evident on radiographs.
- Postoperative 3 months
  - The patient returns for a motion check.
  - Assess for tenderness at the anatomic snuffbox and scaphoid tubercle.
  - Radiographs consist of wrist PA, lateral, and scaphoid views.
  - If the injury is healed and no pain is noted on examination, release the patient to regular activities without restrictions.
  - If no evidence of healing is seen on radiographs, consider use of a bone stimulator and possibly obtain a CT scan to evaluate for healing.
  - Nonunion occurs if there has been no healing by 6 months postoperatively.

Suggested Readings

Buijze GA, Doornberg JN, Ham JS, et al: Surgical compared with conservative treatment for acute nondisplaced or minimally displaced scaphoid fractures, *J Bone Joint Surg Am* 92(6):1534–1544, 2010.

Kawarmura K, Chung KC: Treatment of scaphoid fractures and nonunions, *J Hand Surg Am* 33(6):988–997, 2008.

Mack GR, Bosse MH, Gelberman RH, et al: The natural history of scaphoid non-union, *J Bone Joint Surg Am* 66:504–509, 1984.

DISTAL RADIUS FRACTURES

History

- Fall on an outstretched hand
- Patient-reported radial wrist pain, pain with motion and weight bearing, swelling, and wrist deformity

Physical Examination

- Radial-sided wrist edema and/or ecchymosis
- Tenderness to palpation at the radial aspect of the wrist
- Pain with all motion, especially wrist extension and flexion
- Silver fork wrist deformity: the forearm and wrist have a curve like the back of a fork.

Imaging: Figure 4-17

- Order wrist radiographs: PA, lateral, and oblique views.

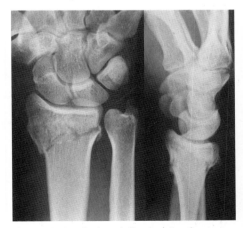

Figure 4-17. Displaced distal radius fracture. *(From Green DP, Hotchkiss RN, Pederson WC, et al, editors: Green's operative hand surgery. In Scott W. Wolf and Diego L. Fernandez, editors:* Distal Radius Fractures, *ed 5, Philadelphia, 2005, Churchill Livingstone p 660.)*

■ MRI or bone scan may be used in rare cases when fracture suspected but plain radiographs do not reveal it.
■ CT scan can be helpful to determine the severity of comminution.

Classification
Describe the fracture in terms of displacement, comminution, radial length, surface tilt, and articular step-off (Figure 4-18 and Table 4-6).

Differential Diagnosis
■ SLL injury
■ Wrist sprain
■ First extensor compartment tendinitis
■ If radiographic findings are negative: wrist splint immobilization and referral to follow-up with an orthopaedic surgeon in 7 to 10 days

Initial Treatment
Patient Education
■ The distal radius is the most commonly fractured bone in the arm. The fracture pattern determines surgical versus nonsurgical treatment. If the fracture is nondisplaced or if the fracture has

been successfully closed reduced and splinted *and* the fingers are sensate with good perfusion, then the injury can wait several days for evaluation by an orthopaedist. If the patient's fingers are numb and/or not well perfused or the fracture is not able to be reduced, the patient should have an immediate surgical evaluation.

First Treatment Steps
■ Immediate closed reduction if the fracture is displaced (to be done in a setting where adequate pain control may be provided, such as an emergency department)
■ **Sugar tong splint** applied until edema subsides
■ Referral to an orthopaedic surgeon to be seen within 7 to 10 days from injury

Treatment Options
Nonoperative Management
■ Conservative management is reserved for nondisplaced fractures or stable reduced fractures or for patients too ill for surgery.

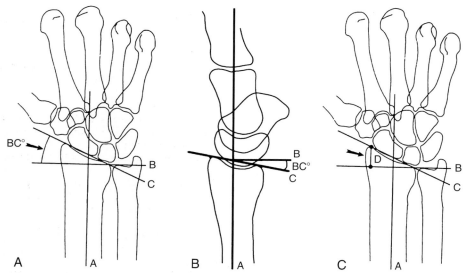

Figure 4-18. How to determine whether a distal radius fracture meets operative criteria. **A,** Radial inclination. **B,** Volar tilt. **C,** Radial height. (Adapted from Baratz ME, Larsen CF. Wrist and hand measurements and classification schemes. In Gilula LA, Yin Y (eds). Imaging of the wrist and hand, Philadelphia, Saunders, 1996.)

Table 4-6. Classification of Distal Radius Fractures

RADIOGRAPHIC ANATOMY	VIEW TO ASSESS	HOW TO MEASURE	NORMAL	ACCEPTABLE
Radial inclination: Figure 4-18A	AP or PA view	Angle BC formed by the following two lines: 1) Line drawn perpendicular to the longitudinal axis of the radius (B) 2) Line drawn from the tip of the radial styloid process to the ulnar corner of the radius (C)	21-23 degrees	16-28 degrees (can accept 5-degree change either way)
Volar/palmar tilt: Figure 4-18B	Lateral view	Angle BC formed by the following two lines: 1) Line drawn across the distal points of the dorsal and volar cortical rims (C) 2) Line drawn perpendicular to the axis of the radius (B)	11-12 degrees	Can accept 10-degree change either way (range, 2-20 degrees)
Radial height/ length: Figure 4-18C	AP view	Distance (D) between lines B and C at the level of the most distal aspect of the radial styloid: 1) Line drawn along the slope of the distal radius that bisects the radial styloid and the ulnar aspect of the radius (C) 2) Perpendicular line (B) to the long axis of the radius that bisects the most ulnar aspect of the radius	10-13 mm	<2 mm loss, may need to compare with uninjured wrist radiograph

AP, anteroposterior; PA, posteroanterior.

- Nondisplaced fractures require casting for 6 to 8 weeks in a short-arm cast.
- Generally, after 6 weeks of immobilization, patients may progress with ROM.
  - Stable reduced fractures require 3 weeks in a sugar tong splint with *weekly radiographs* in the splint to ensure that fracture alignment is maintained. If the reduction is lost, surgery is recommended. If fracture reduction is maintained for 3 weeks, transition the patient to a short-arm cast with radiographs immediately following new cast placement to ensure alignment.
  - The fracture is considered healed if there is radiographic evidence of healing and the patient is nontender over the distal radius. This usually occurs in approximately 2 to 3 months, depending on the severity of the original injury.

Rehabilitation
- Once the fracture is healed, the patient can start active wrist motion and may require formal hand therapy. An off-the-shelf wrist brace may be used to transition from the cast.
- Restrictions: Non–weight bearing is indicated until the injury is healed and pain free.

Operative Management of Acute Distal Radius Fractures
Codes
ICD-9 code: 813.10 Distal radius fracture
CPT codes: 25607 Open treatment of distal radial extra-articular fracture with internal fixation

25608 Open treatment of distal radial intra-articular fracture with internal fixation of 2 fragments

25609 Open treatment of distal radial intra-articular fracture with internal fixation of 3 or more fragments

Operative Indications
- Displaced and/or unstable fractures of the distal radius (see Table 4-6).

Informed Consent and Counseling
- Smoking cessation is important for fracture healing.
- The patient can expect to be immobilized for approximately 6 weeks, but the type of immobilization depends on the surgeon's preference and on fracture fixation.
- The patient may require several sessions of outpatient hand therapy to restore motion and strength.

Anesthesia
- Regional anesthetic such as a brachial plexus block, with sedation or general anesthesia

Patient Positioning
- Supine with the arm extended on a hand table
- Nonsterile tourniquet on the brachium

Surgical Procedures
- May vary; volar approach to the radius most common

Open Reduction, Internal Fixation: See Figure 4-19
- Hardware consists of a volar plate and screws.
- Volar approach: A longitudinal incision is made directly superficial to the flexor carpi radialis (FCR) tendon. An interval is developed between the FCR and the radial artery. Blunt deep dissection is carried down to the pronator quadratus muscle, which is sharply incised on the radial border and elevated off the periosteum of the radius to expose the fracture. Sometimes the brachioradialis tendon insertion must be released to decrease the deforming forces on the fracture. A volar plate and screws are used, and intraoperative fluoroscopy confirms reduction and hardware placement. The patient is placed in a volar short-arm splint postoperatively.

Estimated Postoperative Course
- Postoperative days 10 to 14
  - Sutures are removed, and a wound check is performed.
  - Possible radiographs include wrist PA, lateral, and oblique views.

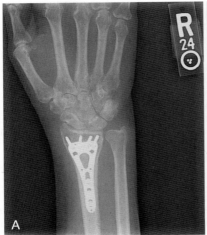
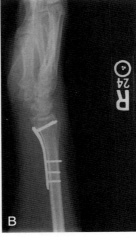

Figure 4-19. Surgical fixation of a displaced distal radius fracture with a volar locking plate. Posteroanterior (**A**) and lateral (**B**) views.

- Immobilization: The patient is placed into a removable spica splint.
- *Therapy referral:* Start edema control and gentle finger and wrist motion only. Some clinicians start therapy at 3 to 5 days postoperatively.
- Note: Some surgeons prefer cast immobilization in a short-arm cast during the initial postoperative period, especially if the fracture was difficult to reduce or especially comminuted.

- Postoperative 6 weeks
  - The patient returns for a motion check.
  - Radiographs consist of wrist PA, lateral, and navicular views.
  - *Therapy:* If healing is present, progress therapy to more aggressive wrist motion, wean the patient from the splint, and start gradual weight bearing and strengthening.
- Postoperative 3 months
  - The patient returns for a motion check.
  - Assess for tenderness to palpation at the fracture site.
  - Radiographs consist of wrist PA, lateral, and oblique views.
  - If the fracture is healed and no pain is noted on examination, release the patient to regular activities without restrictions.

Suggested Readings

Chhabra AB: Wrist and hand. In Miller M, Chhabra B, Hurwitz S, et al, editors: *Orthopaedic surgical approaches,* Philadelphia, 2008, Saunders, pp 145–210.

Juliano JA, Jupiter J: Distal radius fractures. In Trumble TE, Budoff JE, Cornwall R, editors: *Hand, elbow, and shoulder: core knowledge in orthopaedics,* Philadelphia, 2006, Mosby, pp 84–101.

Nesbitt KS, Failla JM, Clifford L: Assessment of instability factors in adult distal radius fractures, *J Hand Surg Am* 29:1128–1138, 2004.

TRIGGER FINGER
Definition
Inflammation of the flexor tendon sheath at the level of the A1 pulley

History
- The patient reports volar finger or hand pain.

- The patient may report painful locking and/or catching of the digit.
- Trigger finger is not directly associated with injury. It may be associated with overuse.
- It can be worse after a period of inactivity, such as on awakening in the morning.

Physical Examination
- Tenderness to palpation directly over the A1 pulley, located at the volar base of each finger just proximal to the metacarpophalangeal (MCP) joint flexion crease
- Palpable or visible locking or catching with flexion (the examiner may need to flex the finger, including the distal interphalangeal [DIP] joint, passively to reproduce triggering)
- Palpable nodularity on the flexor tendon at the level of the A1 pulley

Imaging
- Not necessary for diagnosis

Classification: Figure 4-20
- Grade 1: painful tenderness at the A1 pulley
- Grade 2: uneven finger movements, triggering, unlocks by self

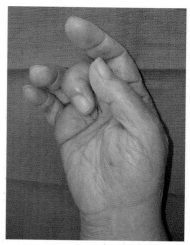

Figure 4-20. Locked trigger finger. *(From Wood MM, Ingari J: Trigger finger. In Miller MD, Hart JA, MacKnight JM, editors:* Essential orthopaedics, *Philadelphia, 2010, Saunders, p 350.)*

- Grade 3: locking, triggering finger, unlocks by outside force
- Grade 4: fixed flexion at the proximal interphalangeal (PIP) joint (Fig. 4-20)

Differential Diagnosis
- Dupuytren disease
- Rheumatoid arthritis
- Infectious flexor tenosynovitis

 ORTHOPAEDIC WARNING

If infectious flexor tenosynovitis (FTS) is suspected, urgent treatment is necessary. FTS is characterized by presence of four Kanavel signs (all four must be present for the diagnosis):
1) Finger held in flexed position for comfort
2) Intense pain with passive extension
3) Uniform swelling involving entire finger (versus localized swelling)
4) Tenderness along the course of the flexor tendon sheath (versus localized inflammation)
If FTS is present or suspected, urgent referral to a surgeon for intravenous antibiotics and incision and drainage is indicated.

Initial Treatment
Patient Education
- Triggering may affect more than one digit, with a higher incidence in patients with diabetes and thyroid disease. There is about an 80% cure rate after the first cortisone injection; if the first injection is unsuccessful, a second injection may be done 3 to 6 weeks later. If triggering is still present after the second injection, consider surgical intervention.

Treatment Options
Nonoperative Management
- If symptoms are mild:
  - Resting
  - Nonsteroidal antiinflammatory drugs (NSAIDs)
  - Nighttime extension splint for the PIP joint (or interphalangeal [IP]

joint of the thumb) to prevent painful night triggering
- If symptoms are painful:
  - Corticosteroid injection into the tendon sheath (see page 167)
  - If necessary, second injection possible 6 weeks following first injection
  - Injections less likely to provide permanent relief in patients with long-term triggering and/or diabetes mellitus

Operative Management
Codes
ICD-9 code: 727.03 Trigger finger
CPT code: 26055 Tendon sheath incision/ A1 pulley release

Operative Indications
- Persistent painful triggering despite conservative measures (including cortisone injections)

Informed Consent and Counseling
- Good results can be expected.
- The patient will have sutures in place for 10 to 14 days.
- The patient will likely be able to move the finger immediately following surgery.
- Depending on the surgeon's preference, the patient may require one to two sessions of outpatient hand therapy.
- Wound sensitivity may occur postoperatively, but it usually improves with time.

Anesthesia
- Local or regional anesthetic, with sedation

Patient Positioning
- Supine with the arm extended on a hand table
- Nonsterile tourniquet on the brachium

Surgical Procedures
A1 Pulley Release
- Local anesthetic can be injected before the skin incision is made.
- A small, transverse incision is made over the level of the A1 pulley.
- The skin and subcutaneous tissues are incised to expose the flexor tendon sheath.

- Identify and protect the neurovascular bundles.
- Identify and release the A1 pulley in its entirety.
- Preserve the A2 pulley to prevent bowstringing.
- Local anesthesia is used so that the patient can actively flex and extend the digit following A1 pulley release, thus confirming successful release of the pulley.
- Place the patient in a soft hand dressing following surgery.

Estimated Postoperative Course
- Postoperative days 10 to 14
  - Sutures are removed, and a wound check is performed.
  - Therapy referral may be necessary in some patients: Start edema control and gentle finger and wrist motion.
- Postoperative 4 weeks
  - The patient returns for final motion and wound checks.

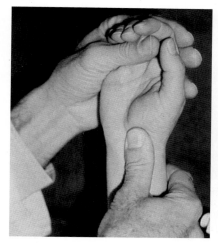

Figure 4-21. Watson maneuver. *(From Green DP, Hotchkiss RN, Pederson WC, et al, editors: Green's operative hand surgery. In Hill Hastings, editor:* Arthrodesis, Partial and Complete, *ed 5, Philadelphia, 2005, Churchill Livingstone, p 493.)*

Suggested Readings
Chhabra AB: Wrist and hand. In Miller M, Chhabra B, Hurwitz S, et al, editors: *Orthopaedic surgical approaches,* Philadelphia, 2008, Saunders, pp 145–210.

Sarris I, Darlis NA, Musgrave D, et al: Tenosynovitis: trigger finger, de Quervain's syndrome, flexor carpi radialis, and extensor carpi ulnaris. In Miller MD, Hart JA, MacKnight JM, editors: *Essential orthopaedics,* Philadelphia, 2010, Saunders, pp 212–221.

Sato ES, Gomes Dos Santos JB, Belloti JC, et al: Treatment of trigger finger: randomized clinical trial comparing the methods of corticosteroid injection, percutaneous release and open surgery, *Rheumatology* 51(1): 93–99, 2012.

SCAPHOLUNATE LIGAMENT TEAR
History
- The patient reports a fall on an outstretched hand, usually in ulnar deviation. The patient reports dorsal wrist pain and pain with weight bearing with the wrist extended.
- The patient may report weakness with lifting or grip.
- In later stages, the patient may report wrist stiffness.

Physical Examination
- Possible dorsal wrist edema
- Tenderness to palpation at the SL interval (palpated on the dorsal wrist approximately 1 to 3 cm distal to Lister tubercle)
- Positive Watson maneuver (Fig. 4-21)
  - **Watson maneuver** tests for SLL instability. The examiner places his or her thumb firmly on the patient's volar wrist over the scaphoid tubercle and applies pressure. With the other hand, the examiner moves the patient's wrist from ulnar to radial deviation. A positive test result occurs when there is a palpable "clunk" *with pain.* The presence of a clunk alone is not a positive test result.
  - The clunk occurs when the scaphoid has dissociated from the lunate because of an SLL tear and hits against the dorsal lip of the radius during the maneuver.

Imaging
- Order wrist radiographs: PA, lateral, oblique, clenched fist, and scaphoid (navicular) views.
- Clenched fist views may show widening of the SL interval (>3 to 4 mm is abnormal; must compare with the contralateral side) (Fig. 4-22).

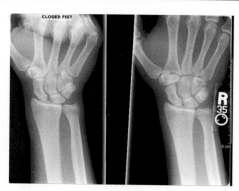

Figure 4-22. Clenched fist view with widening of the scapholunate (SL) interval (left) and non-stress posteroanterior view with a normal SL interval (right). *(From Rynders SD, Chhabra AB: Scapholunate ligament injury. In Miller MD, Hart JA, MacKnight JM, editors: Essential orthopaedics, Philadelphia, 2010, Saunders, p 306.)*

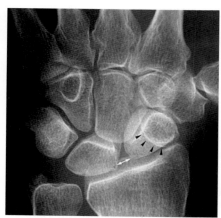

Figure 4-24. Scaphoid ring sign *(arrowheads).* Double arrow, SL interval. *(From Green DP, Hotchkiss RN, Pederson WC, et al, editors: Green's operative hand surgery. In Marc Garcia-Elias and William B. Geissler, editors: Carpal Instability, ed 5, Philadelphia, 2005, Churchill Livingstone p 557.)*

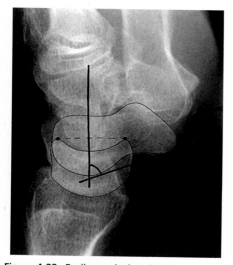

Figure 4-23. Radiograph showing an abnormal scapholunate angle. *(From Green DP, Hotchkiss RN, Pederson WC, et al, editors: Green's operative hand surgery. In Marc Garcia-Elias and William B. Geissler, editors: Carpal Instability, ed 5, Philadelphia, 2005, Churchill Livingstone p 558.)*

- The PA view may reveal a scaphoid ring sign (Fig. 4-24).
- MRI can help to identify SL injuries, but sensitivity and specificity vary depending on the quality of MRI and the expertise and experience of the radiologist.
- The gold standard for diagnosis of a tear is wrist arthroscopy.

Classification
The SLL has three bands: volar, interosseous, and dorsal. The thickest and most supportive is the dorsal band.

Stages of Instability Resulting from Ligament Injury
1) Occult or predynamic instability
   - Partial tear (detected only by MRI or during arthroscopy)
   - Normal radiographs
2) Dynamic instability
   - Partial or complete tear
   - PA and lateral radiographs appearing normal; stress radiograph (clenched fist view) abnormal, with a wide SL interval (compare with the contralateral side)
3) Static instability
   - Complete tear
   - Radiographs demonstrating an SL interval greater than 3 mm and an SL angle greater than 60 degrees

- The lateral view may show an SL angle greater than 60 degrees (an increased SL angle is also known as dorsal intercalated segment instability or DISI). The normal angle is 30 to 60 degrees (Fig. 4-23).

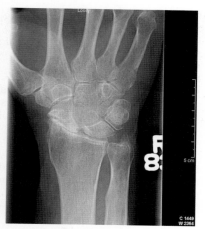

Figure 4-25. Scapholunate advanced collapse. *(From Rynders SD, Chhabra AB: Scapholunate ligament injury. In Miller MD, Hart JA, MacKnight JM, editors: Essential orthopaedics, Philadelphia, 2010, Saunders, p 307.)*

 ORTHOPAEDIC WARNING

If a scapholunate ligament tear is left undiagnosed or untreated, the patient will develop wrist arthritis within 10 to 15 years after the injury.

Scapholunate Advanced Collapse (SLAC): *Figure 4-25*

This term refers to a predictable pattern of osteoarthritis of the wrist that results from a chronic untreated SL tear. The radioscaphoid joint is first affected, followed by the lunatocapitate joint (Fig. 4-26).

Stage 1: radial styloid arthritis and radial styloid beaking
Stage 2: radiocarpal joint arthritis
Stage 3: capitolunate interface arthritis
Stage 4: pan-carpal arthritis

Differential Diagnosis
- Kienbock disease
- Acute fracture of scaphoid
- de Quervain tenosynovitis
- Gout or pseudogout
- Wrist tendinitis (flexor or extensor)

Initial Treatment
Patient Education
- SLL instability is the most common form of carpal instability. Complete tears should be treated surgically within 6 weeks. Complete SLL tears left untreated *will* lead to wrist arthritis (SLAC wrist). Partial SLL tears may be treated with casting and/or cortisone injections. If symptomatic after conservative treatment, patients with partial SLL tears may undergo wrist arthroscopy for staging, débridement, and treatment planning.

First Treatment Steps
- Immobilize in a volar short-arm splint
- Referral to an orthopaedic surgeon to be seen within 7 to 10 days from injury

Treatment Options
Nonoperative Management
- Conservative management is reserved for patients with partial tears or chronic complete tears with evidence

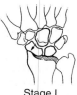
Stage I

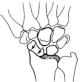
Stage II

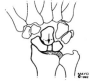
Stage III

Figure 4-26. Stages of scapholunate advanced collapse *(arrows).* Note with advancing stage, capitate migrates proximally. *(From Shin AY, Moran SL: Carpal instability including dislocation. In Trumble T, Budoff J, Cornwall R, editors:* Hand, elbow, and shoulder: core knowledge in orthopaedics, *Philadelphia, 2006, Mosby, p 151.)*

of static instability or patients too ill for surgery.

- Partial tears: Cast immobilization for 4 to 6 weeks is indicated. If immobilization does not provide relief, consider radiocarpal wrist injection.
- Chronic injuries (>6 months) respond poorly to surgical repair. Consider symptom control with splinting and radiocarpal cortisone injections as needed. Patients should be counseled that arthritic changes and loss of motion will be expected.
- Salvage procedures for symptomatic injuries that are identified late (chronic injuries) include proximal row carpectomy and total wrist fusion (for stages 3 and 4). Surgery should be suggested only after conservative treatment has failed.

Operative Management of Acute Scapholunate Ligament Injuries
Codes
ICD-9 code: 842.01 Scapholunate ligament injury
CPT code: 25320 Capsulorrhaphy or reconstruction, wrist, any method (e.g., capsulodesis or ligament repair for carpal instability)

Operative Indications
- Acute/subacute SLL tear

Informed Consent and Counseling
- Surgery will result in decreased wrist ROM but it will prevent arthritis.
- The patient can expect to be immobilized for approximately 3 to 4 months.
- Approximately 1 to 2 months of outpatient hand therapy will be needed to restore motion and strength.

Anesthesia
- Regional anesthetic such as a brachial plexus block, with sedation or general anesthesia

Patient Positioning
- Supine with the arm extended on a hand table
- Nonsterile tourniquet on the brachium

Surgical Procedures
- Surgical options are numerous and include:
  - Débridement of the SLL
  - Pinning of the SL interval
  - Repair of the SLL
  - Ligament reconstruction with dorsal capsulodesis (uses portion of dorsal wrist capsule to tether the scaphoid and prevent it from subluxing)
  - Ligament reconstruction (using ligament-bone constructs)
- Diagnostic wrist arthroscopy is used to confirm the diagnosis, to stage the injury, and to assist with the decision for repair option.

Estimated Postoperative Course
- The postoperative course depends on the type and extent of the procedure.
- If the SL is pinned, the patient is usually casted, and the pins are removed 6 to 8 weeks postoperatively.
- All procedures require postoperative rehabilitation with a hand therapist.

Suggested Readings
Shin AY, Moran SL: Carpal instability including dislocation. In Trumble TE, Budoff JE, Cornwall R, editors: *Hand, elbow, and shoulder: core knowledge in orthopaedics,* Philadelphia, 2006, Mosby, pp 139–176.
Walsh J, Berger R, Cooney W: Current status of scapholunate interosseous ligament injuries, *J Am Acad Orthop Surg* 10(1):32–42, 2002.
Watson HK, Ballet FL: The SLAC wrist: scapholunate advanced collapse pattern of degenerative arthritis, *J Hand Surg Am* 9(3):358–365, 1984.

KIENBOCK DISEASE
Definition
Avascular necrosis of the lunate bone

History
- Pain over the dorsum of the wrist
- Possible swelling in the wrist
- Weakness in grip
- Pain with motion, eventual pain at rest
- Wrist stiffness

Physical Examination
- Pain in the dorsal wrist with possible edema
- Decreased motion with advancing disease
- Possible reduction in grip strength
- Tenderness to palpation over the lunate

Imaging: Figure 4-27
- Order wrist radiographs: PA, lateral, and oblique views.
- Evaluate for negative ulnar variance (defined as the distal ulna being shorter than the distal radius). This finding is a risk factor for Kienbock disease because it increases the amount of force transmitted across the radiolunate joint.
- Consider MRI if the diagnosis not clear on radiographs or to assist in staging the disease.

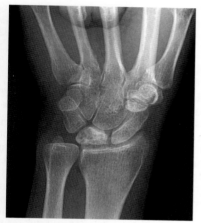

Figure 4-27. Radiograph of stage IIIa Kienbock disease. The lunate shows increased sclerosis and collapse. *(From Thaller JB: Kienbock's disease. In Miller MD, Hart JA, MacKnight JM, editors: Essential orthopaedics, Philadelphia, 2010, Saunders, p 318.)*

- Evaluate for sclerosis and collapse of the lunate.

Classification: Table 4-7
Differential Diagnosis
- Ulnar impaction syndrome (ulna abuts the lunate and causes pain and degenerative changes over time)
- Avascular necrosis of the scaphoid (Preiser's disease)
- SLL injury
- Lunate fracture

Initial Treatment
Patient Education
- Kienbock disease is more common in men than in women and usually affects patients 20 to 40 years old. It is usually unilateral. Although the cause is unknown, isolated or repetitive trauma to a lunate predisposed to the disease may lead to necrosis. Treatment is based on symptoms and stage of the disease, and prognosis is very difficult to predict.

Treatment Options (Based on Stage) Table 4-7
- Stage I: immobilization with cast or external fixator for up to 3 months
  - Progression of disease common despite immobilization
- Stages II and IIIa with negative ulnar variance:
  - Revascularization procedures using insertion of vascularized pedicle bone graft into lunate

Table 4-7. Classification and Treatment of Kienbock Disease

STAGE	RADIOGRAPHIC FINDINGS
Stage I	Normal radiographs or linear fracture; abnormal and nonspecific bone scan; on magnetic resonance imaging, lunate shows low signal intensity on T1-weighted images and high or low signal on T2-weighted images
Stage II	Lunate sclerosis, one or more fracture lines with possible early collapse of lunate on radial border
Stage IIIa	Lunate collapse with normal carpal alignment and height
Stage IIIb	Fixed hyperflexion of scaphoid, carpal height decreased, proximal migration of capitate
Stage IV	Severe lunate collapse with intra-articular degenerative changes seen at midcarpal joint and/or radiocarpal joint

From Allan CH, Joshi A, Lictman DM: Kienbock's disease: diagnosis and treatment, *J Am Acad Orthop Surg* 9: 128–136, 2001.

- Alternative treatment options include radial wedge osteotomy or capitate shortening
- Stage IIIa with negative ulnar variance: foregoing procedures, in addition to radius shortening osteotomy, ulnar lengthening, or capitate shortening
- Stage IIIb: scaphotrapeziotrapezoid (STT) or scaphocapitate joint fusion with or without lunate excision, radius shortening osteotomy, or proximal row carpectomy
- Stage IV: proximal row carpectomy
  - Advantages: preserves ROM; wrist arthrodesis possible at a later date
  - Total wrist arthrodesis: better for heavy laborers or those who fail to improve after other surgical procedures

Operative Management
Codes
ICD-9 code: 732.3 Kienbock disease
CPT codes: 25215 Proximal row carpectomy
25350 Radius shortening osteotomy
25800 Total wrist arthrodesis
25820 Limited wrist arthrodesis, STT joint fusion
25210 Lunate excision

Informed Consent and Counseling
- Even with appropriate treatment and good surgical technique, the disease may progress.
- Smoking cessation is imperative for healing.
- The patient can expect to be immobilized for approximately 6 weeks, but the type of immobilization depends on the surgeon's preference.
- The patient will require approximately 2 to 3 months of outpatient hand therapy to improve motion and strength.

Anesthesia
- Regional anesthetic such as a brachial plexus block, with sedation or general anesthesia

Patient Positioning
- Supine with the arm extended on a hand table
- Nonsterile tourniquet on the brachium

Surgical Procedures
- Multiple surgical procedures are used, with varying indications.

Suggested Readings
Allan CH, Joshi A, Lichtman DM: Kienbock's disease: diagnosis and treatment, *J Am Acad Orthop Surg* 9:128–136, 2001.
Innes L, Strauch RJ: Systematic review of the treatment of Kienbock's disease in its early and late stages, *J Hand Surg Am* 35(5):713–717, 2010.
Salmon J, Stanley JK, Trail IA: Kienbock's disease: conservative management versus radial shortening, *J Bone Joint Surg Br* 82:820–823, 2000.
Thaller JB: Kienbock's disease. In Miller MD, Hart JA, MacKnight JM, editors: *Essential orthopaedics*, Philadelphia, 2010, Saunders, pp 317–320.

TRIANGULAR FIBROCARTILAGE COMPLEX TEAR
Definition
The TFCC is a group of anatomic structures that stabilize the DRUJ and carpus. This complex includes the volar and dorsal radioulnar ligaments, the ulnar collateral and ulnocarpal ligaments, and the articular disc. The articular disc separates the carpal bones from the DRUJ. The complex is important for three biomechanical functions of the wrist: (1) stability of the DRUJ, (2) axial load transmission from the carpus to the ulna, and (3) ulnar-sided carpal stability.

History
- A fall in ulnar deviation or twisting mechanism may cause this injury.
- The patient reports ulnar-sided wrist pain and increased pain with wrist positions that mimic injury.
- The patient may report weakness or sense of instability at the wrist.
- The patient may have a history of distal radius malunion with ulnar positive variance.

Physical Examination
- Examination may reveal a prominent ulnar styloid, edema, or ecchymosis over the ulnar side of the wrist.
- Tenderness to palpation is noted on the ulnar side of the wrist.
- Grip strength is reduced.

- **Positive fovea sign:** This sign consists of palpable tenderness in the soft depression proximal to triquetrum and between the FCU tendon and the ECU tendon.
- **Positive ulnar grind test:** The examiner extends, axially loads, and ulnarly deviates wrist; a positive test result is pain with this motion.
- **Piano key test** for stability of the DRUJ: The examiner places one hand on the patient's radius and then applies dorsal pressure over the ulnar head with the opposite hand. Compare with contralateral side. Increased motion or pain with motion on injured side is a positive test result.

Imaging
- Order wrist radiographs: PA, lateral, and oblique views.
- This injury may be associated with ulnar positive variance (defined as ulna >4 mm longer than the radius) and ulnocarpal impaction syndrome (distal ulna abuts the lunate and causes degeneration of the TFCC over time) (Fig. 4-28).
- Assess for DRUJ widening compared with the uninjured wrist on the PA view.
- MRI, with or without contrast, is recommended for evaluating TFCC injuries. The quality of scans and the radiologist's experience play a role in accurately diagnosing a tear. Studies suggest an accuracy rate of approximately 64% with MRI with an arthrogram. The gold standard for diagnosis is wrist arthroscopy (Fig. 4-29).

Classification*
The vascular supply of the TFCC guides treatment. The peripheral TFCC is vascularized; the central portion of the TFCC is avascular. The poor vascularity of the central aspect of the TFCC makes healing potential poor, and therefore débridement is indicated; peripheral lesions, in contrast, have a high healing potential and can usually be repaired.

---

*This section is adapted from Green DP, Hotchkiss RN, Pederson WC, et al, editors: *Green's operative hand surgery* (vol 1), ed 5, Philadelphia, 2005, Churchill Livingstone.

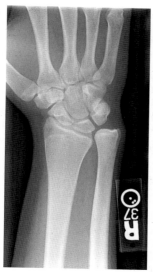

Figure 4-28. Measuring ulnar positive variance. Radiograph shows ulnar positive variance. *(From Rynders SD, Chhabra AB: Triangular fibrocartilage complex injuries. In Miller MD, Hart JA, MacKnight JM, editors:* Essential orthopaedics, *Philadelphia, 2010, Saunders, p 323.)*

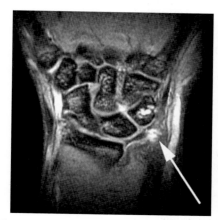

Figure 4-29. Triangular fibrocartilage complex tear *(arrow)* as seen on magnetic resonance imaging. *(From Rynders SD, Chhabra AB: Triangular fibrocartilage complex injuries. In Miller MD, Hart JA, MacKnight JM, editors:* Essential orthopaedics, *Philadelphia, 2010, Saunders, p 324.)*

Class 1: Traumatic
A) Central perforation
B) Ulnar avulsion, which may produce DRUJ instability
   1) With styloid fracture
   2) Without styloid fracture
C) Distal avulsion (from carpus)
D) Radial avulsion
   1) With sigmoid notch fracture
   2) Without sigmoid notch fracture

Class 2: Degenerative (Most Result from the Presence of Ulnocarpal Impaction Syndrome)
A) TFCC degeneration
B) TFCC degeneration
   1) Lunate and/or ulnar head chondromalacia
C) TFCC perforation
   1) Lunate and/or ulnar head chondromalacia
D) TFCC perforation
   1) Lunate and/or ulnar head chondromalacia
   2) Lunotriquetral interosseous ligament perforation
E) TFCC perforation
   1) Lunate and/or ulnar head chondromalacia
   2) Lunotriquetral ligament (LTL) perforation
   3) Ulnocarpal arthritis

Differential Diagnosis
- Extensor or flexor tendinitis
- Pisotriquetral arthritis
- DRUJ arthritis
- Cubital tunnel syndrome
- Ulnar nerve compression at Guyon canal
- Ulnar artery thrombosis
- Hook hamate fracture
- LTL tear
- SLL tear
- Calcium pyrophosphate dihydrate (CPPD) disease, also known as pseudogout

Initial Treatment
Patient Education
The type and location of tear will guide treatment. Often degenerative central tears can be initially treated with splinting and/or injection, whereas peripheral tears frequently require surgical repair.

Immobilization
- **Short-arm volar splint** for acute injury; removable splint for chronic injury
- Referral to an orthopaedic surgeon to be seen within 7 to 10 days from injury

Treatment Options (Based on Classification)
Class 1: Traumatic Tears
- Class 1A: Options include rest, immobilization in a Muenster cast, anti-inflammatory medication, and local steroid injections.
- If symptoms persist, an arthroscopic débridement may be necessary
- Class 1B and 1C: Initial treatment consists of a volar splint, short-arm cast, or Muenster cast for 6 weeks followed by an additional 4 to 6 weeks of activity modification (e.g., no heavy lifting). Most Class 1B injuries respond to conservative measures. If symptoms persist or instability is present, surgery is indicated. Surgery may include open or arthroscopic repair.
- Class 1D: These tears are frequently associated with distal radius fractures. This injury usually heals with appropriate treatment of the fracture.

Class 2: Degenerative Tears
- Severity and progression vary.
- Treatment options include activity modification, anti-inflammatory medications, wrist splinting, and cortisone injection into the wrist joint. If these measures fail, wrist arthroscopy for débridement of the tear is indicated. Often, an ulnar-shortening osteotomy is performed if there is underlying ulnar positive variance.

Operative Management
Codes
ICD-9 code: 842.09 Sprain of distal radioulnar joint
CPT codes: 25107 (Arthrotomy, distal radioulnar joint including repair of triangular cartilage complex)
  29846 (Arthroscopy wrist with excision or repair of triangular fibrocartilage and/or joint débridement)

Operative Indications
■ Conservative measures have failed.
■ An ulnar shortening osteotomy is sometimes indicated when there is significant ulnar positive variance and evidence of ulnocarpal impaction.

Informed Consent and Counseling
■ The patient can expect to be immobilized for approximately 6 weeks, but the type of immobilization depends on the surgical procedure performed.
■ The patient will require approximately 1 to 2 months of outpatient hand therapy to restore motion and strength.

Anesthesia
■ Regional anesthetic such as a brachial plexus block, with sedation or general anesthesia

Patient Positioning
■ Supine with the arm positioned on a traction tower
■ Nonsterile tourniquet on the brachium

Surgical Procedures
Arthroscopic Debridement and Repair
■ The affected arm is positioned in a traction tower with 15 lb of traction across the wrist.
■ Use the 3-4 portal (between third and fourth dorsal extensor compartments) for visualization and classification of the tear while a probe is placed in the 4-5 portal (between the fourth and fifth dorsal extensor compartments).
■ A shaver is used to débride class 1A tears.
■ Many different techniques for TFCC repairs are used. In general, the camera can be placed in 6R portal and the shaver placed in 3-4 portal to débride synovitis. Then an incision is made in line with the 6U portal (just ulnar to the ECU tendon). Sutures are passed through a cannula in the 3-4 portal into the TFCC and out through the capsule into the 6U incision. Tie sutures down over the capsule (take care not to entrap branches of the ulnar dorsal sensory nerve). For TFCC repairs, the patient

should be placed in a long-arm splint with the forearm supinated 45 degrees.

Estimated Postoperative Course
Débridement
■ Postoperative 2 weeks
  • Perform a wound check, and remove the sutures.
  • Apply a removable wrist splint, and start therapy for gentle wrist motion.
■ Postoperative 4 to 6 weeks
  • Wean the patient from the splint, and have the patient return to gradual activities as tolerated.

Repair
■ Postoperative 2 weeks
  • Sutures are removed. A long-arm cast or Muenster cast with the wrist in supination is applied for 4 weeks.
  • Some surgeons prefer a removable long-arm thermoplastic splint so that the patient can start to work on gradual forearm pronation.
■ Postoperative 6 weeks
  • Some surgeons apply a short-arm cast at this point, or they initiate splinting and motion.
■ Postoperative 8 to 9 weeks
  • Apply a removable splint for 4 weeks with therapy for motion and strengthening.

Suggested Readings
Ahn A, Chang D, Plate A: Triangular fibrocartilage complex tears: a review, *Bull Hosp Jt Dis* 64(3-4):114–118, 2006.
Henry MH: Management of acute triangular fibrocartilage complex injury of the wrist, *J Am Acad Orthop Surg* 16:320–329, 2008.
Palmer AK: Triangular fibrocartilage complex lesions: a classification, *J Hand Surg Am* 14; 594–606, 1989.

OSTEOARTHRITIS OF THE WRIST AND HAND
History
■ Osteoarthritis usually affects the first CMC joint, PIP and DIP joints. Less commonly, the MCP joints are affected. Its predilection for the wrist joint is usually the result of a previous injury such as a remote ligament sprain or previous carpal or radius fracture.

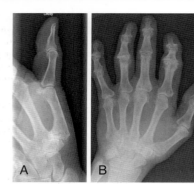

Figure 4-30. A, First carpometacarpal joint osteoarthritis. **B,** Osteoarthritis of the hand. Note the joint space narrowing and periarticular sclerosis.

- The patient may report pain, edema, stiffness, or deformity of the affected joint.
- Pain may be worse in the morning and after repetitive activities.

Physical Examination
- Edema over the affected joint
- Nodules over the DIP joints (Heberden nodes) or PIP joints (Bouchard nodes)
- Mucous or ganglion cysts over the DIP joints
- Tenderness to palpation over the involved joint
- **First CMC grind test:** An axial load placed on the thumb in combination with circumduction eliciting pain and sometimes crepitus
- Pain with joint motion
- Reduced motion
- Weakened grip or pinch strength

Imaging: Figure 4-30
- Order affected wrist, hand, or finger radiographs: PA, lateral, and oblique views.
  - The pisiform oblique view is used to evaluate for pisotriquetral arthritis.
- Radiographic findings of osteoarthritis include joint space narrowing, sub-chondral sclerosis or subchondral cysts, and periarticular osteophytes.
- Symptoms of arthritis can precede radiographic findings.

Classification
First Carpometacarpal Joint Arthritis
- Eaton stages of first CMC joint osteo-arthritis†
  Stage 1: normal joint with exception of possible widening from synovitis
  Stage 2: joint space narrowing with debris and osteophytes smaller than 2 mm
  Stage 3: joint space narrowing with debris and osteophytes larger than 2 mm
  Stage 4: scaphotrapezial joint space involvement in addition to narrowing of the CMC joint

Differential Diagnosis
- Joint sprain or fracture
- Inflammatory arthritis such as rheumatoid arthritis
- Gout

Initial Treatment
Patient Education
- Osteoarthritis is very common and although there is no cure, effective treatment options exist. These include both nonoperative (over-the-counter medication, splinting, cortisone injections) and operative interventions.

†Adapted from Eaton RG, Littler JW: Ligament reconstruction for the painful thumb carpometacarpal joint. *J Bone Surg Am* 55:1655–1666, 1973.

First Treatment Steps
- Temporary immobilization of the affected joint for comfort is indicated for an arthritis flare.
- Refer to an orthopaedic surgeon if patient would like specialized splints, cortisone injections, or surgical intervention.

Treatment Options
Nonoperative Management
- NSAIDs if tolerated; glucosamine chondroitin sulfate (may provide relief but not well studied)
- Intermittent splinting to rest the affected joint
- Activity modification
- Intra-articular cortisone injection into the affected joint (see page 167)

Operative Management of Distal Interphalangeal, Proximal Interphalangeal, Metacarpophalangeal, and First Carpometacarpal Osteoarthritis
Codes
ICD-9 codes: 715.9 Degenerative arthritis of finger
715.34 Thumb CMC degenerative arthritis
CPT codes: 25447: Arthroplasty, interposition, intercarpal or carpometacarpal joints
26860: arthrodesis, interphalangeal joint, with or without internal fixation
26531: Arthroplasty, metacarpophalangeal joint, with prosthetic implant, each joint
26536: Arthroplasty, interphalangeal joint, with prosthetic implant each joint

Operative Indications
- Painful or dysfunctional joint that does not respond to conservative measures
  - Not recommended in fingers that function well and when pain can be controlled by other means

Informed Consent and Counseling
- Arthrodesis or joint fusion is a pain-relieving surgical procedure that renders the joint immobile.

- A risk of nonunion is reported in smokers; smoking is considered a relative contraindication.
- For first CMC joint arthroplasty with interposition, recovery may take up to 3 to 6 months and involves a period of immobilization.
- There is a risk of nail deformity with DIP joint surgical interventions.
- Almost all surgical interventions for arthritis require postoperative therapy.

Anesthesia
- Regional anesthetic such as a brachial plexus block, with sedation or general anesthesia

Patient Positioning
- Supine with the arm extended on a hand table
- Nonsterile tourniquet on the brachium

Surgical Procedures
First Carpometacarpal Joint Arthroplasty
Many surgical options are available, and procedure selection depends on the joint or joints involved, the level of pain and dysfunction, and the severity of the arthritis and deformity. Options include arthrodesis (multiple techniques exist) or arthroplasty (using interposition graft or various implants). Selection of procedures and implants depends on the surgeon.

Suggested Readings
Leit ME, Tomaino MM: Osteoarthritis of the hand and wrist. In Trumble TE, Budoff JE, Cornwall R, editors: *Hand, elbow, and shoulder: core knowledge in orthopaedics*, Philadelphia, 2006, Mosby, pp 325–343.
Matullo KS, Ilyas A, Thoder JJ: CMC arthroplasty of the thumb: a review, *Hand* 2(4):232–239, 2007.
Shuler MS, Luria S, Tumble TE: Basal joint arthritis of the thumb, *J Am Acad Orthop Surg* 16(7):418–423, 2008.

CARPAL TUNNEL SYNDROME
Definition
Carpal tunnel syndrome (CTS) is compression of the median nerve at the wrist and is the most common compression neuropathy of the upper extremity.

History

- Numbness and tingling occur in the thumb, index finger, middle finger, and the radial half of the ring finger.
- Some patients report numbness or tingling in all fingers.
- Symptoms are worse at night, with nocturnal awakening or when driving.
- The patient reports feeling the need to shake out the hands to get relief, also known as the "flick sign."
- The patient may note clumsiness and/ or weak grip.
- Pain radiation to the forearm or hand is possible.

Physical Examination

- Inspect for thenar atrophy of the abductor pollicis brevis (suggestive of severe involvement).
- **Positive Tinel sign:** Percussion over the median nerve at the wrist flexor crease reproduces paresthesias in the fingers.
- **Positive pressure test:** Direct compression over the median nerve reproduces paresthesias in the fingers.
- **Positive Phalen test:** Wrist flexion for 1 to 2 minutes reproduces paresthesias in the fingers (note: keep the elbow extended during this test to prevent compression at the elbow).
- Two-point discrimination may be diminished in the median nerve distribution (5 mm considered normal).
- Weakness with resisted thumb abduction is noted.

Further Diagnostic Testing

- Electrodiagnostic testing: Be sure to evaluate for a differential diagnosis, as listed in the next subsection.
  - Nerve conduction study (NCS) evaluates motor and sensory portions of the nerve.
  - Electromyography (EMG) evaluates either spontaneous or volitional electrical activity in the muscle; fibrillation potentials are early signs of muscle denervation.

Differential Diagnosis

- Cubital tunnel syndrome
- Cervical radiculopathy
- Peripheral neuropathy associated with diabetes, renal failure, or chronic substance abuse

Initial Treatment

Patient Education

- CTS is the most common compression neuropathy and is more common in women and patients with diabetes mellitus. The syndrome is progressive; therefore, it is important to diagnose and treat it appropriately to prevent permanent damage to the nerve and the muscles it innervates.
- CTS may occur during pregnancy and is usually temporary and self-limited after delivery. Carpal tunnel surgery should be avoided during pregnancy.

Treatment Options

Nonoperative Management

- Splinting in an off-the-shelf removable wrist splint, usually worn at night
- Judicious use of NSAIDS
- Cortisone injection (shown to be effective and "mimics" results of surgical intervention)

Operative Management

Codes

ICD-9 code: 354.0 Carpal tunnel syndrome

CPT codes: 64721 Open carpal tunnel release

29848 Endoscopic carpal tunnel release

Operative Indications

- CTS not responsive long-term to cortisone injections
- Evidence of atrophy and/or denervation on nerve testing

Informed Consent and Counseling

- Even with appropriate treatment and good surgical release, there may be residual paresthesias, depending on the severity of disease.
  - If the patient has concomitant cervical nerve root compression in addition to

CTS, he or she may not gain full relief of symptoms in the upper extremity.

- The patient may be immobilized for a period of roughly 2 weeks postoperatively and can return to most strenuous activities by 4 to 6 weeks.
  - The patient may require one to two visits with an outpatient hand therapist postoperatively.
  - Peri-incisional tenderness may occur for up to 3 months postoperatively.
  - This pain is commonly known as "pillar pain".

Anesthesia

- Local or regional anesthetic with sedation; general anesthesia possibly preferable for endoscopic techniques, to limit patient motion

Patient Positioning

- Supine with the arm extended on a hand table
- Nonsterile tourniquet on the brachium

Surgical Procedures

Open Carpal Tunnel Release:
Figure 4-31

- Determine the location of incision: Draw a Kaplan cardinal line from the hook of the hamate to the first web space.
- A volar palmar incision is made along radial border of the ring finger to the ulnar side of the palmaris longus to avoid injury to the palmar cutaneous branch of the median nerve.
- Protect the recurrent motor branch of the medial nerve (the point at which the line from the radial aspect of the middle finger intersects with the Kaplan line). This branch has a variable course.
- Use sharp dissection through the subcutaneous tissues and the longitudinal fibers of the superficial palmar fascia, and expose the transverse fibers of the transverse carpal ligament (TCL).
- Place a blunt instrument such as a Freer or hemostat under the TCL to protect the median nerve beneath, and sharply incise along the entire length.

Endoscopic Carpal Tunnel Release

- May provide earlier return to work and less sensitive scar on palm
- Small, volar transverse incision near the wrist flexor crease
- Carpal canal dilated
- Endoscopic device inserted and TCL incised

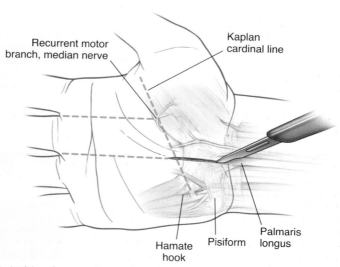

Figure 4-31. Incision for carpal tunnel release. *(From Chhabra AB: Wrist and hand. In Miller MD, Chhabra AB, Hurwitz S, et al, editors:* Orthopaedic surgical approaches, *Philadelphia, 2008, Saunders, p 177.)*

Estimated Postoperative Course
- Postoperative days 3 to 6
  - Some surgeons initiate hand therapy at this point.
- Postoperative days 10 to 14
  - Sutures are removed, and a wound check is performed.
- Postoperative 4 weeks
  - Motion and wound checks are performed; release the patient to regular activities if he or she is minimally symptomatic.

Suggested Readings

Chhabra AB: Wrist and hand. In Miller M, Chhabra B, Hurwitz S, et al, editors: *Orthopaedic surgical approaches*, Philadelphia, 2008, Saunders, pp 145–210.

Dellon L: Compression neuropathy. In Trumble TE, Budoff JE, Cornwall R, editors: *Hand, elbow, and shoulder: core knowledge in orthopaedics*, Philadelphia, 2006, Mosby, pp 234–254.

Keith MW, Masear V, Chung K, et al: Diagnosis of carpal tunnel syndrome, *J Am Acad Orthop Surg* 17(6):389–396, 2009.

Keith MW, Masear V, Chung K, et al: Treatment of carpal tunnel syndrome, *J Am Acad Orthop Surg* 17(6):397–405, 2009.

DE QUERVAIN TENOSYNOVITIS
Definition
de Quervain tenosynovitis is a painful inflammation of the abductor pollicis longus (APL) and the extensor pollicis brevis (EPB) tendons, also known as the first extensor compartment.

History
- This disorder is associated with repetitive tasks involving the thumb and wrist.
- The patient reports pain over the radial wrist and thumb that is worse with thumb abduction and/or extension.
- This condition is often seen in pregnancy or in patients with newborns as a result of cradling infants in arms ("new mom's tendinitis").

Physical Examination
- Edema and tenderness are noted at the first dorsal extensors extending to the radial styloid.

- **Positive Finkelstein test** (Fig. 4-32): The thumb is clasped into the palm, and the wrist is passively ulnarly deviated. A positive test result consists of severe pain.
- Pain occurs with thumb motion or active radial deviation.
- Occasionally, this disorder is associated with a ganglion cyst over the first dorsal compartment.

Imaging
- Not necessary for diagnosis

Differential Diagnosis
- Intersection syndrome (inflammation and pain at the point where the first extensor compartment tendons cross over the second extensor compartment tendons [the extensor carpi radialis longus and the extensor carpi radialis brevis tendons, proximal to Lister tubercle of the distal radius])
- First CMC joint arthritis
- Wrist arthritis
- Scaphoid fracture
- Superficial sensory radial nerve neuroma
- Radial styloid fracture

Initial Treatment
Patient Education
- de Quervain tenosynovitis is more common in female patients, especially after childbirth. It is an inflammatory condition that is exacerbated by overuse. Treatment may include a thumb

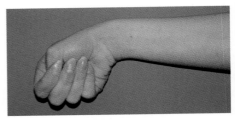

Figure 4-32. Finkelstein test. *(From Schnur D: de Quervain's tenosynovitis. In Miller MD, Hart JA, MacKnight JM, editors:* Essential orthopaedics, *Philadelphia, 2010, Saunders, p 326.)*

spica splint, hand therapy, and/or a cortisone injection. Although effective, cortisone injections in this area may cause subcutaneous fat atrophy and/or skin hypopigmentation at the injection site.

First Treatment Steps
- Short-arm thumb spica removable splint until edema subsides
- Nonurgent referral to an orthopaedic surgeon if the condition does not respond to splinting

Treatment Options
Nonoperative Management
- Splinting in a thumb spica splint or cast with a cortisone injection (see page 169)
- Hand therapy referral for local antiinflammatory modalities and activity modification

Operative Management
Codes
ICD-9 code: 727.04 de Quervain's tenosynovitis
CPT code: 25000 Incision extensor tendon sheath

Operative Indications
- No response to conservative measures and symptoms lasting more than 10 months

Informed Consent and Counseling
- Superficial sensory radial nerve (SSRN) irritation may occur postoperatively and is usually temporary.

Anesthesia
- Regional anesthetic such as a brachial plexus block, with sedation or general anesthesia

Patient Positioning
- Supine with the arm extended on a hand table
- Nonsterile tourniquet on the brachium

Surgical Procedure
First Dorsal Compartment Release
- Approach via the first extensor compartment radially with a short transverse incision.

- Divide the extensor retinaculum longitudinally.
- Protect the SSRN and its branches, and avoid excessive dissection.
- Release the first dorsal compartment on its dorsal margin.
- Identify the EPB and all slips of the APL.
- Be aware of anatomic variations (the compartment may have a longitudinal septum, the APL often has two or more slips with various insertions, and the EPB is absent in 5% to 7% of extremities).

Estimated Postoperative Course
- Postoperative days 10 to 14
  - Sutures are removed, and a wound check is performed.
  - A thumb spica cast or splint is applied.
- Postoperative 4 weeks
  - Remove the cast or splint.
  - Initiate thumb and wrist motion.
- Postoperative 3 months
  - Release the patient to all regular activities.

Suggested Readings
Sarris I, Darlis NA, Musgrave D, et al: Tenosynovitis: trigger finger, de Quervain's syndrome, flexor carpi radialis, and extensor carpi ulnaris. In Trumble TE, Budoff JE, Cornwall R, editors: *Hand, elbow, and shoulder: core knowledge in orthopaedics*, Philadelphia, 2006, Mosby, pp 212–221.

Schnur D: de Quervain's tenosynovitis. In Miller MD, Hart JA, MacKnight JM, editors: *Essential orthopaedics, Philadelphia,* 2010, Saunders, pp 326–328.

Witt J, Pess G, Gelberman RH: Treatment of de Quervain's tenosynovitis: a prospective study of the results of injection of steroid and immobilization in a splint, *J Bone Joint Surg Am* 73:219–222, 1991.

NAIL BED INJURY
The nail bed is made of the following structures: germinal matrix, sterile matrix, and dorsal nail bed. The germinal matrix is proximal to the lunula and contains specialized cells that generate the nail plate. The sterile matrix is located distal to the germinal matrix and functions to adhere the nail plate to the nail bed.

History

- Traumatic, crush-type injury to the finger
- Painful finger

Physical Examination

- Assess vascularity and sensation.
- Inspect for edema, erythema, drainage, and hematoma.

Imaging

- Order finger radiographs: PA, lateral, and oblique to evaluate for an associated distal phalanx fracture.

Initial Treatment

Patient Education

- Inadequate or delayed treatment can lead to functional and/or cosmetic nail deformities. Patients should be educated that the nail plate grows at a rate of 0.1 mm/day with quicker growth in summer than in winter. After injury, nail growth does not normalize until approximately 100 days.

Treatment Options

Hematoma

- If the hematoma involves less than 50% of the nail plate, trephine the nail plate with a sterile needle to allow the hematoma to drain.

Laceration

- If the nail is lacerated or has a hematoma larger than 50%, proceed with nail bed repair immediately (can be done in a well-equipped emergency department or outpatient office).

Operative Management

Codes
ICD-9 code: 883.0 Open wound of finger, includes fingernail
CPT codes: 11730 Removal of nail plate
11760 Repair of nail bed

Operative Indications
- If nail is lacerated or has hematoma larger than 50%

Informed Consent and Counseling
- Even with appropriate treatment and good surgical repair, there is still a possibility of nail plate deformity.

Anesthesia

- Digital block

Patient Positioning

- Seated, with the finger placed on a stable surface

Surgical Procedures: Figure 4-33

Nailbed Repair

- After performing a digital block, exsanguinate the digit with a finger tourniquet (e.g., a sterile Penrose drain wrapped around the base of finger and held tight with a hemostat), and scrub or cleanse digit to remove debris.
- Remove the remaining nail with a hemostat, with care taken not to avulse or injure additional areas of the nail bed. If necessary, repair the skin surrounding the nail bed with 5.0 nylon sutures first. Next, repair the nail bed itself with 6.0 chromic suture under loupe magnification.
- After the nail bed has been repaired, the proximal nail fold (or cuticle) must be stented open with the original minimally injured nail plate, a piece of nonadherent gauze, or a silicon sheet. Once in place, a nylon suture is placed distally through the nail plate or synthetic material to secure it in place. Wrap with nonadherent dressing. A small splint across the DIP joint may be applied if an associated distal phalanx fracture is present.

Estimated Postoperative Course

- Postrepair days 5 to 7
  - The dressing is changed.
- Postrepair 2 to 3 weeks
  - Suture through the nail plate is removed. The nail plate or other

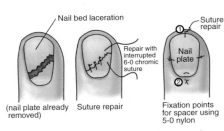

Figure 4-33. Nail bed repair technique. *(From Fledman M, Isaacs JE: Nail bed injuries. In Miller MD, Hart JA, MacKnight JM, editors:* Essential orthopaedics, *Philadelphia, 2010, Saunders, p 370.)*

material will adhere to matrix for 1 to 3 months until it is pushed off by the new nail.
- If a fracture is present, splint for 6 weeks with repeat radiographs at 6 weeks.

Suggested Readings

Feldman M, Isaacs JE: Nail bed Injuries. In Miller MD, Hart JA, MacKnight JM, editors: *Essential orthopaedics,* Philadelphia, 2010, Saunders, pp 369–371.

Richards A, Crick A, Cole R: A novel method of securing the nail following nail bed repair, *Plast Reconstr Surg* 103(7):1983–1985, 1999.

BENNETT FRACTURE

Definition

This injury is an intra-articular, oblique fracture-dislocation of the ulnar-volar metacarpal base. Proximal and radial subluxation of the metacarpal base from the CMC articulation results from the pull created by the insertion of the abductor pollicis brevis tendon on the radial side of the metacarpal base.

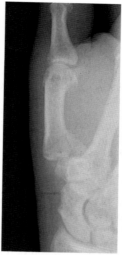

Figure 4-34. Radiograph of a Bennett fracture. *(From Rynders SD, Chhabra AB: Thumb fractures. In Miller MD, Hart JA, MacKnight JM, editors:* Essential orthopaedics, *Philadelphia, 2010, Saunders, p 404.)*

History
- Axial loading and abduction force to the thumb (usually from fall or sporting event)
- Patient-reported thumb pain and reduced motion

Physical Examination
- Edema and/or ecchymosis in the thenar region
- Thumb possibly appearing deformed or malrotated
- Tenderness over the base of the thumb

Imaging: Figure 4-34
- Order thumb radiographs: PA, lateral, and oblique views.

Differential Diagnosis
- Rolando fracture (three-part intra-articular fracture at the base of the thumb metacarpal; in addition to the ulnar-volar fragments seen in a Bennett fracture, also a large dorsal fragment resulting in a Y- or T-shaped fracture)
- Thumb CMC joint dislocation
- CMC joint osteoarthritis
- Thumb MCP joint sprain
- Scaphoid fracture

Initial Treatment

Patient Education
- Most Bennett fractures are resistant to closed reduction and nonoperative treatment and often require open reduction and fixation. Additionally, surgical treatment is more likely to produce reliable results than casting. A mismanaged Bennett fracture will result in traumatic arthritis and cause impairment of thumb function. Even with surgical intervention, the injured joint is more likely to develop arthritis.

First Treatment Steps
- Short-arm thumb spica splint until edema subsides
- Referral to an orthopaedic surgeon to be seen within 3 to 5 days from injury

Treatment Options

Nonoperative Management
- Conservative management is reserved for fractures with less than 1 mm displacement. The patient requires frequent follow-up with radiographs to ensure that reduction is maintained.
- Immobilize in a thumb spica splint for 1 to 2 weeks to reduce edema. Then

apply a thumb spica cast for 4 to 6 weeks.

Rehabilitation
- After 6 weeks of splint and cast immobilization and with evidence of healing on a radiograph, the patient can start thumb motion.
- An off-the-shelf wrist brace may be used to transition from the cast.
- The patient can return to a preinjury activity level at 6 to 8 weeks.

Operative Management
Codes
ICD-9 code: 815.01 Closed fracture base of thumb metacarpal
CPT codes: 26665 Open reduction, internal fixation of a Bennett's fracture
26650 Closed reduction percutaneous pinning of a Bennett's fracture

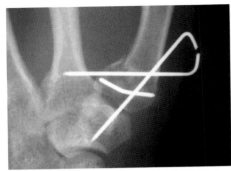

Figure 4-35. Bennett fracture treated with closed reduction, percutaneous pinning. *(From Markiewitz AD: Fractures and dislocations involving the metacarpal bone. In Trumble T, Budoff J, Cornwall R, editors: Hand, elbow, and shoulder: core knowledge in orthopaedics, Philadelphia, 2006, Mosby, p 42.)*

Operative Indications
- Bennett fracture with at least 1 mm of displacement

Informed Consent and Counseling
- The affected joint is more likely to develop osteoarthritis.
- The patient can expect to be immobilized for roughly 4 to 6 weeks postoperatively.
- The patient will require a short course of outpatient hand therapy to restore motion and strength.
- Pins will stay in for 4 to 6 weeks.

Anesthesia
- Regional anesthetic such as a brachial plexus block, with sedation or general anesthesia

Patient Positioning
- Supine with the arm extended on a hand table
- Nonsterile tourniquet on the brachium

Surgical Procedures
Closed Reduction, Percutaneous
Pinning: *Figure 4-35*
- Because this technique is minimally invasive, it may be used preferentially for treatment of Bennett fractures.

- Wires are placed through the metacarpal shaft and into the trapezium. It is not always necessary to capture the Bennett fragment because reduction of the joint should reapproximate the fracture fragment.
- Place a thumb spica splint.

Estimated Postoperative Course
- Postoperative days 10 to 14
  - Splint and sutures are removed, and a wound check is performed.
  - Radiographs are obtained: thumb PA, lateral, and oblique views.
  - Immobilization: The patient is given a thumb spica cast, padded to protect pin sites.
- Postoperative 4 weeks
  - Radiographs are obtained: thumb PA, lateral, and oblique views.
  - Wires are removed if present.
  - *Therapy:* If healing is present, progress therapy to more aggressive wrist motion, wean the patient from the splint, and have the patient start gradual weight bearing.
  - If no healing occurs, the patient should continue gentle motion exercises and wear the brace at all times until healing is evident on radiographs.

- Postoperative 3 months
  - The patient returns for a motion check and radiographs.

Suggested Readings

Soyer AD: Fractures of the base of the first metacarpal: current treatment options, *J Am Acad Orthop Surg* 7:403–412, 1999.

Stern PJ: Fractures of the metacarpals and phalanges. In Green DP, Hotchkiss RN, Pederson WC, et al, editors: *Green's operative hand surgery,* ed 5, Philadelphia, 2005, Churchill Livingstone, pp 330–339.

Taras JS, Hankins SM: Fractures and dislocations of the thumb. In Trumble TE, Budoff JE, Cornwall R, editors: *Hand, elbow, and shoulder: core knowledge in orthopaedics,* Philadelphia, 2006, Mosby, pp 56–68.

BABY BENNETT FRACTURE
Definition
A fracture-dislocation of the fifth CMC joint

History
- High-energy trauma, falls, direct blows
- Axial loading to the hand with hyperextension or hyperflexion of the hand. (i.e., fist striking a firm, immobile object)
- Possible patient-reported sense of instability

Physical Examination
- Edema and/or ecchymosis at and near the base of the small finger
- Motion reduced secondary to pain
- Tenderness to palpation at the fifth CMC joint
- Loss of grip strength

Imaging: Figure 4-36
- Order hand radiographs: PA, lateral, and oblique (30-degree oblique view with pronation can accentuate the fifth CMC joint) views.
- If the diagnosis is suspected and cannot be confirmed on radiographs, consider a CT scan.

Differential Diagnosis
- Metacarpal fracture
- Contusion
- ECU tendinitis
- Triquetrum or hamate fracture

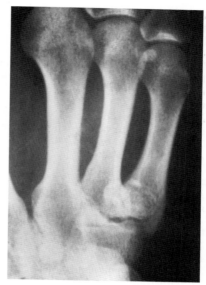

Figure 4-36. Radiograph of a baby Bennett fracture-dislocation. *(From Green DP, Hotchkiss RN, Pederson WC, et al, editors: Green's operative hand surgery. In Peter J. Stern, editor: Fractures of the Metacarpals and Phalanges, ed 5, Philadelphia, 2005, Churchill Livingstone, p 288.)*

Initial Treatment
Patient Education
- The fifth digit CMC joint is a highly mobile joint; minor subluxation is not usually well tolerated. Residual subluxation and articular step-off are associated with posttraumatic arthritis, so most of these injuries require surgery. A delay in treatment can result in chronic pain, weakness, and stiffness of the joint. Treatment for late presentation of these injuries includes conservative management with the option for CMC joint fusion.

First Treatment Steps
- **Ulnar gutter splint** until edema subsides
- Referral to an orthopaedic surgeon to be seen within 3 to 5 days from injury

Treatment Options
Nonoperative Management
- Usually, this injury is unstable and nonoperative management is not recommended.

Operative Management

Codes
ICD-9 code: 815.02 Closed fracture base of metacarpal

CPT codes: 26676: percutaneous skeletal fixation of carpometacarpal dislocation, other than thumb, with manipulation, each joint
26685: Open treatment of carpometacarpal dislocation, other than thumb; includes internal fixation, when performed, each joint

Operative Indications
- All unstable fifth CMC joint fracture-dislocations

Informed Consent and Counseling
- The joint is more likely to develop osteoarthritis.
- The patient can expect to be immobilized for roughly 4 to 6 weeks.
- The patient will require a short course of outpatient hand therapy to restore motion and strength.

Anesthesia
- Regional anesthetic such as a brachial plexus block, with sedation or general anesthesia

Patient Positioning
- Supine with the arm extended on a hand table
- Nonsterile tourniquet on the brachium

Surgical Procedures

Closed Reduction, Percutaneous Pinning: Figure 4-37
- The fifth CMC joint is reduced, and fractures are aligned.
- The reduction is stabilized with two wires. One wire should be directed across the metacarpohamate joint, and other is directed into the base of the fourth metacarpal.
- The patient is placed in an ulnar gutter splint to include the MCP joints of the fourth and fifth digits, but still allow PIP joint motion.

Estimated Postoperative Course
- Postoperative days 10 to 14
  - Sutures are removed, and a wound check is performed.

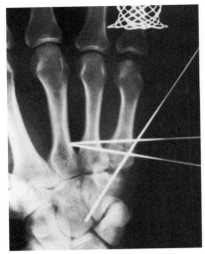

Figure 4-37. Closed reduction, percutaneous fixation of a baby Bennett fracture. *(From Green DP, Hotchkiss RN, Pederson WC, et al, editors: Green's operative hand surgery. In Peter J. Stern, editor: Fractures of the Metacarpals and Phalanges, ed 5, Philadelphia, 5, 2005, Churchill Livingstone p 288.)*

- Radiographs are obtained: hand PA, lateral, and oblique views.
- Immobilization: An outrigger cast covers the MCP joints of digits 4 and 5 but allows PIP joint motion.
- Postoperative 4 to 6 weeks
  - The patient returns for a motion check.
  - Pins are removed if evidence of healing is noted.
  - Radiographs are obtained: wrist PA, lateral, and oblique hand views.
  - *Therapy:* If healing is present, progress therapy to more aggressive wrist ROM, wean the patient from the splint, and have the patient start gradual weight bearing.

Suggested Readings
Markiewitz AD: Fractures and dislocations involving the metacarpal bone. In Trumble TE, Budoff JE, Cornwall R, editors: *Hand, elbow, and shoulder: core knowledge in orthopaedics,* Philadelphia, 2006, Mosby, pp 38–55.

Starnes T, Chhabra AB: Metacarpal fractures. In Miller MD, Hart JA, MacKnight JM, editors: *Essential orthopaedics,* Philadelphia, 2010, Saunders, pp 273–275.

Yoshida R, Shag MA, Patterson RM, et al: Anatomy and pathomechanics of ring and small finger carpometacarpal joint injuries, *J Hand Surg Am* 28:1035–1043, 2003.

METACARPAL FRACTURES

History
- Trauma, often striking an object with a closed fist
- Patient-reported pain and reduced motion of the affected digit

Physical Examination
- Inspect for any open injuries or a "fight bite" when the patient was involved in an altercation.
- Edema or ecchymosis is seen surrounding the affected area.
- Tenderness to palpation is noted over the affected metacarpal.
- Perform a neurovascular examination.
- Examine the affected metacarpal's finger in flexion and extension to evaluate for angulation or rotation. It may be helpful to compare digital cascade with that of the uninjured hand. A local field block may help to obtain an accurate examination.
- Evaluate for tendon injury if a wound is present.

Imaging: Figures 4-38 and Figure 4-39
- Order hand radiographs: PA, lateral, and oblique views.

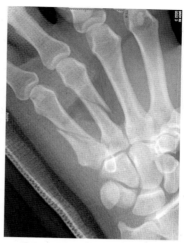

Figure 4-39. Fourth and fifth metacarpal shaft fractures. This is considered an unstable fracture pattern.

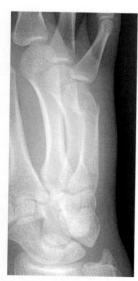

Figure 4-38. Fifth metacarpal neck fracture or Boxer fracture.

Classification
- Alignment is key to determining intervention.
- Describe the location of the fracture:
  - Intra-articular or extra-articular?
  - Simple or comminuted?
  - Displaced or nondisplaced?
- Measure displacement and/or angulation on a radiograph.

Initial Treatment

Patient Education
- Closed nondisplaced or minimally displaced fractures can usually be treated with splinting and casting.
- All open injuries require bedside irrigation before splint application, as well as oral antibiotics.
- All "fight bite" injuries, with or without tendon injury, require operative exploration and irrigation to prevent joint infection by human oral flora.

First Treatment Steps
- Reduce the fracture and irrigate any wounds as needed. Apply an ulnar gutter, radial gutter, or volar splint with the MCP joints in flexion, also known as the "intrinsic plus" position.
- Refer the patient to an orthopaedic surgeon to be seen within 3 to 5 days.

Treatment Options
Nonoperative Management
- Conservative management is reserved for nondisplaced or minimally displaced fractures without rotation or angulation or for patients too ill for surgery.
- Most metacarpal fractures will maintain reduction in a cast or splint.
- After 1 to 2 weeks of initial splint immobilization, apply a cast based on the location of the fracture:
  - **Metacarpal base fractures:** A short-arm cast is used for 3 to 4 weeks.
  - **Metacarpal shaft and neck:** A short-arm outrigger cast (include fractured finger and adjacent fingers as necessary for comfort) in the intrinsic plus position is used for 3 to 4 weeks; oblique shaft injuries comprise the most unstable fracture pattern; any fracture at the risk of displacing should be followed with weekly radiographs.
- Evaluate the patient after 4 to 6 weeks of immobilization to obtain repeat radiographs of the fracture and assess healing.
- The fracture is considered healed if there is radiographic evidence of healing and the patient is nontender at the fracture site.

Rehabilitation
- Once the fracture is healed, the patient can start active finger and wrist motion.
- An off-the-shelf wrist brace may be used to transition from the cast.
- Restrictions: The patient is non–weight bearing on the extremity until the injury is healed and pain free.

Operative Management
Codes
ICD-9 codes: 815.0 Fracture of metacarpal bone, closed
  815.1 Fracture of metacarpal bone, open
  815.02 Closed fracture of base of metacarpal
  815.03 Closed fracture of shaft of metacarpal
  815.04 Closed fracture of neck of metacarpal
CPT codes: 26608: percutaneous skeletal fixation of metacarpal fracture, each bone
  26615: open treatment of metacarpal fracture, single, includes internal fixation, when performed, each bone
  26746: open treatment of articular fracture, involving metacarpophalangeal or interphalangeal joint, includes internal fixation, when performed, each bone

Operative Indications: Table 4-8
- Metacarpal fractures with an associated fight bite or suspected or known extensor tendon injury
- Fractures meeting operative criteria as defined in Table 4-8

Informed Consent and Counseling
- The patient can expect to be immobilized for approximately 4 weeks, but the type of immobilization depends on the surgeon's preference and the fracture fixation.
- The patient will require outpatient hand therapy to restore motion and strength.

Anesthesia
- Regional anesthetic such as a brachial plexus block, with sedation or general anesthesia

Patient Positioning
- Supine with the arm extended on a hand table
- Nonsterile tourniquet on the brachium

Surgical Procedures
Open Reduction, Internal Fixation: Figure 4-40
- **For shaft fractures:** longitudinal incision just lateral to the extensor tendon
  - Use lag screws or plate fixation.
- **For head fractures:** curvilinear incision made over the MCP joint
  - Protect the extensor tendon.
  - Avoid injury to the collateral ligaments.
  - If fragments are large enough, use wires for fixation; otherwise, a headless screw can be used.
  - Initiate early controlled motion to allow extensor mechanism to heal without stretching out.

Closed or Open Reduction, Percutaneous Pinning
- Transverse wires are placed proximal and distal to the fracture line.

Table 4-8. Indications for Surgery in Metacarpal Fractures

METACARPAL FRACTURE LOCATION	SURGICAL INDICATION	COMMENTS
Head	1-mm step-off Fracture involving >20% articular surface	Collateral ligament injuries common in thumb, index finger, and small finger; also assess for "fight bite"
Neck	Index and long fingers: >15 degrees of angulation Ring and small fingers: >45 degrees of angulation (some surgeons allow up to 70 degrees angulation of small finger) Rotation unacceptable and treated with surgery	Acceptable degree of angulation contested in literature
Shaft	Index and long fingers: >15 degrees of angulation Ring and small fingers: >40 degrees of angulation All fingers: shortening: >5 mm	Every 10-degree shaft rotation = 2 cm of fingertip overlap with flexion
Base	Usually indicated in thumb and small finger	See section on Bennett fracture and baby Bennett fracture for thumb and small finger metacarpal base fractures

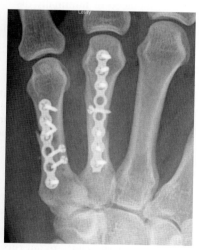

Figure 4-40. Open reduction and internal fixation of fourth and fifth metacarpal shaft fractures.

Estimated Postoperative Course
- Postoperative days 10 to 14
  - A wound check is performed, and sutures are removed as necessary.
  - Radiographs are obtained: hand PA, lateral, and oblique views.

- Immobilization: A short-arm or outrigger cast is used for approximately 4 weeks, depending on the fixation.
- *Therapy referral:* Early controlled motion with therapy is indicated, depending on the surgical procedure.
- Postoperative 4 weeks
  - Pins are removed as necessary.
- Postoperative 6 to 8 weeks
  - The patient returns for a motion check.
  - Radiographs are obtained: hand PA, lateral, and oblique views.

Suggested Readings

Henry MH: Fractures of the proximal phalanx and metacarpals in the hand: preferred methods of stabilization, *J Am Acad Orthop Surg* 16(10):586–595, 2008.

Koval KJ, Zuckerman JD: *Handbook of fractures,* Philadelphia, 2006, Lippincott Williams & Wilkins, pp 257–274.

Markiewitz AD: Fractures and dislocations involving the metacarpal bone. In Trumble TE, Budoff JE, Cornwall R, editors: *Hand, elbow, and shoulder: core knowledge in orthopaedics,* Philadelphia, 2006, Mosby, pp 38–55.

Stern PJ: Fractures of the metacarpals and phalanges. In Green DP, Hotchkiss RN, Pederson WC, et al, editors: *Green's operative hand surgery,* ed 5, Philadelphia, 2005, Churchill Livingstone, pp 277–341.

PHALANX FRACTURES

History
- Trauma to the finger, often during sports, is reported.
- The patient may report a "jammed" finger.

Physical Examination
- Inspection of the skin and nail
- Edema, ecchymosis
- Tenderness at the fracture site
- Painful and reduced finger ROM
- Evaluate neurovascular status, with a check of each digital nerve

Imaging: Figure 4-41
- Order radiographs of the affected finger: PA, lateral, and oblique views.

Classification: Table 4-9
- Alignment is key to determining intervention.
- Describe the location of the fracture (base, shaft, condyles):
  - Intra-articular or extra-articular?
  - Simple or comminuted?
  - Displaced or nondisplaced?
- Measure displacement and/or angulation.

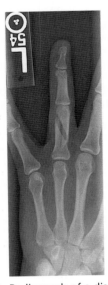

Figure 4-41. Radiograph of a displaced, rotated, extra-articular long oblique fracture of the middle phalanx.

Initial Treatment

Patient Education
- Phalanx fractures are common and affect all age groups. Even with timely treatment, loss of ROM may occur. Whether these fractures are treated operatively or nonoperatively, prolonged immobilization should be avoided, to minimize loss of motion.

Immobilization
- Close reduce the fracture if necessary.
- Splint with a **radial or ulnar gutter splint** with the MCP joints in the intrinsic plus position.
  - Do not splint with the MCP joints in extension because this can result in tightness of the hand intrinsics.
- Refer the patient to an orthopaedic surgeon to be seen within 3 to 6 days from injury.

Treatment Options

Nonoperative Management
- Nonoperative management is reserved for nondisplaced or minimally displaced fractures that do not cause change in finger rotation or angulation through finger ROM.

Proximal and Middle Phalanx Fractures
- Minimally displaced fractures: Splint in a radial or ulnar gutter splint or cast with the MCP joints in the intrinsic plus position for 2 to 3 weeks and then transition to buddy-taping fingers and begin ROM.
  - Obtain weekly radiographs to ensure the alignment is maintained.

Distal Phalanx Fractures
- Tuft fracture:
  - Immobilize only the DIP joint in a splint for 2 to 3 weeks. Begin DIP joint motion at 3 weeks, but protect the joint during active use until pain resolves.
- Shaft fracture:
  - Transverse: For a nondisplaced fracture, use a DIP joint splint for 3 to 4 weeks.
  - Displaced: The fracture may require percutaneous pinning; splint in a DIP joint splint.

Rehabilitation
- Except for mallet fingers, most phalanx fractures should be immobilized in some fashion for 2 to 3 weeks with focus on early return to motion.
- Hand therapy may be necessary to improve finger motion after splinting.

Operative Management
Codes
ICD-9 codes: 816.1 Middle or proximal phalanx fracture
   816.2 Distal phalanx fracture
CPT codes: 26727: percutaneous skeletal fixation of unstable phalangeal shaft fracture, proximal or middle phalanx, finger or thumb, with manipulation, each
   26735: open treatment of phalangeal shaft fracture, proximal or middle phalanx, finger or thumb, includes internal fixation, when performed, each
   26756: percutaneous skeletal fixation of distal phalangeal fracture, finger or thumb, each
   26765: open treatment of distal phalangeal fracture, finger or thumb, includes internal fixation, when performed, each

Operative Indications: Table 4-9

Informed Consent and Counseling
- Even with appropriate treatment and good surgical fixation, ROM may be reduced.
- A period of immobilization after surgery is required, and the patient will require hand therapy postoperatively.

Anesthesia
- Digital block, or regional anesthetic such as a brachial plexus block, with sedation or general anesthesia

Patient Positioning
- Supine with the arm extended on a hand table
- Nonsterile tourniquet on the brachium

Surgical Procedures: Figure 4-42
Open Reduction Internal Fixation, Phalanx Fracture
The operative goal is to reduce and stabilize the fracture with as minimally invasive a procedure as possible. Wire fixation, when an option, is preferable to internal fixation because of the risk of tendon adhesions and finger stiffness with open procedures. Many different surgical techniques have been described, and procedure selection is based on the

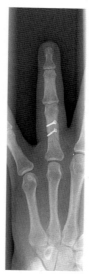

Figure 4-42. Open reduction and internal fixation with lag screws of the same fracture as in Figure 4-41.

Table 4-9. Surgical Indications for Phalanx Fractures

PHALANX	INDICATIONS FOR SURGERY	COMMENTS
Proximal	Articular step-off >2-mm shortening	Oblique, comminuted, spiral fractures are unstable
Middle	Articular step-off >2-mm shortening Irreducible dislocation Injury to central slip (in volar dislocations)	Oblique, comminuted, spiral fractures are unstable
Distal	Irreducible fractures Unstable transverse fracture	See also mallet finger/jersey finger

location and character of the fracture. Regardless of the procedure, the patient can expect to participate in a postoperative rehabilitation program to restore ROM.

Estimated Postoperative Course
- Wires are left in place for 3 to 4 weeks.
- All patients will require extensive hand therapy to restore ROM.

Suggested Readings

Henry MH: Fractures of the proximal phalanx and metacarpals in the hand: preferred methods of stabilization, *J Am Acad Orthop Surg* 16(10):586–595, 2008.

Koval KJ, Zuckerman JD: *Handbook of fractures,* Philadelphia, 2006, Lippincott Williams & Wilkins, pp 257–274.

Ng CY, Oliver CW: Fractures of the proximal interphalangeal joints of the fingers, *J Bone Joint Surg Br* 91(6):705–712, 2009.

Slade JF, Magit DP: Phalangeal fractures and dislocations. In Trumble TE, Budoff JE, Cornwall R, editors: *Hand, elbow, and shoulder: core knowledge in orthopaedics,* Philadelphia, 2006, Mosby, pp 22–37.

Starnes T, Chhabra AB: Phalangeal fractures. In Miller MD, Hart JA, MacKnight JM, editors: *Essential orthopaedics,* Philadelphia, 2010, Saunders, pp 416–423.

THUMB ULNAR COLLATERAL LIGAMENT SPRAIN
History
- Also known as skier's thumb (acute injury) or gamekeeper's thumb (chronic injury)
- Abrupt, forced, radial deviation of the thumb at the MCP joint
- Fall on an outstretched hand with the thumb abducted
- Often associated with sports such as skiing and contact and ball-handling athletics

Physical Examination
- Edema and ecchymosis at the thumb MCP joint
- Tenderness at the ulnar aspect of the thumb MCP joint

Ulnar Collateral Ligament (UCL)
Stress Test: Figure 4-43
Apply valgus stress across the thumb MCP joint in extension *and* 30 degrees of flexion. Laxity of more than 30 degrees when compared with the contralateral thumb with or without pain is diagnostic of a complete

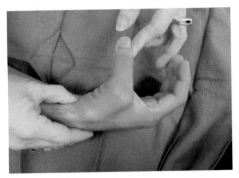

Figure 4-43. Ulnar collateral ligament stress test. *(From Ignore J, Blum G: Ulnar collateral ligament injuries of the thumb [gamekeeper's thumb, skier's thumb]. In Miller MD, Hart JA, MacKnight JM, editors: Essential orthopaedics, Philadelphia, 2010, Saunders, p 346.)*

rupture. Another method is to assess for the presence or absence of an end point to valgus stress across the joint. A complete rupture is suspected when the joint can be opened completely with valgus stress. If there is a definitive end point with pain, the injury is likely partial.

 ORTHOPAEDIC WARNING

Always obtain radiographs before the stress test to evaluate for the presence of an avulsion fracture. If a fracture is present, the injury is considered a complete ligament tear even though the defect is at the bony insertion and is not within the substance of the ligament. If stressed before radiography, the bony fragment could displace, and a nonoperative injury could become operative.

Imaging: Figure 4-44
- Order thumb radiographs: PA, lateral, and oblique views.
- The image may appear normal or may have an associated avulsion fracture.
- If no fracture is present, stress views can be helpful. Obtain a radiograph while applying radial stress to the thumb MCP and compare it with the uninjured thumb. A positive stress view will reveal opening at the ulnar MCP.

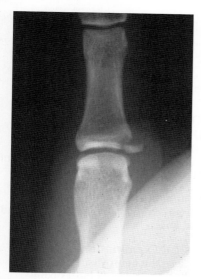

Figure 4-44. Avulsion fracture associated with an ulnar collateral ligament sprain.

■ MRI may be helpful if the radiograph is negative for an avulsion fracture and the physical examination does not differentiate between a complete or partial tear. Some institutions may use ultrasound as a diagnostic tool, but its sensitivity and specificity are user dependent.

Classification
■ Complete tear
■ Partial tear
■ With or without avulsion fracture
■ Stener lesion: A palpable mass just proximal to the MCP joint may represent a Stener lesion. This occurs when the torn aspect of the ulnar collateral ligament displaces outside the adductor aponeurosis. A Stener lesion does not occur with partial tears and can be diagnosed only by MRI or intraoperatively. When this lesion occurs, it always requires operative intervention.

Differential Diagnosis
■ Radial collateral ligament injury
■ Proximal phalanx fracture without ligament injury
■ MCP joint capsular sprain
■ Trigger finger

Initial Treatment
Patient Education
Nonoperative treatment is highly successful in partial tears. If surgery is required, it should be performed within 10 to 14 days. Postoperatively, patients will require therapy because joint stiffness is to be expected. If left untreated, chronic complete tears are associated with persistent pain, instability, and early arthritis.

First Treatment Steps
■ Short-arm thumb spica splint
■ Referral to a hand surgeon to be seen within 7 to 10 days from injury

Treatment Options
Nonoperative Management
■ Conservative treatment is reserved for partial ligament tears and stable nondisplaced avulsion fractures that do not involve more than 10% of the articular surface.
■ After an initial 2 weeks of thumb spica splint immobilization, apply a thumb spica cast for 2 to 4 weeks. At 4 to 6 weeks after injury, replace the cast with a removable thumb spica splint and allow the patient to start gentle thumb motion.

Operative Management
Codes
ICD-9 code: 842.12 Thumb UCL sprain
CPT codes: 26540: repair of collateral ligament, metacarpophalangeal or interphalangeal joint
26541: Reconstruction, collateral ligament, metacarpophalangeal joint, single; with tendon or fascial graft (includes obtaining graft)
26542: Reconstruction, collateral ligament, metacarpophalangeal joint, single; with local tissue e.g., adductor advancement)

Operative Indications
■ Acute, complete tear of the thumb MCP joint UCL
■ Partial tear that does not respond to nonoperative management
■ A displaced avulsion fracture at the ulnar base of proximal phalanx that involves more than 10% of the articular surface

155

- Chronic tears, which may require reconstruction with a tendon graft

Informed Consent and Counseling
- The patient can expect to be immobilized for roughly 3 to 4 weeks.
- The patient will require outpatient hand therapy to restore motion and strength.

Anesthesia
- Regional anesthetic such as a brachial plexus block, with sedation or general anesthesia

Patient Positioning
- Supine with the arm extended on a hand table
- Nonsterile tourniquet on the brachium

Surgical Procedures
Thumb Ulnar Collateral Ligament Repair
- An incision is made on the midlateral ulnar thumb, curved over the MCP joint, and extended proximally, just ulnar to the extensor pollicis longus tendon.
- If present, a Stener lesion may be visible at this point. Care is taken to protect the ulnar digital nerve.
- Repair of the ligament may be direct or with suture anchors, and any fracture fragment is stabilized with a screw or wire.

Estimated Postoperative Course
- Postoperative days 10 to 14
  - Sutures are removed, and a wound check is performed.
  - Immobilization: The patient will be given a thumb spica cast for 4 weeks.
- Postoperative 4 weeks
  - The cast is removed, and a support splint is applied. The patient will start therapy for thumb motion.
  - The wire is removed, if present.
- Postoperative 3 months
  - Return to activities is unrestricted.

Suggested Readings
Heymen P: Injuries to the ulnar collateral ligament of the thumb metacarpophalangeal joint, *J Am Acad Orthop Surg* 5:224–229, 1997.
Ingari J, Blum G: Ulnar collateral ligament injuries of the thumb (gamekeeper's thumb, skier's thumb). In Miller MD, Hart JA, MacKnight JM, editors: *Essential orthopaedics,* Philadelphia, 2010, Saunders, pp 345–348.
Taras JS, Hankins SM: Fractures and dislocations of the thumb. In Trumble TE, Budoff JE, Cornwall R, editors: *Hand, elbow, and shoulder: core knowledge in orthopaedics,* Philadelphia, 2006, Mosby, pp 56–68.

EXTENSOR TENDON INJURIES
History
- Injury or laceration to the dorsum of the wrist, hand, or finger
- Often associated with bone, skin, or joint injuries
- Possible reported inability to extend the finger

Physical Examination
- Assess the neurovascular status.
  - Be sure to check both digital nerves.
- Inspect the wound for the presence of a foreign body.
- Often, the patient will have an extension lag in the affected digit.
- Examine the hand with wrist in the neutral position.
- Examine the patient's ability to extend each finger individually while the adjacent fingers remain flexed at the MCP joint. This maneuver eliminates pull from a juncturae tendinum that can confuse the examination:
  - Juncturae tendinum are variable interconnections between the extensor tendons at the level of the hand metacarpals. If an extensor tendon laceration is proximal to the juncturae, the adjacent intact extensor tendon can extend the finger, and an extensor tendon laceration can be missed.
- An extensor tendon injury may also be indicated by loss of hyperextension or relative weakness and pain in one finger compared with the other fingers.
- Perform an **Elson test** (Fig. 4-45) for injuries in zone III:
  - Rest the patient's hand on a table with the affected finger flexed at the PIP joint over the edge of the table.
  - Hold the PIP joint fixed at 90 degrees while the patient attempts to extend at the PIP joint.

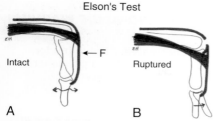

Elson's Test

Intact ←F Ruptured

A   B

Figure 4-45. A and **B,** The Elson test for acute rupture of the central slip. F, static force. *(From Lattanza LL, Hattwick EA: Extensor tendon repair and reconstruction. In Trumble T, Budoff J, Cornwall R, editors: Hand, elbow, and shoulder: core knowledge in orthopaedics, Philadelphia, 2006, Mosby, p 206.)*

- If the DIP joint is supple during active extension, the central slip is intact.
- If the DIP joint is rigid during active extension, the central slip is likely completely ruptured. This occurs because the patient will inadvertently try to extend the finger by using the intact lateral bands and terminal extensor tendon that inserts onto the distal phalanx, thereby making the DIP joint rigid (see Fig. 4-5 for anatomy).

Imaging
- Order wrist, hand, and finger radiographs based on the zone of injury: PA, lateral, and oblique views to evaluate for concomitant fracture.
- MRI or ultrasound can help evaluate for tendon ruptures or lacerations if the diagnosis cannot be made based on physical examination alone.

Classification
- Describe the zone of injury (see Fig. 4-46).

Initial Treatment
Patient Education
All extensor tendon lacerations must be repaired acutely to restore function. It is important to ensure early, protected postoperative motion with an experienced hand therapist to decrease the risk of tendon adhesions. Even with good surgical repair and compliance with therapy, tenolysis surgery may be necessary if significant stiffness persists.

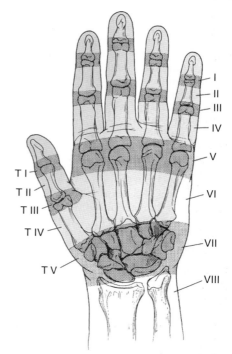

Figure 4-46. Zones of the extensor tendon system. T, thumb. *(From Trumble T, Budoff J, Cornwall R, editors: Hand, elbow, and shoulder: core knowledge in orthopaedics. In Lattanza, Lisa L and Hattwick, Emily A, editors: Extensor tendon tepair and reconstruction, Philadelphia, 2006, Mosby, p 203.)*

First Treatment Steps
- Update tetanus immunization as necessary.
- Irrigate and débride the wound as needed.
- Explore the wound, and identify the extensor tendons and any lacerations.
- If able to see both ends of the tendon and a surgeon is available, the provider may be able to repair the tendon at the time of injury while in the office or emergency department (see operative management in the next subsection). Otherwise, apply a volar extension splint that includes the fingers.
- Refer the patient to a hand surgeon urgently to be seen within 3 to 5 days of injury.

Treatment Options

Operative Management

- Extensor tendons have less excursion than flexor tendons, so minimal shortening can result in great loss of motion (6 mm of shortening = 18-degree motion loss at the MCP and PIP joints).
- Modified Kessler and modified Bunnell suture techniques are thought to be the best.

Codes

ICD-9 codes: 727.63 Rupture of hand/wrist extensor tendon
- 883.2 Open finger wound with tendon involvement
- 882.2 Open hand wound with tendon involvement
- 905.8 Late effect tendon injury

CPT codes: 25270 Repair tendon or muscle extensor, forearm and/or wrist; primary, single,
- 25272 Repair tendon or muscle extensor, forearm and/or wrist; secondary, single
- 26410 Extensor tendon repair, dorsum of hand, single, primary or secondary
- 26418 Extensor tendon repair, dorsum of finger, single, primary or secondary
- 26426 Extensor tendon repair, central slip repair, secondary (boutonnière deformity); using local tissue

Zone I Injuries

- Also known as mallet finger (see page 159)

Zone II Injuries

- These injuries also usually result in mallet deformity.
- If the laceration is less than 50% of the width of the tendon, splint the finger in extension for 7 to 10 days and then start active ROM.
- If the laceration is more than 50% of the tendon width, repair with nonabsorbable suture in a running fashion to minimize tendon shortening.

Zone III Injuries

- Disruption of the central slip.

 ORTHOPAEDIC WARNING

If left untreated, zone III tendon injuries can result in a permanent boutonnière deformity.

Nonoperative Management Zone III Injuries

- Conservative management may be an option for an acute closed injury only.
- Treat with the PIP joint in an extension splint for 6 weeks, and allow DIP and MCP joint motion.

Operative Management Zone III Injuries

- Indications
  - Displaced avulsion fracture
  - Instability of the PIP joint with loss of extension
  - Failure of nonoperative treatment
- **Central slip repair:** The insertion of the central slip is repaired using suture or suture anchors. The finger is splinted in extension, and the patient will require extensive postoperative hand therapy to restore motion (often full flexion or extension is not obtained postoperatively).

Zone IV Injuries

- Partial lacerations: Splint the entire finger in extension and wrist in the neutral position for 3 to 4 weeks.
- Complete lacerations: Surgical repair is indicated.

Zone V Injuries

- Primary tendon repair is indicated.
- Repair the sagittal bands to prevent lateral migration of the extensor digitorum communis tendon at the level of the MCP joint
- **"Fight bites"** occur in zone 5 and refer to a skin and possible tendon laceration that occurs during an altercation and results in an open, contaminated wound. Typical isolated organisms are *Eikenella, Streptococcus, or Staphylococcus* species. If the patient is presenting early, thorough irrigation and débridement and initiation of broad spectrum antibiotics are key to preventing infection. A

thorough evaluation for tendon injury and subsequent repair is also indicated. Monitor the wound closely for infection after repair. Remember to culture an active infection and request antibiotic sensitivities if a patient is presenting late.

Zone VI Injuries
- Exploration of the wound is the gold standard for diagnosis.
- To repair the injury, use a four-strand core suture technique.
- Splint the wrist and the affected digit in extension after repair.
- Postoperative therapy protocol depends on the surgeon.

Zone VII Injuries
- Laceration is present at the level of the extensor retinaculum.
- Tendons retract significantly at this level and are prone to adhesion development after repair.
- Sensory branches of the radial nerve are at risk and should be repaired or resected to prevent a neuroma.
- Immobilization should be limited to a short period with the wrist in 10 to 20 degrees of extension.

Zone VIII Injuries
- Identify the proximal and distal tendon ends.
- Muscle bellies can be repaired with multiple figure-of-eight suture technique.
- Repair the posterior interosseous nerve if it is lacerated.
- Splint the wrist in extension and the MCP joints in 15 to 20 degrees of flexion for 4 to 6 weeks.

Thumb Extensor Tendon Injuries
- Treatment is similar to that described for the foregoing zones.

Suggested Readings
Abrams RA, Botte MJ: Hand infections: treatment recommendations for specific types, *J Am Acad Orthop Surg* 4(4):219–230, 1996.

Hanz KR, Saint-Cyr M, Semmler M, et al: Extensor tendon injuries: acute management and secondary reconstruction, *Plast Reconstr Surg* 121:109e–120e, 2008.

Lattanza LL, Hattwick EA: Extensor tendon repair and reconstruction. In Trumble TE,

Budoff JE, Cornwall R, editors: *Hand, elbow, and shoulder: core knowledge in orthopaedics,* Philadelphia, 2006, Mosby, pp 201–211.

Matzon JL, Bozentka DJ: Extensor tendon injuries, *J Hand Surg Am* 35:854–861, 2010.

Newport ML: Extensor tendon injuries in the hand, *J Am Acad Orthop Surg* 5(2): 59–66, 1997.

Rockwell WB, Butler PN, Byrne BA: Extensor tendon: anatomy, injury and reconstruction, *Plast Reconstr Surg* 106:1592–1603, 2000.

MALLET FINGER
Definition
Disruption of the terminal extensor tendon insertion from the distal phalanx that results in an inability to extend the finger actively at the DIP joint

History
- The mechanism of injury is forced flexion of an extended finger at the DIP joint.
- The injury may be associated with an open laceration dorsally.
- The injury may or may not be associated with fracture.

Physical Examination:
Figure 4-47
- The finger may be edematous, ecchymotic, and painful at the DIP joint.
- Loss of active extension is noted at the DIP joint, but passive extension is intact.

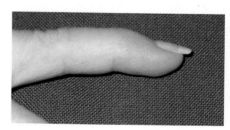

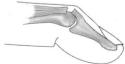

Figure 4-47. Mallet finger position resulting from rupture of the terminal extensor tendon. *(From Henry SL, Ingari J: Mallet finger. In Miller MD, Hart JA, MacKnight JM, editors:* Essential orthopaedics, *Philadelphia, 2010, Saunders, p 362.)*

- The finger is often held in a flexed position at the DIP joint.
- Nail hematoma is possible.

Imaging
- Order finger radiographs: PA, **unsupported** lateral, and oblique views.

Classification: Figures 4-48 and 4-49
- Soft tissue or bony
- Type 1: closed mallet finger
- Type 2: open mallet finger (laceration at the dorsum of the DIP joint)
- Type 3: open with loss of skin and tendon
- Type 4: involving large mallet fragments

Differential Diagnosis
- Arthritis of the DIP joint

Initial Treatment
Patient Education
This common injury usually can be treated without surgery. Even with appropriate treatment, a small extensor lag may persist, and a less than 15-degree extensor lag after treatment is acceptable.

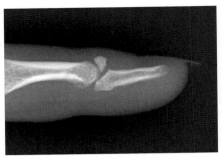
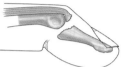

Figure 4-49. Bony mallet finger with a large fracture fragment that encompasses 50% of the articular surface with subluxation of the distal phalanx. This requires operative intervention. *(From Henry SL, Ingari J: Mallet finger. In Miller MD, Hart JA, MacKnight JM, editors: Essential orthopaedics, Philadelphia, 2010, Saunders, p 363.)*

 ORTHOPAEDIC WARNING

If left untreated, a mallet finger will result in a permanent swan neck deformity.

First Treatment Steps
- For type 1 injuries: Splint with the DIP joint in extension (allow PIP joint motion) and refer to a hand surgeon to be seen within 7 to 10 days (Fig. 4-50).
- For all others, generate an urgent referral to an orthopaedic surgeon, and treat open wounds.

Treatment Options
Nonoperative Management
- Conservative management is reserved for closed mallet fingers or bony mallets with an articular fragment smaller

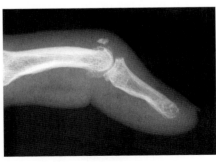
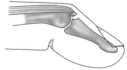

Figure 4-48. Bony mallet finger involving a small avulsion fracture. This injury will usually heal with splinting.*(From Henry SL, Ingari J: Mallet finger. In Miller MD, Hart JA, MacKnight JM, editors: Essential orthopaedics, Philadelphia, 2010, Saunders, p 362.)*

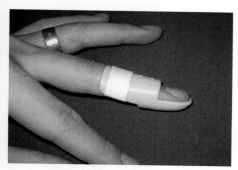

Figure 4-50. Stack splint used to hold the distal interphalangeal joint in extension while allowing proximal interphalangeal joint motion. *(From Henry SL, Ingari J: Mallet finger. In Miller MD, Hart JA, MacKnight JM, editors:* Essential orthopaedics, *Philadelphia, 2010, Saunders, p 364.)*

than 40% of the joint surface and no joint subluxation.

- Immobilize type 1 injuries for 6 to 8 weeks in a DIP joint hyperextension splint, and allow PIP motion (Fig. 4-50).
  - The finger must remain in the splint at all times for 6 weeks. If the splint is removed at any point, the clock is restarted for splinting.
  - Education regarding skin care and the importance of keeping the finger extended at all times is essential.
  - Mallet injuries up to 3 months old may be treated in a splint.
  - If an extensor lag is still present after 6 weeks of splinting, an additional 2-week period of nighttime splinting in extension is indicated.

Rehabilitation
- After 6 to 8 weeks of splinting, the patient can start gradual ROM and use the splint intermittently.

Operative Management
Codes
ICD-9 code: 736.1 Mallet finger
CPT codes: 26432 Closed treatment of distal extensor tendon with or without percutaneous pinning
    26433 Tendon repair, distal insertion (mallet finger), open, primary, or secondary repair; without graft

Operative Indications
- Surgery is indicated if there is subluxation of the distal phalanx or if there is a bony articular fragment greater than 40% of joint surface (both seen on lateral radiograph).
- Type 2 injuries:
  - Acute primary repair is performed with nonabsorbable suture sewn in a figure-of-eight fashion. This repair can often be done by incorporating the skin and tendon into the repair. A DIP joint extension splint is still required for 6 to 8 weeks.
- Type 3 injuries:
  - These injuries require soft tissue coverage in the operating room.
- Type 4 injuries:
  - These injuries require open reduction, internal fixation with screw or wire.

Informed Consent and Counseling
- The wire may stay in place for 4 to 6 weeks.
- Stiffness of the DIP joint can develop after surgery, and the patient will require hand therapy to improve terminal finger flexion.

Anesthesia
- Digital block with sedation

Patient Positioning
- Supine with the arm extended on a hand table
- Nonsterile tourniquet on the brachium

Surgical Procedure
Closed Reduction, Percutaneous Pinning of the Distal Interphalangeal Joint
- The DIP joint is hyperflexed, and a wire is inserted into the head of the middle phalanx.
- The distal phalanx is then extended until the fracture fragment abuts the wire. The wire acts as an extension block and facilitates reduction.
- Following reduction, a second wire is driven through the end of the finger and across the DIP joint for internal fixation. The patient is placed in a hyperextension finger splint.

Estimated Postoperative Course
- Splinting and wires remain in place for approximately 6 weeks.
- In some cases, nighttime splinting is recommended for an additional 4 weeks after the wire is removed.

Suggested Readings
Henry SL, Ingari J: Mallet finger. In Miller MD, Hart JA, MacKnight JM, editors: *Essential orthopaedics*, Philadelphia, 2010, Saunders, pp 361–366.

Lattanza LL, Hattwick EA: Extensor tendon repair and reconstruction. In Trumble TE, Budoff JE, Cornwall R, editors: *Hand, elbow, and shoulder: core knowledge in orthopaedics*, Philadelphia, 2006, Mosby, pp 201–211.

Matzon JL, Bozentka DJ: Extensor tendon injuries, *J Hand Surg Am* 35:854–861, 2010.

FLEXOR TENDON INJURIES
History
- Laceration to the volar surface of the wrist, hand, or finger is present.
- The patient may report an inability to flex a digit or digits.
- The patient may report decreased sensation if there is concomitant nerve injury.
- Ruptures may occur in the setting of chronic attrition (seen in inflammatory conditions such as rheumatoid arthritis).

Physical Examination
- Inspect the wound (do not probe).
- Assess capillary refill in the digits.
- Assess sensation to light touch on *both* ulnar and radial sides of the digits *before* digital block anesthetic is administered.
- Evaluate the flexor tendons (Figs. 4-51 and 4-52). There are two tendons to each finger, and each must be tested individually. (See the note later in this section about the thumb tendon.)

Flexor Digitorum Profundus Tendon (Figure 4-52)
- The flexor digitorum profundus (FDP) tendon controls motion of the DIP joint.
- Place the patient's hand on the examining table with the palm up. Apply pressure over the middle phalanx, and ask the patient to flex the DIP joint.

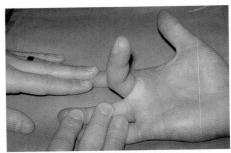

Figure 4-51. Testing for flexor digitorum superficialis tendon injury. *(From Chadderdon RD, Isaacs, JE: Flexor tendon injuries. In Miller MD, Hart JA, MacKnight JM, editors:* Essential orthopaedics, *Philadelphia, 2010, Saunders, p 354.)*

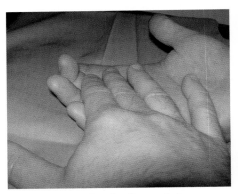

Figure 4-52. Testing for flexor digitorum profundus tendon injury. *(From Chadderdon RD, Isaacs, JE: Flexor tendon injuries. In Miller MD, Hart JA, MacKnight JM, editors:* Essential orthopaedics, *Philadelphia, 2010, Saunders, p 354.)*

If the FDP is injured, the patient will not be able to flex the DIP joint. (If the FDS is still intact, the patient will be able to flex at the PIP joint.)

Flexor Digitorum Superficialis Tendon (Figure 4-51)
- The *flexor digitorum superficialis* (FDS) tendon controls motion of the PIP joint.
- Isolated FDS injuries may be more difficult to identify because the FDP will flex the entire digit. Again, place the patient's hand on the examining table with the palm up. Ask the patient to

flex the digit. The patient will often have pain, weakness, or incomplete flexion if the FDS is injured.

Flexor Pollicis Longus Tendon
- **Note:** There is only one flexor tendon to the thumb: the flexor pollicis longus (FPL).
- Test the FPL by applying pressure over the proximal phalanx and asking the patient to flex the thumb at the IP joint. An inability to flex the distal phalanx indicates an FPL injury.
- Pain with flexion against resistance may indicate a partial tendon injury.

Imaging
- Order wrist, hand, and finger radiographs: PA, lateral, and oblique views to evaluate for concomitant fracture.

Classification: Figure 4-53
Initial Treatment
Patient Education
- Complete tendon injuries require immediate repair within 7 to 10 days.
- Successful outcomes depend on the patient's compliance with postoperative therapy.

First Treatment Steps
- Update tetanus immunization as necessary.
- Irrigate and débride the wound.
- Suture the wound.

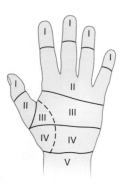

Figure 4-53. Zones of the flexor tendons. *(From Green DP, Hotchkiss RN, Pederson WC, et al, editors: Green's operative hand surgery. In Martin I. Boyer, editor: Flexor Tendon Injuries, ed 5, Philadelphia, 2005, Churchill Livingstone. Copyright Elizabeth Martin, p 221.)*

- Splint the wrist in the neutral position and the MCP in 60 to 70 degrees flexion, and refer the patient to a hand surgeon to be seen within 3 to 5 days.

Treatment Options
Operative Management
Ideal Repairs
- Easy placement of sutures
- Secure suture knots
- Smooth juncture at tendon ends
- Minimal gapping at the repair site
- Minimal interference with tendon vascularity
- Sufficient strength throughout healing to allow early motion

Codes
ICD-9 codes: 727.64 Rupture of hand/ wrist flexor tendon
    883.2 Open wound, finger, with tendon involvement
    882.2 Open wound, hand, with tendon involvement
CPT codes: 25260 Repair, flexor tendon primary
    25263 Repair, tendon, secondary
    26350 Repair, flexor tendon not in "no man's land"
    26356 Repair, flexor tendon in no man's land
    26370 Profundus tendon repair, with intact sublimis, primary

Zone I Injuries
- Jersey finger (see the next section, on jersey finger)

Zone II Injuries
- This zone is referred to as "no man's land" because stiffness after injury is very common, and surgery in this area is difficult because of the relationship of the two flexor tendons within the flexor tendon sheath:
  - Camper chiasm occurs at this level (the FDS splints to allow the FDP to continue distally), as does the A2 pulley, which must be repaired to prevent bowstringing of the tendons. Tendon adhesions occur very easily in this area.
- Many techniques have been described, and the type of repair is based on the surgeon's preference.

Zone III Injuries

■ Surgical exposure of tendons in this area is easier than in zone II because of the lack of the tendon sheath at this level. Surgical repairs at this level are usually less prone to the stiffness seen in zone II injuries.

Zone IV Injuries

■ The tendon is repaired in similar fashion to zone III injuries.
■ Repair of the median nerve may also be necessary at this level.

Zone V Injuries

■ These injuries can be difficult to repair because muscle tissue will not hold suture.
■ Often, mattress sutures are used.

Thumb Flexor Pollicis Longus Tendon Injuries

■ Preserve the oblique pulley and the A2 pulley.
■ If the FPL tendon has retracted proximally, an incision at the level of the wrist is recommended rather than an incision in the thenar region.
■ Repair is similar to that of other flexor tendons, based on the level of injury.

Estimated Postoperative Course

A successful outcome of flexor tendon repair is directly related to strict compliance with a hand therapy program. Many postoperative rehabilitation protocols exist, and the one chosen is based on the experience and preference of the surgeon.

Suggested Readings

Boyer M, Taras JS, Kaufman RA: Flexor tendon injury. In Green DP, Hotchkiss RN, Pederson WC, et al, editors: *Green's operative hand surgery,* ed 5, Philadelphia, 2005, Churchill Livingstone, pp 219–276.

Chadderdon RC, Isaacs JE: Flexor tendon injuries. In Miller MD, Hart JA, MacKnight JM, editors: *Essential orthopaedics,* Philadelphia, 2010, Saunders, pp 352–356.

Lilly SI, Messer TM: Complications after treatment of flexor tendon injuries, *J Am Acad Orthop Surg* 14(7):387–396, 2006.

Rekant M: Flexor tendon injuries. In Trumble TE, Budoff JE, Cornwall R, editors: *Hand, elbow, and shoulder: core knowledge in orthopaedics,* Philadelphia, 2006, Mosby, pp 189–200.

Strickland, JW: Development of flexor tendon surgery: twenty-five years of progress, *J Hand Surg Am* 25(2):214–235, 2000.

JERSEY FINGER

Definition

Rupture of the FDP tendon from its insertion on the distal phalanx results in an inability to flex the finger at the DIP joint.

History

■ Forced hyperextension of the distal phalanx from a flexed position (Fig. 4-54).
■ Jersey finger often results from an athletic injury.
■ The patient may report hearing a "pop" in the finger.
■ The ring finger is the most commonly injured.

Physical Examination

■ Tenderness to palpation at the volar base of the DIP joint
■ Edema and/or ecchymosis surrounding the volar DIP joint
■ Inability to flex at the DIP joint actively, with intact passive flexion
■ Possible tenderness to palpation at the location of a retracted tendon stump

Imaging

■ Order finger radiographs: PA, lateral, and oblique views.

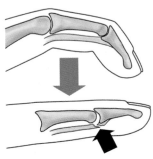

Figure 4-54. Jersey finger: flexor digitorum profundus rupture. Tendon rupture occurs when a flexed digit in forcibly extended. *(From Ingari J: Jersey finger [flexor digitorum profundus avulsion]. In Miller MD, Hart JA, MacKnight JM, editors:* Essential orthopaedics, *Philadelphia, 2010, Saunders, p 368.)*

- Avulsion fracture can accompany tendon injury.
- *Pearl:* Ultrasonography or MRI can help differentiate the type of avulsion if necessary.

Classification
- Type 1: The FDP stump has retracted into the palm.
- Type II: The FDP stump has retracted to the level of the PIP joint.
- Type III: The FDP avulsion is attached to a large fracture fragment.

Differential Diagnosis
- Fracture not associated with an FDP avulsion
- Nerve injury or palsy (e.g., anterior interosseous nerve palsy)
- Flexor tendon rupture outside zone 1

Initial Treatment
Patient Education
- A jersey finger requires surgical intervention. The urgency of the intervention depends on the type of avulsion.
- Nonoperative intervention results in lack of flexion at the DIP joint and a potentially painful mass at the tendon stump.

First Treatment Step
- Apply a dorsal blocking splint with the finger in flexion and refer the patient to a hand surgeon.

Treatment Options
Nonoperative Management
- Not usually indicated

Operative Management of Acute Flexor Digitorum Profundus Avulsion
Codes
ICD-9 code: 842.13 FDP tendon avulsion
CPT code: 26350 Repair of flexor tendon

Type 1 Injury
- The blood supply is compromised, and the tendon should be repaired within 7 days.

Type II and III Injuries
- These injuries can be repaired even after a delay in treatment of several weeks.

Informed Consent and Counseling
- The patient can expect to be immobilized in some fashion for 4 to 6 weeks.
- The patient will require approximately 3 to 4 months of outpatient hand therapy to restore motion and strength. This therapy is essential for a good outcome.
- Even with good surgical repair and compliance with a therapy program, stiffness may persist.

Anesthesia
- Regional anesthetic such as a brachial plexus block, with sedation or general anesthesia

Patient Positioning
- Supine with the arm extended on a hand table
- Nonsterile tourniquet on the brachium

Surgical Procedures
Flexor Digitorum Profundus Repair with Button Technique or Suture Anchor
- A Bruner-type incision is made on the volar aspect of the finger.
- The proximal end of the tendon is retrieved, and core sutures are placed in the tendon stump for subsequent passage into the tendon sheath.
- Protect the A2 and A4 pulleys.
- Tie suture over a button on the top of the nail plate, or, alternatively, use a suture anchor instead of a button.
- Place the patient in dorsal blocking splint with wrist in slight flexion, with the MP joints at 70 degrees, and the PIP and DIP joints in extension.

Estimated Postoperative Course
- Postoperative days 10 to 14
  - Sutures are removed from the volar finger incision; the button or suture over the nail remains in place for 4 to 6 weeks.
  - Immobilization: The patient is given a dorsal blocking splint.
  - *Therapy referral:* Start a flexor tendon protocol (many exist, it will be the surgeon's choice).
- Postoperative 4 to 6 weeks
  - The button or suture is removed, and the therapy protocol progresses.

- Postoperative 12 and 16 weeks
  - The patient returns for a motion check.
  - Progress with therapy is made according to the protocol.

Suggested Readings

Ingari J: Jersey finger (flexor digitorum profundus avulsion). In Miller MD, Hart JA, MacKnight JM, editors: *Essential orthopaedics*, Philadelphia, 2010, Saunders, pp 367–368.

Murphy BA, Mass DP: Zone 1 flexor tendon injuries, *Hand Clin* 21:167–171, 2005.

Rekant M: Flexor tendon injuries. In Trumble TE, Budoff JE, Cornwall R, editors: *Hand, elbow, and shoulder: core knowledge in orthopaedics*, Philadelphia, 2006, Mosby, pp 189–200.

Tuttle HG, Oley SP, Stern PJ: Tendon avulsion injuries of the distal phalanx, *Clin Orthop Relat Res* 445:157–168, 2006.

ORTHOPAEDIC PROCEDURES
Carpal Tunnel Injection
Code
CPT code: 20526

Indications
- Median nerve compression (i.e., CTS) that has not responded conservative treatment

Contraindications
- Allergy to an intended medication
- Local skin rash or active skin lesion over the injection site

Equipment Needed
- Alcohol swabs and povidone-iodine swab sticks or other antiseptic of choice
- 5-mL syringe
- 25-gauge needle, 1 to 1.5 inches
- Injectate: 3 mL 1% lidocaine without epinephrine and 1 mL 20 or 40 mg/ml triamcinolone (Kenalog) or other corticosteroid
- Adhesive bandage
- Optional: ethyl chloride spray

Procedure
1) Identify anatomic landmarks.
   - Have the patient pinch all fingertips together while the wrist is in a neutral position to identify the palmaris longus (PL) tendon.
   - Identify the proximal wrist crease.

- In patients without a PL tendon, use the ulnar midline of the wrist.
2) Clean and prepare skin at the site of injection.
3) Spray with ethyl chloride.
4) Wipe once more with an alcohol pad.
5) Insert the needle just ulnar to the PL tendon at the level of the proximal wrist crease at a 30- to 45-degree angle, directed toward the ring finger (Fig. 4-55).
6) If the needle meets obstruction or the patient experiences nerve pain, withdraw the needle and redirect in a slightly more ulnar location.
7) Inject slowly with constant pressure.
8) Remove the needle, and hold pressure with gauze.
9) Place a bandage over the injection site.

Aftercare Instructions
1) If the patient has diabetes mellitus, caution that glucose levels may increase for up to 5 to 7 days.
2) The patient should avoid strenuous activity with the hand for 24 to 48 hours after injection.
3) Pain or discomfort at the injection site may occur, but it typically subsides within 24 to 48 hours. This pain may be treated with ice and/or NSAIDs.

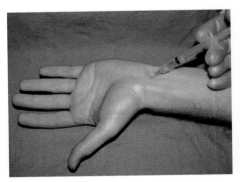

Figure 4-55. Carpal tunnel wrist injection. The needle is inserted just ulnar to Palmaris longus at the wrist crease. *(From Schnur D: Carpal tunnel injection. In Miller MD, Hart JA, MacKnight JM, editors: Essential orthopaedics, Philadelphia, 2010, Saunders, p 441.)*

Trigger Finger Injection
Code
CPT code: 20526

Indications
- Symptomatic trigger finger
- Noninfectious flexor tenosynovitis (found in rheumatoid arthritis)

Contraindications
- Allergy to intended medication
- Local skin rash or active skin lesion over the injection site

Equipment Needed
- Alcohol swabs and povidone-iodine swab sticks or other antiseptic of choice
- 3-mL syringe
- 25- or 27-gauge needle, 1 to 1.5 inches
- Injectate: 1 mL 1% lidocaine without epinephrine and 1 mL of 20 or 40 mg/mL triamcinolone (Kenalog) or other corticosteroid
- Adhesive bandage
- Optional: ethyl chloride spray

Procedure: *Figures 4-56 and 4-57*
1) Identify anatomic landmarks, and inject at the level of the A1 pulley.
2) Clean and prepare the skin at the site of injection.
3) Spray with ethyl chloride.
4) Wipe once more with an alcohol pad.

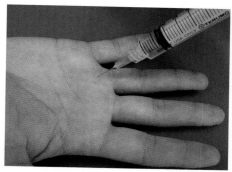

Figure 4-57. Trigger finger injection. *(From Ingari J: Trigger finger injection. In Miller MD, Hart JA, MacKnight JM, editors:* Essential orthopaedics, *Philadelphia, 2010, Saunders, p 446.)*

5) Insert the needle at the level of the A1 pulley with the needle pointing toward the affected finger.
6) If the needle meets obstruction or the patient experiences nerve pain, withdraw the needle slightly and inject again.
7) Inject slowly with constant pressure.
8) Remove the needle, and hold pressure with gauze.
9) Place a bandage on the injection site.

Aftercare Instructions
1) If the patient has diabetes mellitus, caution that glucose levels may increase for up to 5 to 7 days.
2) The patient should avoid strenuous activity with the hand for 24 to 48 hours after injection.
3) Pain or discomfort at the injection site may occur, but it typically subsides within 24 to 48 hours. This pain may be treated with ice and/or NSAIDs.

First Carpometacarpal Joint Injection
Code
CPT code: 20526

Indications
- First CMC joint osteoarthritis not responsive to conservative measures

Contraindications
- Allergy to intended medication
- Local skin rash or active skin lesion over the injection site

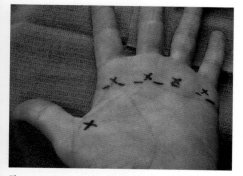

Figure 4-56. X marks the sites of injection for trigger digits. *(From Ingari J: Trigger finger injection. In Miller MD, Hart JA, MacKnight JM, editors:* Essential orthopaedics, *Philadelphia, 2010, Saunders, p 446.)*

Equipment Needed
- Fluoroscopy to help guide the injection site, if available
- Alcohol swabs and povidone-iodine swab sticks or antiseptic of choice
- 3-mL syringe
- 25- or 27-gauge needle, 1 to 1.5 inches
- Injectate: 1 mL 1% lidocaine without epinephrine and 1 mL of 20 or 40 mg/mL triamcinolone (Kenalog) or other corticosteroid
- Adhesive bandage
- Optional: ethyl chloride spray

Procedure: Figures 4-58 and 4-59
1) Identify anatomic landmarks.
   - Place the patient's hand dorsal side down.
   - Palpate the joint space between the trapezium and the first metacarpal.

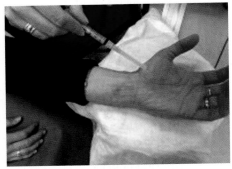

Figure 4-58. Volar approach to first carpometacarpal (CMC) injections.

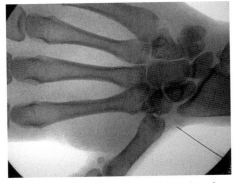

Figure 4-59. Fluoroscopic confirmation of needle placement for a first CMC injection.

2) Clean and prepare the skin at the site of injection.
3) Spray with ethyl chloride.
4) Wipe once more with an alcohol pad.
5) Insert the needle at the first CMC joint; use fluoroscopy if available. Traction may be applied to the thumb to open the joint space further.
6) If the needle meets obstruction, withdraw the needle slightly and inject again.
7) Inject slowly with constant pressure.
8) Hold pressure with gauze.
9) Place a bandage on the injection site.

Aftercare Instructions
1) If the patient has diabetes mellitus, caution that glucose levels may increase for up to 5 to 7 days.
2) The patient should avoid strenuous activity with the hand for 24 to 48 hours after injection.
3) Pain or discomfort at the injection site may occur, but it typically subsides within 24 to 48 hours. This pain may be treated with ice and/or NSAIDs.

Wrist Injection and Aspiration
Code
CPT code: 20605

Indications
- Injection
  - Radiocarpal wrist arthritis
  - SLAC
  - Scaphoid nonunion advanced collapse
  - Kienbock disease
  - Hematoma block for fracture reduction
- Aspiration to aid in diagnosis of:
  - Septic arthritis
  - Crystalline arthropathy (i.e., gout or pseudogout)

Contraindications
- Allergies to cortisone or its derivative
- Local skin rash or active skin lesion over the injection site
- Suspected wrist infection

Equipment Needed
- Alcohol swabs and povidone-iodine swab sticks or antiseptic of choice

- Bandage strip and gauze pad
- Optional: ethyl chloride spray

Injection
- 5-mL syringe
- 25- or 27-gauge needle, 1 to 1.5 inches
- Injectate: 3 mL 1% lidocaine without epinephrine and 1 mL of 20 or 40 mg/mL triamcinolone (Kenalog) or other corticosteroid

Aspiration
- 10-mL empty syringe
- 18- to 21-gauge needle

Procedure: *Figures 4-60 and 4-61*
1) Identify anatomic landmarks for the radiocarpal joint.
2) Palpate Lister tubercle; about 1 to 2 cm distal to this is the SL interval.
3) Clean and prepare the skin at the site of injection.
4) Spray with ethyl chloride.
5) Wipe once more with an alcohol pad.
6) Insert the needle into the radiocarpal joint at the previously described interval. Traction may be applied to wrist to open the joint space further.

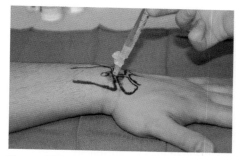

Figure 4-61. Injection of the radiocarpal joint. *(From Zlotolow DA: Radiocarpal joint injection. In Miller MD, Hart JA, MacKnight JM, editors:* Essential orthopaedics, *Philadelphia, 2010, Saunders, p 438.)*

7) If the needle meets obstruction, withdraw the needle slightly and redirect it.
8) Inject slowly with constant pressure.
9) Hold pressure with gauze.
10) Place a bandage on the injection site.
   - Aspiration is performed in a similar manner.

Aftercare Instructions
1) If the patient has diabetes mellitus, caution that glucose levels may increase for up to 5 to 7 days.
2) The patient should avoid strenuous activity with the wrist for 24 to 48 hours after injection.
3) Pain or discomfort at the injection site may occur, but it typically subsides within 24 to 48 hours. This pain may be treated with ice and/or NSAIDs.

De Quervain Tenosynovitis Injection
Code
CPT code: 20550

Indications
- Pain from de Quervain's tenosynovitis that has not responded to conservative measures

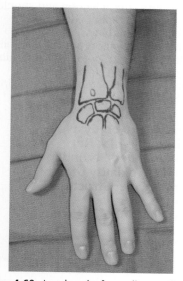

Figure 4-60. Landmarks for radiocarpal injection. *(From Zlotolow DA: Radiocarpal joint injection. In Miller MD, Hart JA, MacKnight JM, editors:* Essential orthopaedics, *Philadelphia, 2010, Saunders, p 438.)*

Contraindications
- Allergy to intended medication
- Local skin rash or active skin lesion over the injection site

Equipment Needed

- Alcohol swabs and povidone-iodine swab sticks or other antiseptic of choice
- 5-mL syringe
- 25- or 27-gauge needle, 1 to 1.5 inches
- Injectate: 2 mL 1% lidocaine without epinephrine and 1 mL of 20 or 40 mg/mL triamcinolone (Kenalog) or other corticosteroid
- Adhesive bandage
- Optional: ethyl chloride spray

Procedure: Figures 4-62 and 4-63

1) Identify anatomic landmarks.
   - With the patient's thumb abducted and extended, palpate the APL and EPB.
2) Clean and prepare the skin at the site of injection.
3) Spray with ethyl chloride.
4) Wipe once more with an alcohol pad.
5) Place the needle in the first extensor compartment, direct it proximally toward the radial styloid, and slide it parallel to the abductor and extensor tendons; observe filling in the sheath.
6) Inject slowly with constant pressure.
7) Hold pressure with gauze.
8) Place a bandage at the injection site.

Aftercare Instructions

1) If the patient has diabetes mellitus, caution that glucose levels may

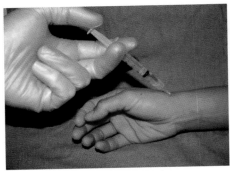

Figure 4-63. The first dorsal compartment injected at the level of the radial styloid. *(From Zlotolow DA: Radiocarpal joint injection. In Miller MD, Hart JA, MacKnight JM, editors: Essential orthopaedics, Philadelphia, 2010, Saunders, p 436.)*

increase for up to 5 to 7 days. Subcutaneous fat atrophy and skin hypopigmentation may occur at the injection site. These changes are usually reversible but may take up to 1 year to resolve.

2) The patient should avoid strenuous activity with the wrist for 24 to 48 hours after injection and should wear a wrist splint continuously except for bathing.
3) Pain or discomfort at the injection site may occur, but it typically subsides within 24 to 48 hours. This pain may be treated with ice and/or NSAIDs.

Dorsal Ganglion Cyst Aspiration (Volar Not Recommended Secondary to Close Proximity of Neurovascular Structures)

Code
CPT code: 20612

Indications
- Painful dorsal wrist or hand cyst
- Cosmetically displeasing cyst

Contraindications
- Allergy to intended medication
- Local skin rash or active skin lesion over the injection site

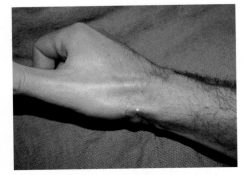

Figure 4-62. With the thumb abducted and extended, note the tendons of the first dorsal compartment make up the radial border of the snuffbox. *(From Zlotolow DA: Radiocarpal joint injection. In Miller MD, Hart JA, MacKnight JM, editors: Essential orthopaedics, Philadelphia, 2010, Saunders, p 436.)*

Equipment Needed

- Alcohol swabs and povidone-iodine swab sticks or antiseptic of choice
- 10- to 20-mL empty syringe
- 18-gauge needle for aspiration
- Local anesthetic: 2-5mL 1% lidocaine without epinephrine
- 3-mL syringe with 25- or 27-gauge needle, 1 to 1.5 inches for lidocaine administration
- Adhesive bandage
- Compressive wrap
- Optional: ethyl chloride spray

Procedure: *Figure 4-64*

1) Identify anatomic landmarks.
   - Palpate the cyst boundaries.

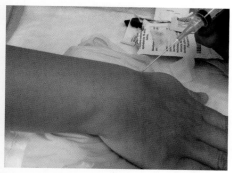

Figure 4-64. Aspiration of a dorsal ganglion cyst.

2) Clean and prepare the skin at the site of aspiration.
3) Spray with ethyl chloride.
4) Wipe once more with an alcohol pad.
5) Anesthetize the area just proximal to the cyst with 2-5 mL 1% lidocaine without epinephrine.
6) Using an 18-gauge needle and a 10- to 20-mL syringe, aspirate the ganglion cyst. The practitioner may need to encourage aspiration of fluid with digital pressure over the cyst. After the needle is removed, deep palpation may be used for continued release of the cyst.
7) Hold pressure with gauze.
8) Place an adhesive bandage at the injection site, and apply a compressive dressing.

Aftercare Instructions

1) Remove the pressure dressing after 12 to 24 hours.
2) Patients should be aware of the risk of possible cyst recurrence after aspiration.
3) Patients should avoid strenuous activity with the wrist for 24 to 48 hours after aspiration.
4) Pain or discomfort at the injection site may occur, but it typically subsides within 24 to 48 hours. This pain may be treated with ice and/or NSAIDs.

5 Pelvis
Deana Bahrman and Katherine Sharpe

ANATOMY
- See Chapter 6 (Hip and Femur) for additional images.

Ligaments: Figure 5-1

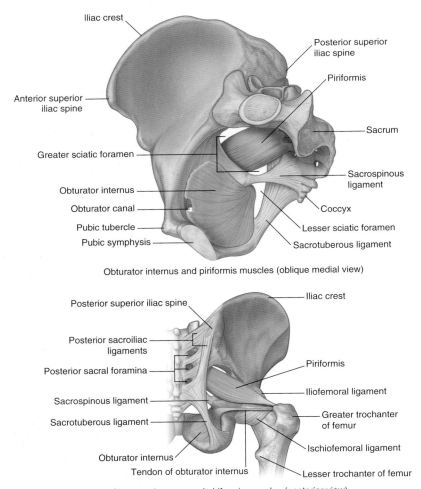

Obturator internus and piriformis muscles (oblique medial view)

Obturator internus and piriformis muscles (posterior view)

Figure 5-1. Pelvis ligaments. *(Elsevier illustration from* www.elsevierimages.com. *Copyright, Elsevier Inc. All rights reserved.)*

Physical Examination

Inspect for deformity, lower extremity malrotation, leg length discrepancy, increased/decreased lordosis, pelvic obliquity.

Palpate anterior and posterior landmarks:

- Iliac crest
- Iliac tubercle
- Pubic tubercle
- Anterior superior iliac spine (ASIS)
- Posterior superior iliac spine (PSIS)
- Sacroiliac (SI) joint
- Coccyx
- Ischial tuberosity
- Greater trochanter
- Iliopsoas tendon
- Piriformis
- Inguinal ligament
- Symphysis
- Pubic rami

Palpate the abdomen for masses or hernias.

Neurovascular Examination: Table 5-1.

Special Tests

- Fabere test: Test for SI joint or hip pathology. With the patient lying supine, place the foot of the involved side on the opposite knee. Inguinal pain, in this position, suggests hip pathology. With one hand on the knee and the other hand on the ASIS, apply pressure; increased pain suggests SI joint pathology.
- Trendelenburg sign: Ask the patient to stand and lift one leg (flex hip). The flexed side of the pelvis should elevate. If the pelvis falls, there is abductor or gluteus medius dysfunction.
- FAIR test: Flexion Adduction Internal Rotation with patient in the lateral recumbent position with the affected side up reproduces gluteus pain, suggesting piriformis syndrome.

Differential Diagnosis: Table 5-2

SACROILIAC DYSFUNCTION
History

- Most common etiology:
  - Pregnancy (hormones and pelvic stress increase mobility in SI joint)
  - Limb length discrepancy
  - Scoliosis
  - Trauma/motor vehicle collision (foot on the brake during collision)
- Less common etiology:
  - Inflammatory arthritis (rheumatoid arthritis, gout, psoriatic arthritis, ankylosing spondylitis)
  - Bacterial infection
  - Malignancy

Table 5-1. Neurovascular Examination

NERVE/VESSEL	LOCATION
Femoral artery	Inferior to inguinal ligament; halfway between the anterior superior iliac spine and the pubic tubercle
Cluneal nerve	Iliac crest between the posterior superior iliac spine and the iliac tubercle
Sciatic nerve	Midway between the greater trochanter and the ischial tuberosity

Table 5-2. Differential Diagnosis

Anterior pelvic pain	Pubic rami fracture, acetabular fracture, femur fracture, pubic symphysis disruption, iliopsoas tendonitis/bursitis, hip arthritis, femoral acetabular impingement (FAI), lumbar radiculopathy, nonorthopaedic causes (e.g., intra-abdominal, gynecologic, genitourinary)
Lateral pelvic pain	Greater trochanter bursitis, FAI
Posterior pelvic pain	Sacral fractures, sacroiliac joint arthritis/dislocation/fracture, piriformis syndrome, lumbar radiculopathy

- Complaints of pain in the lower back exacerbated by prolonged sitting, twisting, or hyperextending the back
- Difficulties getting in or out of a car, putting on shoes, or turning over in bed
  - Pain is usually unilateral
  - ± Radiation to groin or buttocks

Physical Examination
- Thrombotic thrombocytopenic purpura (TTP) is evident at the SI joint.
- Perform a Gillet or "stork" test. (Ask the patient to stand with his or her back to the examiner while the examiner places his or her thumbs at the SI joint and has the patient flex each hip, individually. A positive test will cause the thumb ipsilateral to the flexed hip to either remain still or move cranially. If the thumb moves caudally, this indicates a negative test.)

Imaging
- Order a radiograph of the pelvis (Fig. 5-2): anteroposterior (AP) and lateral to evaluate for sclerosis.
- Bone scans may indicate areas of stress; magnetic resonance imaging (MRI) may reveal synovitis or tumors.
- *The gold standard is a lidocaine/steroid injection under fluoroscopy to the SI joint, which may be both diagnostic and therapeutic.*

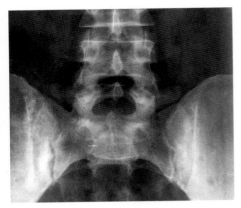

Figure 5-2. Sclerosis and pseudowidening at the sacroiliac joint. (*From Goldman L, Schafer AI: In* Goldman's cecil medicine, *ed 24, Philadelphia, 2012, Saunders.*)

Initial Treatment
Patient Education
- The junction of the sacrum with the right and left ilea forms the SI joint. It is designed for stabilization, twisting, and load transference to the lower body. It is a small joint and only allows for minimal movements. Pain is usually derived from hypermobility or instability of the joint. Treatment is geared toward stabilization of the joint and relieving pain and inflammation.

Treatment Options
Nonoperative Management
- Most patients will recover with conservative therapy that includes the following:
  - Ice for acute injury
  - Heat if initial onset of pain is > 48 hours
  - Nonsteroidal antiinflammatory drugs (NSAIDs)
  - Physical therapy (PT) for massage, electrical stimulation therapy, stretching and strengthening exercises
  - Steroid injections under fluoroscopy
  - Follow-up in 3 months for reevaluation

Operative Management
- Criteria for SI joint stabilization
  - Conservative measures must be tried and must have failed.
  - Pain relief from fluoroscopically guided lidocaine/steroid injection must be documented.
  - Other causes such as herniated disk, spinal stenosis, degenerative disk disease, piriformis, or hip disorders must be ruled out.
  - If criteria are met, the patient will undergo an SI joint fusion, which involves the manual manipulation of the SI joint into anatomic position and then using screws across the joint to fuse the R and L ilea to the sacrum using a posterior approach. Obtain a postoperative radiograph of the AP pelvis and lateral hip and lumbar spine.
  - The patient does not need to be immobilized and will start PT at 3 weeks for rehabilitation. Follow up with the patient in 6 weeks for repeat radiographs.

Suggested Readings

Eck JC: Sacroiliac joint dysfunction. *MedicineNet. com* (website). http://www.medicinenet.com/ sacroiliac_joint_pain/article.htm. Accessed November 26, 2011

OSTEITIS PUBIS

Osteitis pubis is the inflammation of the pubic symphysis. The etiology is unclear, although it was first described in patients who had undergone subrapubic surgery and later linked to athletes. Inflammation is caused by microtrauma to the adductors or lower rectus muscles, which increases shear forces across the pubis symphysis.

- It can follow urologic surgery.
- It is associated with athletes involved in soccer, track (sprinters), ice hockey, and football.
- The patient will complain of pain in the groin, hip, perineum, or testicles. The pain may also manifest as lower abdominal pain that radiates to the pubis.
- The pain is worse with running, kicking, or pushing off.

Physical Examination

- A waddling gait is noticeable.
- Tenderness to palpation presents over the pubic symphysis.
- A "single leg hop" may reproduce pain.
- Compression of greater trochanters bilaterally causes pain at the pubic symphysis.
- Weakness at hip adductors or flexors is evident.
- Evaluate for SI joint dysfunction, which can contribute to instability of the pubic symphysis.

Imaging

- A bone scan of the pelvis may be helpful in early diagnosis because a radiograph does not typically demonstrate findings early. Unilateral findings on a bone scan are inconclusive, however, and a stress fracture must be considered.
- Order an MRI for suspicion of bone tumor, muscle, or tendon disruption.
- AP radiographs of the pelvis may show sclerotic bone, osteolysis,

widening or instability, but positive findings are not seen until more than 4 weeks after the onset of symptoms.
- Widening of cleft = 10 mm
- Instability = >2 mm cephalad translation with the patient standing alternately on one leg

Initial Treatment
Patient Education

Osteitis pubis is due to inflammation of the pubic symphysis and surrounding musculature. Males are more commonly affected than females. A study in Sweden has shown that approximately 80% of athletes develop this condition. It is self-limiting but can take an average of 9 months to recover and has a 25% chance of recurrence.

Treatment Options
Nonoperative Management

- **REST:** Athletes need to be pulled from sports for at least 1 week.
- Start NSAIDs to reduce inflammation and PT for pain relief using ice massage, ultrasound (if no suspicion of infection), and stretching to improve flexibility of the pelvis.
- If there is no improvement of pain, corticosteroid injections to the pubic symphysis may be considered. After injection, the athlete must continue to rest and refrain from activity for another week.

Operative Management

- Surgery is rarely indicated for osteitis pubis.

Rehabilitation

- Follow up in 4 weeks and reevaluate pain. If pain free, begin PT for strengthening exercises and occupational therapy (OT) for evaluation and correction of biomechanics. Begin to wean NSAIDs, if possible.
- Recovery can take 6 to 12 months.
- Athletes especially should be cautioned that 25% of patients will be unable to continue playing due to this condition.

Differential Diagnosis

- If the patient has fevers, you must rule out osteomyelitis. Refer to gynecology, urology, or infectious disease to evaluate for pelvic inflammatory disease (PID), prostatitis, or other causes of pelvic pain.

 ORTHOPAEDIC WARNING

If a patient presents with fevers, lymphadenopathy, nausea/vomiting, or anorexia, you must rule out osteomyelitis. Biopsy and cultures are required for definitive diagnosis, but if you see fluid on an MRI or bony lesions on radiograph, suspect osteomyelitis.
　　Most common pathogen in athletes: *Staphylococcus aureus*
　　Most common pathogen in IV drug users: *Pseudomonas aeruginosa*

Suggested Readings

Allen KL, Lorenzo C: Physical medicine and rehabilitation for osteitis pubis follow-up. *Medscape* (website). http://emedicine.medscape.com/article/308384-followup#a2649. Accessed November 26, 2011

Disabella V, Young C: Osteitis pubis treatment and management. *Medscape* (website). http://emedicine.medscape.com/article/87420-treatment#aw2aab6b6b1aa. Accessed November 26, 2011

Pham D, Scott K: Presentation of osteitis and osteomyelitis pubis as acute abdominal pain, *Permanente J* 11:2, 2007.

APOPHYSITIS AND HIP POINTERS
History

- *Apophysitis:* overloading injury at a tendon insertion site; may be acute/chronic and may be associated with avulsion fracture. Mechanism of injury (MOI) is a sudden contraction of the muscle followed by acute pain, swelling, and weakness at the insertion point. Symptoms are usually acute but may develop gradually. Apophysitis is rarely due to a direct blow (Table 5-3).
- *Hip pointers:* contusions due to direct blow or fall, usually at iliac crest or greater trochanter. The patient will complain of pain, swelling, or bruising at the site of injury. Symptoms are acute, although they may take 24 to 48 hours to develop after initial injury.

Physical Examination
- TTP, edema, or ecchymosis along insertion site of hip tendons or bony landmarks
- + Antalgic gait
- Pain may limit range of motion
- Pain reproduced with imitation of MOI in apophysitis

Imaging
- Order a radiograph of the AP/lateral pelvis. It may show an avulsion fracture or myositis ossificans.
- The bone scan may show a stress/avulsion fracture.

Table 5-3. Apophysitis and Hip Pointers

INSERTION	MOI/MUSCLE CONTRACTION	ACTIVITY EXAMPLE
Anterior superior iliac spine	Sartorius when hip is extended and knee flexed	Sprinter at starting line
Anterior inferior iliac spine	Rectus femoris	Forceful kicking
Ischial tuberosity	Hamstrings when hip flexed and knee extended	Hurdles
Iliac crest	Simultaneous abs, gluteus medius, and tensor fasciae latae	Forceful arm swinging or quick change of direction while running
Lesser trochanter	Iliopsoas	Running

Initial Treatment
Patient Education
These injuries are common to athletes, and most will resolve with conservative management.
- Apophysitis usually presents in boys 12 to 18 years of age due to continued development of the apophysis.

Treatment Options
Nonoperative Management
- Recommend ice, rest, NSAIDs, and the use of crutches to facilitate walking if pain prohibits.
- Avoidance of aggravating activity. Athletes need to refrain from play until they are pain free to avoid further injury.
- See the patient in follow-up at 2-week intervals until he or she is pain free with ambulation and range of motion.
- A potential complication with hip pointers is development of a hematoma within the first 24 hours. If hematoma causes neurovascular compromise, the patient needs emergent surgery to decompress. If pain persists more than 2 weeks or an avulsion fracture is suspected, refer the patient to an orthopedic surgeon.

Rehabilitation
- Once the pain resolves, the patient may start PT or sport-specific strengthening to return to his or her level of play.
- The patient needs to pad hip pointers with ¼- to ½- inch padding to prevent further injury.
- Emphasize stretching techniques and massage for apophysitis.

Suggested Readings
Iliac apophysitis, *OrthoInfo* (website). www.pedortho.com. Accessed September 9, 2012.
Martinez J: Hip pointer, *Medscape* (website). 2009. http://emedicine.medscape.com/article/87322-overview. Accessed September 9, 2012.

PIRIFORMIS SYNDROME
History
- Increase in seated or forward-moving activities such as running or cycling
- Patient reports pain in gluteal region

- Symptoms can include numbness and tingling but may improve with external rotation of hip

Physical Examination
- No obvious signs on inspection
- Palpable tenderness along piriformis and sciatic notch
- Positive FAIR test
- May have positive straight leg raise
- Pertinent negatives include no palpable tenderness, painless ROM of hip, normal dermatomal sensation

Imaging
- Limited applicability in diagnosis, but MRI is helpful to rule out lumbar pathologies

Initial Treatment
Patient Education
The piriformis is a muscle in the gluteus region. It crosses the nerve that runs down the buttock to the leg, called the sciatic nerve. The piriformis muscle can become inflamed or hypertrophied, causing irritation of the sciatic nerve. There may also be a developmental variant of the piriformis, making it more prone to irritate the sciatic nerve. Differences in leg length can also cause piriformis syndrome. It usually resolves with activity modification, physical therapy, or medication and typically does NOT require surgery.

First Treatment Step
- While in the office the patient should be reassured that this is not a dangerous condition and it usually gets better.

Treatment Options
Nonoperative Management
- Nonoperative management is the mainstay of treatment.
- PT helps to stretch the piriformis and related muscles and induce relaxation of these muscle groups.
- NSAIDs, muscle relaxants, and neuropathic pain agents can be used.
- Steroid injections under radiographic guidance may be helpful.

Operative Management
- Surgical exploration and release of the piriformis have been reported, but the

outcomes have not been shown to be predictive.

Suggested Readings

Benson ER, Schutzer SF: Posttraumatic piriformis syndrome: diagnosis and results of operative treatment, *J Bone Joint Surg* 81:941–949, 1999.

Halpin RJ, Ganju A: Piriformis syndrome: a real pain in the buttock? *Neurosurgery* 65:197–202, 2009.

Kirschner JS, Foye PM, Cole JL: Piriformis syndrome, diagnosis and treatment. *Muscle Nerve* 41:428–430, 2010.

PELVIC FRACTURES

History

- High-velocity trauma or low-energy injury is the cause.
- Patients report pain and inability to ambulate. There is a high rate of associated injuries with high-energy trauma.
- Specific symptoms depend on the location of the fracture.

Physical Examination

- The patient experiences pain or inability to ambulate.
- Inspect the patient and palpate the skin, perineum, and rectum for potential open fractures.
- Palpation of the bony pelvis is painful.
- Use compression-distraction to determine the stability of the fracture pattern. If the iliac crests can be pressed together or pulled apart, the pelvis is unstable.
- High velocity is usually associated with other injuries.

Imaging: Figure 5-3

- Obtain radiographs to evaluate pelvic ring. Inlet and outlet views should also be obtained.
- Obtain a CT scan to evaluate the fracture pattern.

Classification

- Unstable (disruption of pelvic ring) versus stable (no disruption of pelvic ring) pelvic fractures
- Young-Burgess classification: lateral compression (type I-III), anteroposterior compression (type I-III), vertical shear, mixed pattern
- Other classification systems used: Bucholz, Letournel

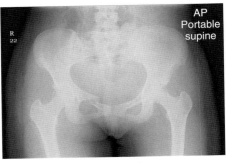

AP Portable supine

R 22

Figure 5-3. Pelvic fracture.

Initial Treatment

Patient Education

Half of all pelvic fractures occur in the elderly and are a result of low-energy forces as with a ground-level fall. Pelvic fractures related to high-energy forces often have multiple additional injuries. Disruption of the pelvic ring often requires surgery for stabilization. Stable pelvic fractures usually do not require surgery and will likely heal on their own, with time. Nonoperative treatment includes analgesics and bed rest with early mobilization.

First Treatment Steps

- Determine if the patient is stable or unstable with a radiograph and/or CT scan.
- If unstable fracture pattern, patient to be transferred to the hospital for further evaluation and possible surgical management.
- Determine hemodynamic stability and trauma workup if warranted, including CT chest, abdomen, pelvis, and abdominal ultrasound to evaluate the source of bleeding.

Treatment Options

Nonoperative Management

- This is reserved for stable fracture patterns or when a patient is too ill for surgery.
- Most stable pelvic fractures will go on to heal without surgery.
- Pain management may require hospitalization; otherwise, manage the pain with oral analgesics.

- Initially the patient should be on bed rest to manage the pain.
- The patient may bear weight as tolerated with an assistive device.
- He or she will need to avoid falls and will require assistance with activities of daily living.

Operative Management
Codes
ICD-9: 808.8 without disruption of pelvic ring, 808.43 with disruption of pelvic ring
CPT: 27215-27220 ORIF pelvic fracture

Operative Indications
- Fractures resulting in a pubic symphysis diastasis of more than 2.5 cm
- Fracture of the pubic rami resulting in more than 2 cm of displacement
- Rotationally unstable fractures causing more than a 1.5-cm leg length discrepancy

Informed Consent and Counseling
- Surgical fixation will provide the best outcome for mobility and decreased pain, although some people will develop chronic low back pain and posterior sacroiliac pain.
- There is a risk of bleeding, which may require a blood transfusion.
- Damage to the great vessels or bladder may occur.
- Another risk is leg length discrepancy, resulting in a gait abnormality.
- Weight bearing will begin with a walker or crutches when the pain is well controlled.

Anesthesia
- General anesthesia is most appropriate.

Patient Positioning
- Supine with legs internally rotated on a radiolucent table for external fixation or anterior approach
- Prone on a radiolucent table for sacroiliac fixation

Surgical Procedures
- External fixation for the acute phase treatment for temporary stabilization to allow access to abdomen or perineum

- Anterior approach for fixation of pubic symphysis
- Posterior approach for fixation of sacral fractures and sacroiliac dislocation

1) External fixation
Hardware: Fluoroscopy, guidewire, #2 5-mm pins.
Place the patient in a supine position on a radiolucent table. Palpate the iliac wing 2 to 4 cm proximal to the anterior superior iliac spine. The incision should be made perpendicular to the iliac wing. A guidewire should be placed along the inner table to determine the pelvic slope. Manually drill a starting point along the inner third of the iliac wing. Aiming toward the hip joint, place a 5-mm pin between the iliac cortical tables. A second pin should be placed in a converging pattern. Using fluoroscopy, confirm pin placement. Connect the pins and apply the crossbars, compressing the iliac wings or greater trochanters if reduction is necessary.
2) Open reduction, internal fixation of the pubic symphysis
Hardware: Fluoroscopy, malleable and Hohmann retractors, Weber pointed reduction clamp, 6-holed, curved, 3-mm reconstruction plate.
Place the patient in the supine position. An incision is made with a Pfannenstiel incision, just distal to the pubic tubercles. The rectus should be incised longitudinally. A malleable retractor should be placed in Retzius' space to protect the bladder. A narrow sharp Hohmann retractor should be placed under the rectus and over the pubis in order to expose the pubic symphysis. Anterior on the body of the pubis, a Weber pointed reduction clamp should be placed for reduction. Apply traction to achieve reduction. Once reduced, place a 6-holed, curved, 3-mm reconstruction plate on the superior surface of the symphysis. Use fluoroscopy to confirm reduction and fixation. A closed suction drain should be placed in the space of Retzius.
3) Open reduction, internal fixation of sacral fractures and sacroiliac dislocation

Hardware: Fluoroscopy, pointed reduction forceps

Place the patient in the prone position. Make a standard vertical incision 2 cm lateral to the posterior superior iliac spine. The posterior portion of the gluteal muscles is reflected from the posterior iliac wing. The greater sciatic notch should then be exposed to evaluate the reduction. The multifidus muscle should be elevated in sacral fractures to expose the posterior sacral lamina. For both sacral fractures and sacroiliac dislocation, reduction is achieved by placing pointed reduction forceps from the iliac wing to the sacrum. Use palpation and direct observation to evaluate reduction. For sacroiliac dislocations, using close fluoroscopic guidance, insert screws perpendicular to the iliac wing across the sacroiliac joint into the sacral ala. For sacral fractures, insert one to two screws from the lateral surface of the iliac wing into the S1 vertebral body. The gluteal fascia should be sutured to the sacral spine before closure.

Estimated Postoperative Course

- The postoperative hospital course will include bed rest, IV/oral analgesic medication, deep vein thrombosis prophylaxis, and physical therapy.
- If an external fixation frame is placed, it will remain for 8 to 12 weeks, and the pin site should be cleaned twice daily and watched closely for signs of infection.
- Ambulation may begin when patient's pain is managed and should start with toe-touch weight bearing on the affected side with assistance from crutches or a walker.
- At 10 to 14 days postoperative, evaluate the incision and obtain radiographs.
- At 6 weeks postoperative, the evaluation should include repeat radiographs. If evidence of healing is seen, advance weight bearing as tolerated.
- At 3 months postoperative, the evaluation should include repeat radiographs to ensure fracture healing.

Suggested Readings

Beaty LH, Canale ST: *Campbell's operative orthopaedics*, ed 11, Philadelphia, 2007, Mosby.

Bramos A, Velmahos GC, Butt UM, et al: Predictors of bleeding from stable pelvic fractures, *Arch Surg* 146:407–411, 2011.

Greene WB: *Netter's orthopaedics*, ed 1, Philadelphia, 2006, Saunders.

Hansen JT: *Netter's clinical anatomy*, ed 2, Philadelphia, 2010, Saunders.

Henry SM, Pollak AN, Boswell S, et al: Pelvic fracture in geriatric patients: a distinct clinical entity, *J Trauma Inj Infect Crit Care* 53:15–20, 2002.

Lotke PA, Abboud JA: *Lippincott's primary care: orthopaedics*, ed 1, Philadelphia, 2008, Lippincott Williams & Wilkins.

Slater SJ, Barron DA: Pelvic fractures—a guide to classification and management, *Eur J Radiol* 7:16–23, 2010.

Hip and Femur 6
Katherine Sharpe and Deana Bahrman

ANATOMY
Bones: Figures 6-1 **and** 6-2

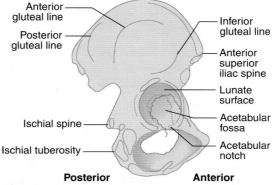

Anterior gluteal line
Posterior gluteal line
Inferior gluteal line
Anterior superior iliac spine
Lunate surface
Ischial spine
Acetabular fossa
Ischial tuberosity
Acetabular notch

Posterior   **Anterior**

Figure 6-1. **External surface of the hip bones.** *(From Bogart Bl, Ort VH:* Elsevier's integrated anatomy and embryology, *Philadelphia, 2007, Mosby.)*

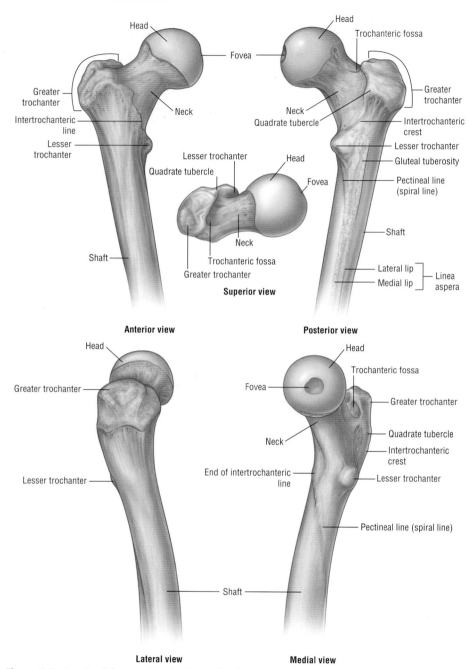

Figure 6-2. Proximal femur. *(Elsevier illustration from* www.elsevierimages.com. *Copyright, Elsevier Inc. All rights reserved.)*

Ligaments: Figure 6-3

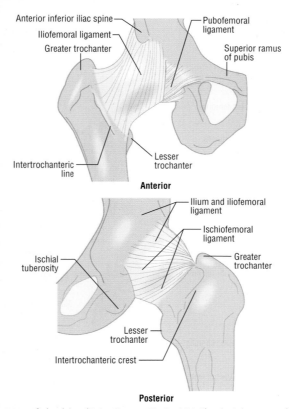

Anterior inferior iliac spine
Iliofemoral ligament
Greater trochanter
Pubofemoral ligament
Superior ramus of pubis
Intertrochanteric line
Lesser trochanter

Anterior

Ilium and iliofemoral ligament
Ischiofemoral ligament
Ischial tuberosity
Greater trochanter
Lesser trochanter
Intertrochanteric crest

Posterior

Figure 6-3. Ligaments of the hip. *(From Bogart BI, Ort VH:* Elsevier's integrated anatomy and embryology, *Philadelphia, 2007, Mosby.)*

183

Muscles and Tendons:
Figures 6-4 **and** 6-5

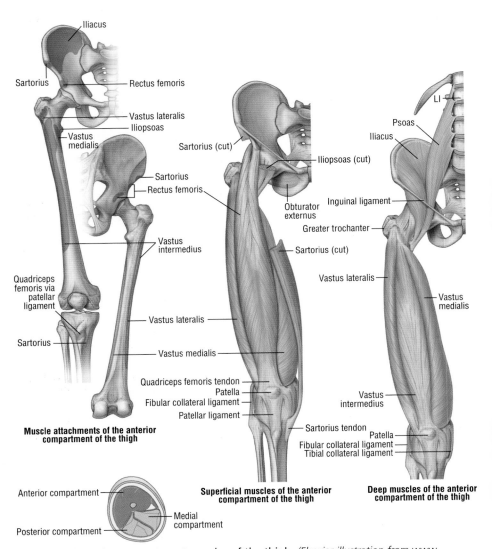

Iliacus

Sartorius

Rectus femoris

Vastus lateralis
Iliopsoas

Vastus
medialis

Sartorius (cut)

LI

Psoas

Iliacus

Iliopsoas (cut)

Sartorius
Rectus femoris

Inguinal ligament

Obturator
externus

Greater trochanter

Vastus
intermedius

Sartorius (cut)

Vastus lateralis

Vastus
medialis

Quadriceps
femoris via
patellar
ligament

Sartorius

Vastus lateralis

Vastus medialis

Vastus
intermedius

Quadriceps femoris tendon
Patella
Fibular collateral ligament
Patellar ligament

Sartorius tendon
Patella
Fibular collateral ligament
Tibial collateral ligament

**Muscle attachments of the anterior
compartment of the thigh**

**Superficial muscles of the anterior
compartment of the thigh**

**Deep muscles of the anterior
compartment of the thigh**

Anterior compartment

Medial
compartment

Posterior compartment

Figure 6-4. Anterior compartment muscles of the thigh. *(Elsevier illustration from* www.
elsevierimages.com. *Copyright, Elsevier Inc. All rights reserved.)*

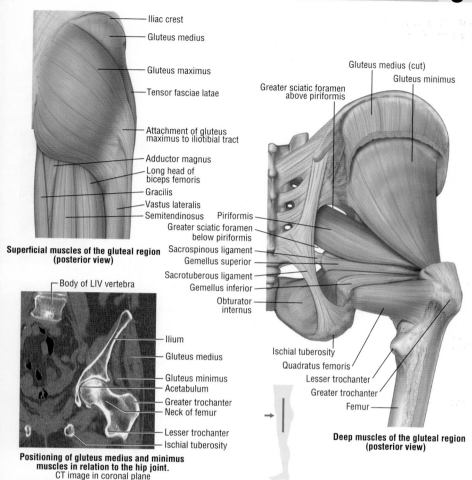

Iliac crest
Gluteus medius
Gluteus maximus
Tensor fasciae latae

Attachment of gluteus maximus to iliotibial tract

Adductor magnus
Long head of biceps femoris
Gracilis
Vastus lateralis
Semitendinosus

Superficial muscles of the gluteal region (posterior view)

Gluteus medius (cut)
Gluteus minimus
Greater sciatic foramen above piriformis

Piriformis
Greater sciatic foramen below piriformis
Sacrospinous ligament
Gemellus superior
Sacrotuberous ligament
Gemellus inferior
Obturator internus

Ischial tuberosity
Quadratus femoris
Lesser trochanter
Greater trochanter
Femur

Deep muscles of the gluteal region (posterior view)

Body of LIV vertebra

Ilium
Gluteus medius
Gluteus minimus
Acetabulum
Greater trochanter
Neck of femur
Lesser trochanter
Ischial tuberosity

Positioning of gluteus medius and minimus muscles in relation to the hip joint.
CT image in coronal plane

Figure 6-5. Gluteal region: superficial and deep muscles. CT, computed tomography. *(Elsevier illustration from* www.elsevierimages.com. *Copyright, Elsevier Inc. All rights reserved.)*

Nerves and Arteries:
Figure 6-6 **and** Table 6-1

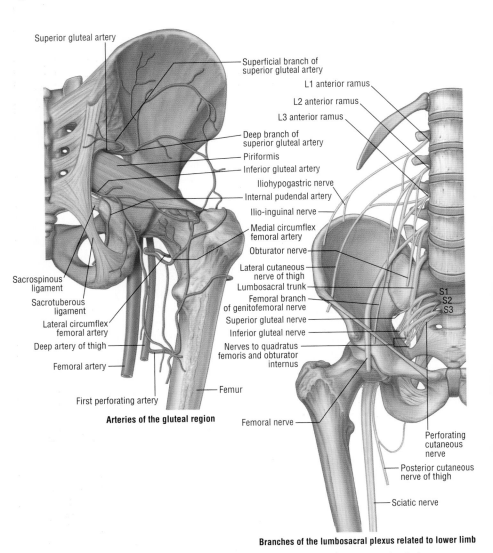

Superior gluteal artery

Superficial branch of superior gluteal artery

L1 anterior ramus

L2 anterior ramus

L3 anterior ramus

Deep branch of superior gluteal artery

Piriformis

Inferior gluteal artery

Iliohypogastric nerve

Internal pudendal artery

Ilio-inguinal nerve

Medial circumflex femoral artery

Obturator nerve

Lateral cutaneous nerve of thigh

Lumbosacral trunk

Femoral branch of genitofemoral nerve

Superior gluteal nerve

Inferior gluteal nerve

Nerves to quadratus femoris and obturator internus

Sacrospinous ligament

Sacrotuberous ligament

Lateral circumflex femoral artery

Deep artery of thigh

Femoral artery

First perforating artery

Femur

Arteries of the gluteal region

Femoral nerve

S1
S2
S3

Perforating cutaneous nerve

Posterior cutaneous nerve of thigh

Sciatic nerve

Branches of the lumbosacral plexus related to lower limb

Figure 6-6. Gluteal region: arteries and nerves. *(Elsevier illustration from* www.elsevierimages.com. *Copyright, Elsevier Inc. All rights reserved.)*

Table 6-1. Nerves of the Hip and Thigh

NERVE	BRANCH	MOTOR	TEST	SENSORY
Lumbar plexus (anterior division) L1-2	Genitofemoral	None		Proximal anteromedial thigh
Lumbar plexus (anterior division) L2-4	Obturator	Gracilis (anterior division) Adductor longus (anterior division) Adductor brevis (anterior and posterior divisions) Adductor magnus (posterior division) Obturator externus	Hip adduction, flexion, internal and external leg rotation	Inferomedial thigh; via cutaneous branch of obturator nerve
Lumbar plexus (posterior division) L2-3	Lateral femoral cutaneous	None		Lateral thigh
Lumbar plexus (posterior division) L2-4	Femoral	Psoas Sartorius Articularis genu Pectineus Quadriceps (rectus femoris, vastus lateralis, vastus intermedius, vastus medialis)	Hip flexion, leg external rotation, leg extension, leg adduction	Anteromedial thigh; via anterior and intermediate cutaneous nerves
Sacral plexus (anterior division) L4-S3	Tibial (descends as sciatic in posterior thigh)	Posterior thigh (biceps femoris [long head], semitendinosus, semimembranosus)	Hip extension, leg flexion	None
Sacral plexus (posterior division) L4-S1	Common peroneal (descends as sciatic in posterior thigh)	Biceps femoris (short head)	Hip extension, leg flexion	None (in thigh)
Sacral plexus (posterior division) S1-3	Posterior femoral cutaneous	None		Posterior thigh

Surface Anatomy: Figure 6-7

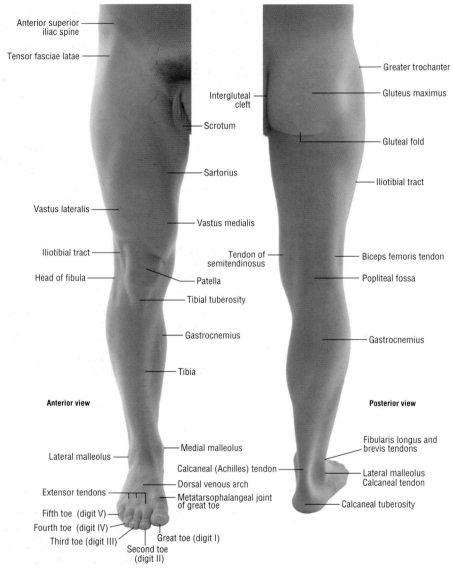

Anterior superior iliac spine

Tensor fasciae latae

Intergluteal cleft

Scrotum

Sartorius

Vastus lateralis

Vastus medialis

Iliotibial tract

Tendon of semitendinosus

Head of fibula

Patella

Tibial tuberosity

Gastrocnemius

Tibia

Anterior view

Lateral malleolus

Medial malleolus

Calcaneal (Achilles) tendon

Dorsal venous arch

Extensor tendons

Metatarsophalangeal joint of great toe

Fifth toe (digit V)

Fourth toe (digit IV)

Third toe (digit III)

Second toe (digit II)

Great toe (digit I)

Greater trochanter

Gluteus maximus

Gluteal fold

Iliotibial tract

Biceps femoris tendon

Popliteal fossa

Gastrocnemius

Posterior view

Fibularis longus and brevis tendons

Lateral malleolus
Calcaneal tendon

Calcaneal tuberosity

Figure 6-7. Hip surface anatomy. *(Elsevier illustration from* www.elsevierimages.com. *Copyright, Elsevier Inc. All rights reserved.)*

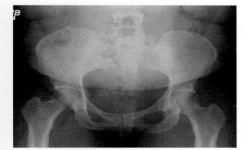

Figure 6-8. Normal radiograph of the hip.

Table 6-2. Normal Range of Motion of the Hip

Extension	115 degrees
Flexion	125 degrees
External rotation	45 degrees
Internal rotation	45 degrees
Abduction	45 degrees
Adduction	45 degrees

Normal Radiographic Findings: Figure 6-8

PHYSICAL EXAMINATION
Inspect the patient's gait and look for deformity.

Palpate
- Greater trochanter
- Iliopsoas tendon
- Sacroiliac joint
- Iliotibial band

Normal Range of Motion (ROM): Table 6-2

Neurovascular Examination: Table 6-3

Special Tests
- FABERE test: This maneuver tests for hip osteoarthritis (OA). The patient lies supine while the examiner flexes hip and knee and places the lateral malleolus across the contralateral knee. The examiner then extends the hip by pushing the flexed knee toward the table. A positive test result is when this maneuver elicits severe pain or restriction. The name of this test is an acronym for flexion abduction external rotation and extension.

Differential Diagnosis: Table 6-4

Suggested Readings
Eustice C: *Osteoarthritis* (website). http://osteoarthritis.about.com/od/osteoarthritisdiagnosis/a/range_of_motion.htm. Accessed September 11, 2012.
Greene WB: *Netter's orthopaedics,* Philadelphia, 2006, Saunders.
Hansen JT: *Netter's clinical anatomy,* ed 2, Philadelphia, 2010, Saunders.

HIP OSTEOARTHRITIS
History
- Causes of hip arthritis
  - Elevated bone density

Table 6-3. Neurovascular Examination

NERVES AND ARTERIES	LOCATION OF TEST	TESTS
Femoral nerve		Check of dorsiflexion, plantar flexion, extensor hallucis longus, inversion, eversion of foot
Sciatic nerve		Numbness and tingling at low back radiating to foot
Femoral artery	Groin; medial to femoral nerve	Palpation
Dorsalis pedis and posterior tibial arteries	Along the dorsal first metatarsal and posterior to medial malleolus	Palpation and comparison with contralateral side

Table 6-4. Differential Diagnosis of Hip and Thigh Pain

Buttock pain	Ischial bursitis Sciatica Hamstring strain Piriformis syndrome Gluteal tear Sacroiliac dysfunction
Groin pain	Hip arthritis Avascular necrosis Femoral acetabular impingement Adductor strain Femoral neck fracture Sacroiliac dysfunction Osteitis pubis
Lateral hip pain	Trochanteric bursitis
Posterior thigh pain	Sciatica
Anterior thigh pain	Iliopsoas tendinitis/bursitis Hip arthritis Hamstring strain Femoral shaft fracture

- Femoral acetabular impingement (FAI)
- Congenital dysplasia (~80% female)
- Trauma (three times more likely to develop)
- Slipped capital femoral epiphysis (SCFE)
- Legg-Calvé-Perthes disease
- Avascular necrosis (AVN) (likely from alcohol or systemic steroid use)
- Inflammatory disorders (rheumatoid arthritis, juvenile rheumatoid arthritis, ankylosing spondylitis)
- Sepsis (complaint of sharp pain in the groin or anterior hip, worse with weight bearing; night pain in in patients with severe OA)

Physical Examination
- Antalgic gait; posture and use of assistive devices
- Limb length discrepancy (LLD)
- Positive Trendelenburg test result: difficulty standing on one leg on the affected side because of abductor weakness
- Pain with active and passive ROM especially with hip flexion and internal rotation
- Check of distal pulses (dorsalis pedis and posterior tibial)
- Positive heel tap with occult fracture

Imaging: Figure 6-9
- Order radiographs: pelvis and OR lateral of hip. OR lateral requires the patient to rotate the hip internally approximately 10 to 15 degrees to provide a true lateral view because of the natural anteversion of the femoral head in the acetabular cup. Consider a frog leg view to assess for FAI.
- FAI: Order magnetic resonance imaging (MRI) without contrast to assess for soft tissue and labral damage. If labral damage is present, the patient will need total hip arthroplasty (THA); if not, consider surgical débridement of the femoral head.
- AVN: Order MRI with and without contrast to assess the extent of necrosis. If the femoral head has collapsed, the patient will need THA; if not, consider core decompression and bone graft to restore the blood supply.
- Order a computed tomography (CT) scan for complex cases to assess the acetabular cup.

Initial Treatment
Patient Education
OA is a progressive condition with three main risk factors: aging, obesity, and trauma. OA is nonreversible; treatment is geared toward pain control with conservative methods, and surgery is a last resort. THA is contraindicated in patients with a body mass index (BMI) greater than 40.

Treatment Options
Nonoperative Management
- Nonsteroidal antiinflammatory drugs (NSAIDs)
- Weight loss
- Physical therapy (PT): possibly helpful for muscle weakness and gait, but discontinued if symptoms increase
- Steroid or hyaluronic acid injections (may repeat at most every 3 months to prevent cartilage damage)

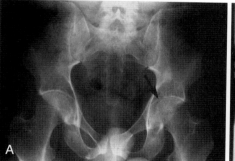 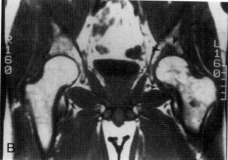

Figure 6-9. Osteoarthritis of the left hip on radiography (**A,** *arrow*) and magnetic resonance imaging (**B,** *arrowheads*). *(From Haaga JR, Lanzieri CF, Gilkeson RC, editors: CT and MR imaging of the whole body, ed 4, St. Louis, 2003, Mosby.)*

- Follow-up in 3 months to assess effectiveness

Operative Management
Codes
ICD-9 code: 715.15 Hip osteoarthritis
CPT code: 27130 Total hip arthroplasty

Operative Indications
- Night pain
- BMI lower than 40
- Failed conservative treatment
- Pain affecting activities of daily living (ADLs) and quality of life (QOL)

Informed Consent and Counseling
- Risks include bleeding, infection, blood clots, and LLD.
- The patient will need medical clearance.
- The average hospital stay lasts 3 days.
- Patients require 2 to 6 weeks of anticoagulation treatment.
- Expect 6 weeks of healing, PT, and strict hip precautions to prevent dislocation (no flexion >90 degrees or adduction) if the posterolateral approach is used; if the anterolateral approach is chosen, no hip precautions are necessary.
- Expect to wait about 3 months before returning to work. Work restrictions include no prolonged sitting or standing and a 40-lb lifting limit.
- It may take 1 year to recover fully.

Anesthesia
- Regional anesthetic, such as spinal block or femoral block with sedation, or general endotracheal

Patient Positioning
- Lateral decubitus, with the operative side up

Surgical Procedures
Posterolateral Approach
- Hardware consists of an acetabular cup, femoral head, femoral stem, polyethylene liner, and acetabular screws. Femoral and acetabular components may be made of titanium, stainless steel, or cobalt chrome (metal-on-polyethylene THA). Ceramic-on-ceramic components may also be used.
- Posterolateral approach: An 8- to 10-cm incision is made along the posterior border of the greater trochanter to the vastus tubercle. Deep dissection is performed using a Cobb elevator through the gluteus maximus over the posterior border of the greater trochanter, and thus the posterior capsule is entered.
- The hip is then dislocated, and the femoral neck is exposed and débrided. A transverse cut is made at the preoperative templated level on the femoral neck with an oscillating saw, and the femoral head is removed. The femur is then reamed, and trial components are placed.

- The acetabulum is then exposed using long Hohmann retractors. The acetabular cup is reamed to create appropriate anteversion (ideally approximately 40 degrees, but no more than 45 degrees) while preserving appropriate bone coverage to ensure that the hip does not impinge, which may increase risk of dislocation. Osteophytes are removed using a rongeur, and soft tissue is débrided. Trial components are placed in the acetabulum.
- The hip is then reduced with trial components and checked to ensure that there is no impingement, LLD, or dislocation at the extremes of flexion or extension.
- When trials are satisfactory, the actual components are placed. The capsule is then closed by using Tycron suture to secure the piriformis to the capsule, while avoiding injury to the sciatic nerve that runs directly posterolateral to the piriformis. A drain is placed in deep layer, and local anesthetic is injected. Deep layers are closed with Vicryl suture, and either nylon horizontal mattress or Monocryl subcutaneous sutures close the superficial layers. Use petrolatum gauze (Xeroform) and 4 × 4 gauze pads or Steri-Strips for a bandage, and affix a hip abduction pillow before extubation.

Estimated Postoperative Course
- Postoperative day 14
  - Sutures are removed, and a wound check is performed.
  - PT is begun for hip ROM, strengthening, balance, and gait training. The patient is weight bearing as tolerated.
- Postoperative 6 weeks
  - The patient returns to the clinic for radiographs of the pelvis and the lateral hip. Check for ROM, as well as abductor and quadriceps strength.
  - Continue to wean the patient off assistive devices (walker, cane) with progressive PT.
  - The patient may drive, if he or she is not taking narcotics. Stop anticoagulation.

- Postoperative 3 months, 6 months, and 1 year
  - The patient returns to the clinic for radiographs of the pelvis and hip.
  - Assess for continued improvement in pain, gait, and strengthening. Assess for trochanteric bursitis or LLD. After 1 year of PT, if the patient complains of LLD, referral for a shoe lift fitting may be indicated.

Suggested Readings
Boettner F, Altneu EI, Sculco TP: Mini-posterior total hip arthroplasty. In Brown TE, Cui Q, Mihalko WM, et al, editors: *Arthritis and arthroplasty: the hip,* Philadelphia, 2009, Saunders, pp 204–210.

McCarthy M, Brown TE, Saleh KJ: Etiology of hip arthritis. In Brown TE, Cui Q, Mihalko WM, et al, editors: *Arthritis and arthroplasty: the hip,* Philadelphia, 2009, Saunders, pp 3–11.

Miller CD, Stiltner AR, Cui Q: Preoperative planning for hip surgery. In Brown TE, Cui Q, Mihalko WM, et al, editors: *Arthritis and arthroplasty: the hip,* Philadelphia, 2009, Saunders, pp 24–36.

MUSCLE STRAINS AND INJURIES (ADDUCTORS, HAMSTRING, QUADRICEPS)
History
- Higher risk in active individuals and athletes
- Typically the result of eccentric contraction
- Patient-reported acute onset, popping sound, or snapping sensation at point of injury, followed by severe pain, possible swelling, tenderness to palpation, and ecchymosis.

Physical Examination
- Antalgic gait
- Pain reproduced with active ROM of the affected muscle
- Ecchymosis evident
- Swelling, palpable mass, or gap in muscle noted
- Tenderness to palpation noted at the point of injury

Imaging
- MRI may assess for fluid collections or severity of tear, but the diagnosis is based on history and clinical presentation.

Classification
Point of Injury
- Origin of muscle
- Musculotendinous junction
- Muscle belly
- Insertion of muscle

American Medical Association Grades for Muscle Strain
- First-degree: tears of a few muscle fibers
- Second-degree: more severe tear
- Third-degree: complete disruption of the musculotendinous unit

Initial Treatment
Patient Education
The hamstrings (three muscles), quadriceps (four muscles), and adductors (four muscles) comprise the musculature of the thigh. Strains are tears in the muscle and are quite common in active individuals. The hamstrings and quadriceps are especially prone to injury because they cross the knee joint. These injuries are managed well with conservative treatment, and surgical intervention is exceedingly rare.

Treatment Options
Nonoperative Management
- Acute phase (up to 5 days)
  - Rest, ice, compression, elevation
- Subacute phase (3 weeks)
  - Beginning active ROM exercises
- Remodeling phase (6 weeks)
  - When the patient can do active ROM without pain, start increasing sport-specific activity and strengthening.
  - Massage, ultrasound, and STIM treatment help prevent scar tissue buildup.
- Functional phase (2 weeks to 6 months)
  - When the patient can run for 20 to 30 minutes and perform sport movements without disability
  - Patients with second- and third-degree strains unlikely to return to play before 5 weeks

Rehabilitation
- Therapy is geared toward prevention by improving balance between opposing muscles (i.e., hamstrings and quadriceps), stretching techniques, and muscle conditioning.

Pearl:
The two most common indicators of required rehabilitation until the patient may return to play are previous muscle strain and the length of time to ambulate without pain. A history of muscle strain increases the risk of recurrent strain.

Suggested Readings
Heftler JM: Hamstring strain. *Medscape* (website). http://emedicine.medscape. com/article/307765-followup. Accessed September 11, 2012.
American Academy of Orthopedic Surgeons: Muscle strains in the thigh. *OrthoInfo* (website). http://orthoinfo.aaos.org/topic. cfm?topic=a00366. Accessed September 11, 2012.

FEMUR FRACTURE
History
- High-kinetic trauma (male patients <25 years old)
- Low-impact injury (female patients >65 years old)
- Acute, severe pain, with possible deformity in the thigh or leg shortening on the affected side

Physical Examination
- Remember the ABCs (airway, breathing, and circulation). The patient can bleed out from a femoral fracture, and 40% of patients with femoral fractures will require blood transfusion.
- Obvious deformity and ecchymosis are evident.
- Patients have severe pain with movement of the affected limb or with palpation.
- Check distal pulses, and assess for hematoma or bruits indicating vascular injury.
- Check for neurologic injury.
- Check for fracture of the ipsilateral knee and for femoral neck fracture.

Imaging
- Anteroposterior (AP) and lateral radiographs of the femur, hip, and knee are obtained.
- CT scan may give further information.

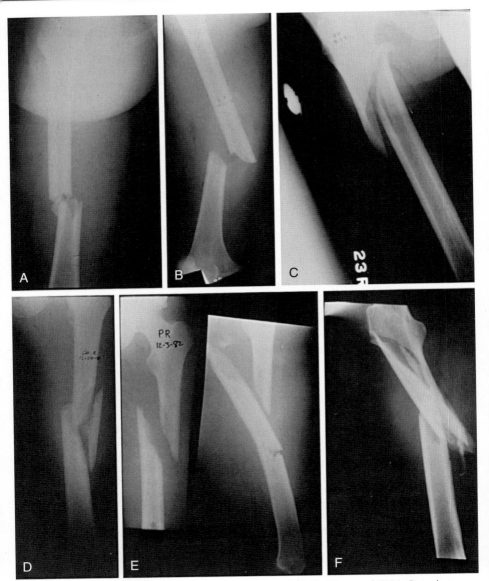

Figure 6-10. A to **F,** Classification of femoral shaft fractures. *(From Townsend CM Jr, Beauchamp RD, Evers BM, et al, editors:* Sabiston textbook of surgery, *ed 18, Philadelphia, 2008, Saunders.)*

- Angiogram is indicated if vascular injury is suspected.

Classification: Figure 6-10
- Transverse, oblique, spiral
- Comminuted
- Open

Initial Treatment
Patient Education
The femur is the longest and strongest bone in the body. A fracture can be life-threatening and requires surgical repair.

Stabilization

- Skeletal traction or an external fixator is applied to keep anatomic alignment and prevent neurovascular injury until surgery is possible (Fig. 6-11).
- Refer the patient to a vascular surgeon or a plastic surgeon in cases of vascular compromise or extensive soft tissue damage, respectively.

Treatment Options

Nonoperative Management

Conservative treatment is rare and is typically reserved only for pediatric patients.

 ORTHOPAEDIC WARNING

Be aware of the risk of *fat embolus* causing acute respiratory distress syndrome (ARDS) in trauma victims with diaphyseal femur fractures.

Operative Management of Diaphyseal Femur Fractures

Codes

ICD-9 code: 821 Closed femur shaft fracture

CPT code: 76000.26 Fluoro-guided ante-grade intramedullary nail

Operative Indications

- Once the patient is hemodynamically stable, the optimal time to surgery is less than 24 hours after fracture occurs.
- Open fractures should be considered emergencies, and surgical intervention is optimal at less than 8 hours.

Informed Consent and Counseling

- Even with appropriate surgical management, there is still a 1% rate of nonunion with intramedullary (IM) nailing.
- Other risks include infection, deep vein thrombosis (DVT), and compartment syndrome.
- The patient should expect 6 weeks of healing with non–weight-bearing status.
- The rate of LLD after femur fracture is 7%.

Anesthesia
- General

Patient Positioning
- Supine

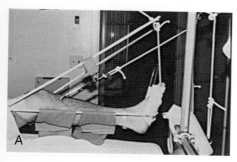

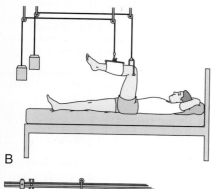

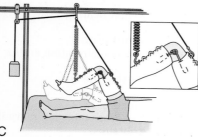

Figure 6-11. A to **C,** Skeletal traction of the femur. *(From Townsend CM Jr, Beauchamp RD, Evers BM, et al, editors: Sabiston textbook of surgery, ed 18, Philadelphia, 2008, Saunders.)*

Surgical Procedures

- Intramedullary (IM) nailing is the gold standard because of its 99% rate of union and 1% rate of infection.
- Plating has more complications and is generally not indicated for diaphyseal fractures.

Intramedullary Nailing

- Hardware includes a titanium IM nail.
- Intraoperative fluoroscopy is required.
- A 2- to 3-cm incision is made about 10 to 15 cm proximal to the greater trochanter. Enter the piriformis fossa medial to the trochanter and posterior to the gluteus medius. Obtain intraoperative radiographs with fluoroscopy at this time.
- The femur is then reamed, a guidewire is placed past the fracture site, and the fracture is reduced. Antegrade IM nailing is the standard, but retrograde placement is becoming more favorable, especially in obese patients. Fluoroscopic pictures should be obtained.
- By using the guidewire, the nail is placed and is advanced past the fracture. Rotate the nail 90 degrees medially during insertion, and then rotate it back. Locking screws are placed distally and proximally on the nail, and fluoroscopic pictures are taken.
- Close the layers of the incision with sutures.

Estimated Postoperative Course

- The patient will need to use crutches and remain non–weight bearing until 6 weeks postoperatively.
- Postoperative days 10 to 14
  - Remove the sutures, and perform a wound check.
- Postoperative 6 weeks
  - The patient returns to the clinic for AP and lateral femur radiographs.
  - Callus formation, union of fracture, the absence of radiolucency around screws, and the patient's lack of pain with touch toe weight bearing indicate that the fracture is healed or has healing. The patient may progress to touch toe weight bearing and PT for ROM and strengthening.

- Postoperative 3 months
  - The patient returns to the clinic for repeat radiographs.
  - If the patient has no pain with touch toe weight bearing, progress to weight bearing as tolerated. PT is given if needed.
- Postoperative 6 months
  - Nonunion occurs at 6 months. If the fracture is not healing radiographically or the patient has pain with weight bearing, consider further surgical intervention.
- Postoperative 1 year
  - Repeat the radiographs.

Suggested Readings

Aukerman DF: Femur injuries and fractures. *Medscape* (website). http://emedicine.medscape.com/article/90779-treatment#aw2aab6b6b2. Accessed September 11, 2012.

Eastwood B: Diaphyseal femur fractures. *Medscape* (website). http://emedicine.medscape.com/article/1246429-treatment#a1128. Accessed September 11, 2012.

Femoral shaft fracture. OrthoInfo (website). http://eorif.com/HipThigh/femoralshaftfx%20ImAnt.html#Anchor-Antegrade-2821. Accessed September 11, 2012.

Femoral shaft fractures. OrthoInfo (website). http://www.rcsed.ac.uk/fellows/lvanrensburg/Femoral.htm. Accessed September 11, 2012.

Femur shaft fractures. OrthoInfo (website). http://orthoinfo.aaos.org/topic.cfm?topic=A00521. Accessed September 11, 2012.

HIP FRACTURES

History

- Fall
- Pain in the groin, lateral hip, buttock, or low back
- Pain with weight bearing

Physical Examination

- Lower extremity malrotation and/or shortening
- Pain with ROM of the hip

Imaging: Figure 6-12

- AP pelvis and cross-table lateral radiographs are obtained.
- If radiographic findings are negative but suspicion is high, proceed with MRI.

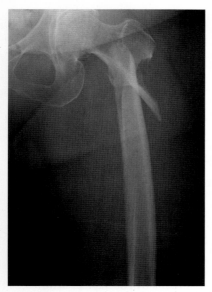

Figure 6-12. Radiographic appearance of classic hip fracture.

Classification
- The Garden classification for femoral neck fractures is based on the degrees of displacement and has a prognostic value for the incidence of osteonecrosis.
  - Type 1: valgus impaction of the femoral head
  - Type 2: nondisplaced, but complete
  - Type 3: displaced and complete, but less than 50%
  - Type 4: displaced, complete and greater than 50%
- The Boyd and Griffin classification is used for intertrochanteric fractures.
  - Type 1: fracture extending from the lesser to the greater trochanter along the intertrochanteric line
  - Type 2: comminuted fracture along the intertrochanteric line with multiple fractures in the cortex
  - Type 3: subtrochanteric fractures with at least one fracture crossing the proximal femur just distal to or at the lesser trochanter
  - Type 4: fracture in the trochanteric region and the proximal shaft in at least two planes, one usually in the sagittal plane

- The Seinsheimer classification for subtrochanteric fractures is based on the number of fragments and the location and configuration of the fracture lines.
  - Type 1: nondisplaced fracture or less than 2 mm of displacement
  - Type 2: two-part fracture
  - Type 2a: transverse fracture
  - Type 2b: spiral fracture with the lesser trochanter attached to the proximal fragment
  - Type 2c: spiral fracture with the lesser trochanter attached to the distal fragment
  - Type 3: three-part fracture
  - Type 3a: three-part spiral fracture with the lesser trochanter as part of the third fragment
  - Type 3b: three-part spiral fracture with the part being a butterfly fragment
  - Type 4: comminuted fracture with four or more parts
  - Type 5: subtrochanteric-intertrochanteric pattern

Initial Treatment
Patient Education
Hip fractures are the most frequent operative fracture and can be very debilitating. Only 25% of patients with hip fractures regain their prefracture function. Hip fractures include fractures in the femoral neck and in the intertrochanteric and subtrochanteric regions. If these injuries are not treated appropriately, they have a 10% to 45% rate of osteonecrosis and a 10% to 30% rate of nonunion.

First Treatment Steps
- Referral to an orthopaedic surgeon and transfer for hospital admission
- Immediate non–weight bearing

Treatment Options
Nonoperative Management
- Reserved for nonambulators or patients too ill to undergo surgical intervention
- Non–weight bearing
- Attentive care for position change to prevent skin breakdown
- Careful attention to pain management and nutrition

- DVT prophylaxis based on the patient's other comorbidities
- Follow-up to nonoperative management variable, based on disposition
- Follow-up in 2 weeks to evaluate pain management
- Follow-up at 6 weeks (patient should be pain free)

Rehabilitation
- The patient should begin ROM and strengthening of other extremities.

 ORTHOPAEDIC WARNING

Among patients with hip fracture who are more than 70 years old, 20% to 30% will die in the first year after fracture.

Operative Management
Codes
ICD-9 codes: 820.8 Femoral neck fracture
820.21 Intertrochanteric fracture
820.22 Subtrochanteric fracture
CPT codes: 27235 Percutaneous fixation
27244 Open reduction internal fixation

Operative Indications
- Fractures in ambulators who are medically stable for surgical intervention

Informed Consent and Counseling
- Despite appropriate surgical treatment and good technique, hardware failure, nonunion, malunion, and osteonecrosis may occur.
- Smoking increases the risk of nonunion.
- After surgical fixation, the patient will need to be protecting weight bearing or non–weight bearing, depending on the adequacy of fixation, for a period of 6 to 12 weeks.
- The patient may require PT for strengthening and gait training.

Anesthesia
- General
- Possibility of epidural with sedation in patients unable to tolerate general

Patient Positioning
- The patient is supine position on a fracture table with the uninjured leg flexed and abducted at the hip in a well leg holder with a padded peroneal nerve.
- The C-arm image intensify is positioned between the patient's legs, and the C-arm is kept on the nonsterile side of the transparent drape.
- The straight lateral position is used for hemiarthroplasty.

Surgical Procedures
- Open reduction, internal fixation of femoral neck, intertrochanteric, or subtrochanteric fractures
- Prosthetic replacement for femoral neck fracture with significant displacement or increased concern for nonunion or osteonecrosis; hemiarthroplasty if no evidence of acetabular arthritis; otherwise, THA

Open Reduction, Internal Fixation
- Hardware includes cannulated screws (femoral neck fractures), sliding compression hip screws with side plate (intertrochanteric fractures), and a regular interlocking IM nail (subtrochanteric fractures).
- Lateral approach for femoral neck fixation
  - A standard 1-inch lateral incision is made 2.5 cm distal and lateral to the anterior superior iliac spine and is curved distally and posteriorly over the lateral greater trochanter. Identify the interval between the gluteus medius and the tensor fasciae latae. Dissect proximally to expose the inferior branch of the superior gluteal nerve. Incise the capsule along the anterosuperior surface of the femoral neck. Along the distal incision, the origin of the vastus lateralis can be reflected distally or split to expose the greater trochanter and proximal femoral shaft. Under direct visualization, reduce the fracture. Flexing the hip to 20 to 30 degrees can help with reduction. With use of lateral radiographs and fluoroscopy, drive the first guide pin into the femoral neck

and into the femoral head to within 5 mm of subchondral bone. Proper placement of pins should be 130 to 135 degrees in relation to the femoral shaft. The second pin should be placed in the anterosuperior quadrant, and the third pin should be placed in the posterosuperior quadrant. Use fluoroscopic assistance for all pin placement. All the wires should be kept parallel. A cannulated drill is placed over each pin and drilled down to 5 to 10 mm short of the tip of the pin. Screw length is determined by direct measurement of the guide pins. All the screw threads should pass the fracture to achieve adequate compression. Screws are then tightened simultaneously so that uniform compression is applied across the fracture.

- Postoperative AP and lateral radiographs are obtained in the postanesthesia care unit to confirm reduction and hardware placement.

■ Lateral approach for intertrochanteric fractures
- Traction should be placed longitudinally, with the affected leg abducted and externally rotated. With traction in place, adduct and internally rotate the leg. Adjust traction to obtain reduction while avoiding too much traction, which can cause overreduction. The same lateral approach and dissection are performed as earlier. The insertion point of the guidewire depends on the angle of plate used. When using a 135-degree plate, use the proximal aspect of the osseous insertion of the gluteus maximus and the tip of the lesser trochanter for the entry point. Place the fixed-angle guide midway on the lateral cortex, and aim the pin toward the apex of the femoral head. Determine the lag screw length and reaming distance after the guide pin is in good position. Use the guide pin placement instrument to place a parallel guide pin 13 mm proximal to the primary guide pin. Ream to the examination

lag screw length. Assemble the plate and lag screw onto the insertion device. Place the entire assembly over the guide pin, and insert it into the reamed holes. Verify position and lag screw length with an image. Advance the plate onto the lag screw, and unscrew the lag screw retaining rod. Remove the guide pin. Using a plate clamp, secure the plate to the shaft. Next, drill the bone screw holes, and determine screw length. Insert screws and tighten, at which point traction may be removed. After traction is removed, compress the compression screws to compress the fracture. Drill for remaining screws. A drain to self-suction should be used. Postoperative radiographs should be obtained.

Prosthetic Replacement Hemiarthroplasty
■ Hardware includes the hemiarthroplasty component.
■ Lateral approach for hemiarthroplasty
- See the earlier description for approach details. Extend the incision 10 cm distal to the greater trochanter. Insert a large self-retaining retractor beneath the fascia lata at the level of the greater trochanter. Dissect the interval between the gluteus minimus and the superior capsule. Divide the entire capsule along its femoral attachment, and excise the visible portion, thus preserving it for repair later. Measure the distance between the greater trochanter and the ilium superior to the acetabulum to determine leg lengths. Dislocate the hip posteriorly. Mark the angle and level on the femoral neck for osteotomy. Use the stem and neck length trials predetermined by preoperative templating. Perform the osteotomy with a power saw, and remove the femoral head. Insert the smallest reamer at the point of the piriformis fossa. Ream to the medullary canal. Using the smallest broach, impact and extract and progressively increase

the broach size. Once broaching is complete, choose the templated length. Perform a trial reduction to evaluate leg length and stability. After trial size is chosen, place a bone block or canal plug in the distal canal to prevent cement from migrating. Determine the depth of cement insertion. Shield surrounding tissue and acetabulum, deliver cement, and insert the component. Apply firm pressure on the component as the cement hardens. Remove excess cement. Assemble the component head to the neck once the cement is dry. Reduce the hip, and irrigate to remove any debris. Repair the capsule if possible, and reattach any rotator muscles removed on exposure. Close the layers, and insert a drain. Obtain postoperative hip AP and lateral radiographs.

Estimated Postoperative Course
- Postoperative hospital course
  - Weight bearing will vary.
  - The patient is out of bed with early mobilization to avoid DVT.
  - Postoperative anticoagulation: The length of time and pharmacologic agent vary based on the preference of the surgeon and facility.
  - PT is begun.
- Postoperative 10 to 14 days
  - Suture removal is performed.
  - The incision and lower extremity are evaluated.
  - Continue PT for strengthening and gait training.
- Postoperative 6 weeks
  - AP and lateral pelvis radiographs are obtained to evaluate hardware and component positions.
  - Full weight-bearing is allowed if initial restrictions were placed.
- Postoperative 3 months
  - AP and lateral pelvis radiographs are obtained to evaluate hardware and component positions.
  - A pain-free patient may resume normal activity.
  - If pain persists, evaluate for nonunion or osteonecrosis with MRI of the osseous pelvis.

Suggested Readings
Beaty LH, Canale ST, editors: *Campbell's operative orthopaedics,* ed 11, Philadelphia, 2007, Mosby.
Font-Vizcarra L, Zumbado A, Garcia S, et al: Relationship between hematoma in femoral neck fractures contamination and early postoperative prosthetic joint infection, *Injury* 42:200–203, 2011.
Gjertsen JE, Vinje T, Engesaeter LB, et al: Internal screw fixation compared with bipolar hemiarthroplasty for treatment of displaced femoral neck fractures in elderly patients, *J Bone Joint Surg Am* 92:619–628, 2010.

TROCHANTERIC BURSITIS
History
- Commonly an overuse injury
- Intermittent or constant lateral hip pain that can radiate down the lateral thigh
- Pain when lying on the affected side

Physical Examination
- No obvious skin color changes or swelling
- Tenderness to palpation over the lateral or posterior aspect of the greater trochanter
- Pain with extreme hip abduction and external rotation

Imaging
- AP pelvis and lateral hip radiographs should be performed to rule out other disorders.

Initial Treatment
Patient Education
This disorder is more common in women than in men. It usually resolves with conservative measures. It may be intermittent or chronic. Pain may increase and activity may be impaired if the condition is untreated.

First Treatment Steps
- Initial treatment includes conservative management.
- Referral to PT may be done.

Treatment Options
Nonoperative Management
- NSAIDs
- PT to focus on stretching of the iliotibial band and strengthening of the muscles around the hip

- Trochanteric bursa corticosteroid injection
- Improvement expected within 6 months of conservative management, although symptoms possible
- Follow-up as needed

Operative Management
- Operative intervention is rare.

Suggested Readings
Aaron DL, Patel A, Kayiaros S, et al: Four common types of bursitis: diagnosis and management, *J Am Acad Orthop Surg* 19:359–367, 2011.

Lequesne M, Mathieu P, Vuillemin-Bodaghi V, et al: Gluteal tendinopathy in refractory greater trochanter pain syndrome: diagnostic value of two clinic tests, *Arthritis Rheum* 59(2):241–246, 2008.

Lustenberger DP, Ng VY, Best TM, et al: Efficacy of treatment of trochanteric bursitis: a systematic review, *Clin J Sports Med* 21(5): 447–453, 2011.

SNAPPING HIP
History
- Lateral hip pain associated with an audible "click"
- Associated with young female athletes
- Pain and click noticed with repetitive hip flexion, extension, and abduction

Physical Examination
- Lateral snapping may be reproduced and felt with flexion and extension of the affected hip.
- Anterior snapping may improve with direct pressure over the iliopsoas tendon at the level of the femoral head.
- Pain or snapping with internal or external rotation of the affected hip may suggest an intra-articular process.

Imaging
- No standard imaging is recommended.
- Radiographs and MRI may be helpful in ruling out other disorders.

Initial Treatment
Patient Education
Snapping can be associated with the iliotibial band moving over the greater trochanter (external) or the iliopsoas tendon moving over the iliopectineal eminence (internal). It can also be associated with

a loose body, labral tear or another disorder within the hip joint (intra-articular). Asymptomatic snapping does not require treatment. Painful snapping usually improves with NSAIDs and PT.

First Treatment Steps
- Identification of the cause of snapping (lateral, anterior, or intra-articular)
- NSAIDs
- PT

Treatment Options
Nonoperative Management
- Most cases responsive to conservative management
- NSAIDs
- PT for stretching and strengthening
- Steroid injections to the greater trochanter bursa or intra-articular injection
- Follow-up 6 weeks after initiation of treatment, to determine effectiveness
- Resolution of pain with any of the foregoing conservative modalities an indication for follow-up on an as-needed basis
- Activity continued as tolerated
- Radiographs or MRI considered if no improvement with conservative management or a suspect intra-articular process

Operative Management
- Surgical treatment is not usually indicated.

Suggested Readings
Bancroft LW, Blankenbaker DG: Imaging of the tendons about the pelvis, *AJR Am J Roentgenol* 195:605–617, 2010.

Tibor LM, Sekiya JK: Differential diagnosis of pain around the hip joint, *Arthroscopy* 24: 1407–1421, 2008.

FEMORAL STRESS FRACTURE
History
- Young athletes, typically runners
- Older patients with metabolic bone disorder
- Localized hip pain as the primary complaint
- Pain worse with activity and improved with rest

- Pain typically in the groin and possibly radiating into the thigh and knee
- Possible report of a new activity or an increase in the intensity of activity
- Night pain common

Physical Examination
- No abnormality on visual inspection
- No palpable tenderness
- Possible pain with ROM of the hip

Imaging
- Initial or late radiographs may not reveal fracture. Diagnosis often requires MRI or bone scan.

Classification
- Tension fractures: Superior aspect of the femoral neck causing a transverse fracture across the femoral neck; more common in older patients; more likely to progress and displace
- Compression fractures: Inferior aspect of the femoral neck; more common in younger population and athletes

Initial Treatment
Patient Education
Stress fractures are the result of repetitive loading of the bone. This injury is seen in young athletes and in older persons with osteoporosis. Most stress fractures heal without surgery; however, if the fracture progresses, surgical repair will be required. Compliance with treatment is important to prevent progression of the fracture.

First Treatment Steps
- Non–weight bearing to the affected side
- Crutches or a walker to facilitate ambulation with this restriction

Treatment Options
Nonoperative Management
- The patient is non–weight bearing.
- Follow up every 4 weeks for repeat radiographs to ensure no change in fracture pattern or symptoms and to evaluate callus formation.
- The fracture usually requires 3 to 6 months to heal.
- Bone scan should be performed at 3 to 6 months to confirm complete resolution, at which time patient may resume normal activity.

- A fracture that displaces or progresses should be fixed operatively.
- Osteonecrosis or nonunion may result if a stress fracture progresses or is missed.
- Once the fracture is healed, the patient may begin PT for general strengthening and gait training.

Operative Management
Codes
ICD-9 code: 733.96 Stress fracture of femoral neck
CPT code: 27235 Closed reduction, internal fixation

Operative Indications
- Displacement of the diastasis or no evidence of healing on radiographs
- Nondisplaced fractures in patients who cannot be compliant with conservative management

Informed consent and counseling
- Fixation may be achieved with closed reduction, internal fixation, but it may require open reduction, internal fixation.
- There is still a risk of osteonecrosis despite good reduction and fixation.
- Nonunion may occur despite adequate fixation.
- Smoking increases the risk of nonunion.
- After surgical fixation, the patient will need to be protecting weight bearing or non–weight bearing, depending on the adequacy of fixation, for a period of 6 to 12 weeks.
- The patient may require PT for strengthening and gait training.

Anesthesia
- General

Patient Positioning
- The patient is supine on a fracture table with the uninjured leg flexed and abducted at the hip in a well leg holder with a padded peroneal nerve.
- The C-arm image intensify is positioned between the patient's legs, and the C-arm is kept on the nonsterile side of the transparent drape.

Surgical Procedures

Closed Reduction, Internal Fixation

- Hardware includes cannulated screws.
- If reduction is required, closed reduction can be attempted first and, one hopes, achieves adequate reduction. Before preparing the patient, while the patient is in the supine position on the fracture table, tie the unaffected extremity to the footplate. Tie the fractured extremity to the other footplate in an externally rotated position. While the extremity is externally rotated, abduct approximately 20 degrees, and apply enough traction to regain normal length. The extremity is then internally rotated until the patella is internally rotated 20 to 30 degrees. Anteroposterior and lateral fluoroscopic images should be obtained to ensure proper alignment.
- A standard 1-inch lateral incision is made, centered over the lesser trochanter. Carefully incise the iliotibial band in line with the incision. Under direct visualization, reduce the fracture. With use of lateral radiographs and fluoroscopy, drive the first guide pin into the femoral neck and into the femoral head to within 5 mm of subchondral bone. Proper placement of pins should be 130 to 135 degrees in relation to the femoral shaft. The second pin should be placed in the anterosuperior quadrant, and the third pin should be placed in the posterosuperior quadrant. Use fluoroscopic assistance for all pin placements. All the wires should be kept parallel. A cannulated drill is placed over each pin and drilled down to 5 to 10 mm short of the tip of the pin. Screw length is determined by direct measurement of the guide pins. All the screw threads should pass the fracture to achieve adequate compression. Screws are then tightened simultaneously so that uniform compression is applied across the fracture.
- Postoperative AP and lateral radiographs are obtained in the postanesthesia care unit to confirm reduction and hardware position.

Estimated Postoperative Course

- The patient is out of bed on postoperative day 1, if tolerable.
- Ambulation with weight-protected or non–weight-bearing restrictions depend on the fixation procedure and the patient's bone quality.
- PT should start postoperative day 1 and continue as needed
- Follow up 10 to 14 days after discharge from the hospital to evaluate the incision and remove the sutures or staples.
- Follow up at 4 to 6 weeks for repeat AP and lateral pelvic radiographs. If the patient has no pain, gradually advance weight-bearing status to weight bearing as tolerated.
- Follow up at 3 months for repeat AP and lateral pelvic radiographs.
- If pain persists, consider an MRI or CT scan for evaluation of osteonecrosis or nonunion.

Suggested Readings

Beaty LH, Canale ST, editors: *Campbell's operative orthopaedics,* ed 11, Philadelphia, 2007, Mosby.

DeLee JC, Drez D, Miller MD: *DeLee and Drez's orthopaedic sports medicine,* ed 3, Philadelphia, 2009, Saunders.

Pihlajamak HK, Ruohola JP, Wechstrom M, et al: Long-term outcome of undisplaced fatigue fractures of the femoral neck in young male adults, *J Bone Joint Surg Br* 88:1574–1579, 2006.

ANATOMY
Bones: Figure 7-1

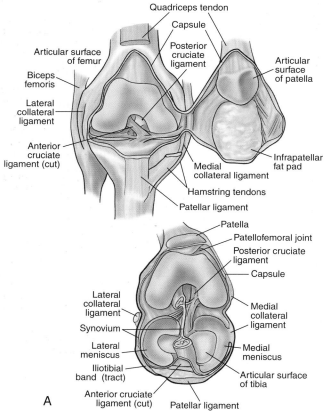

Figure 7-1. A, Knee joint structures.

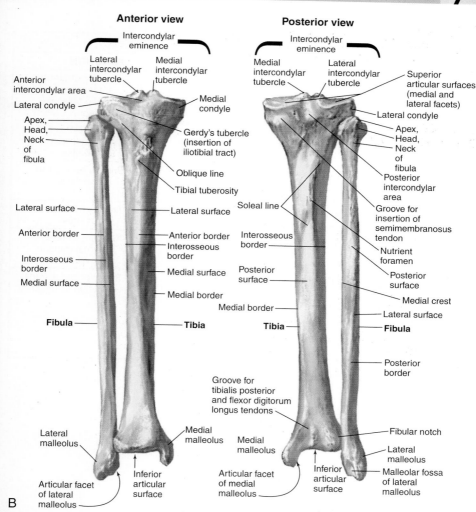

Anterior view

Intercondylar eminence

Lateral intercondylar tubercle
Medial intercondylar tubercle

Anterior intercondylar area
Lateral condyle
Medial condyle

Apex,
Head,
Neck
of
fibula

Gerdy's tubercle (insertion of iliotibial tract)

Oblique line

Tibial tuberosity

Lateral surface
Lateral surface

Anterior border
Anterior border
Interosseous border

Interosseous border
Medial surface

Medial surface
Medial border

Fibula
Tibia

Lateral malleolus
Medial malleolus

Inferior articular surface

Articular facet of lateral malleolus

Posterior view

Intercondylar eminence

Medial intercondylar tubercle
Lateral intercondylar tubercle

Superior articular surfaces (medial and lateral facets)

Lateral condyle

Apex,
Head,
Neck
of
fibula

Posterior intercondylar area

Groove for insertion of semimembranosus tendon

Nutrient foramen

Soleal line
Interosseous border

Posterior surface

Posterior surface

Medial crest

Medial border
Lateral surface

Tibia
Fibula

Posterior border

Groove for tibialis posterior and flexor digitorum longus tendons

Medial malleolus
Medial malleolus

Fibular notch

Lateral malleolus

Malleolar fossa of lateral malleolus

Articular facet of medial malleolus
Inferior articular surface

B

Figure 7-1, cont'd B, The tibia and fibula are the bones in the leg. *(From Miller MD, Hart JA, MacKnight JM, editors:* Essential orthopaedics, *Philadelphia, 2010, Saunders.)*

Ligaments: Table 7-1

Table 7-1. Location and Function of Knee Ligaments		
LIGAMENT	**LOCATION**	**FUNCTION**
Anterior cruciate ligament (ACL)	Originates on the tibia just anterior to the area between the tibial eminences and runs obliquely to the lateral femoral condyle	Primary restraint to anterior translation of the tibia; also rotational stability
Posterior cruciate ligament (PCL)	Originates on lateral border of the medial femoral condyle and inserts on the posterior rim of the tibia	Primary restraint to posterior translation of the tibia
Medial collateral ligament (MCL)	Originates on the medial femoral epicondyle and inserts on the medial proximal tibia	Primary restraint to valgus force
Lateral collateral ligament (LCL)	Originates on the lateral femoral epicondyle and inserts on the anterolateral fibula	Primary restraint to varus stress
Posteromedial corner (PMC): posterior oblique ligament	Located deep and posterior to the MCL	Restraint to tibial internal rotation and valgus force
Posterolateral corner (PLC): biceps, iliotibial band, popliteus, popliteofibular ligament, and joint capsule	Located posterior to the LCL	Resistance to external rotation of the knee

Muscles, Nerves, and Arteries: Figure 7-2 and Tables 7-2 and 7-3

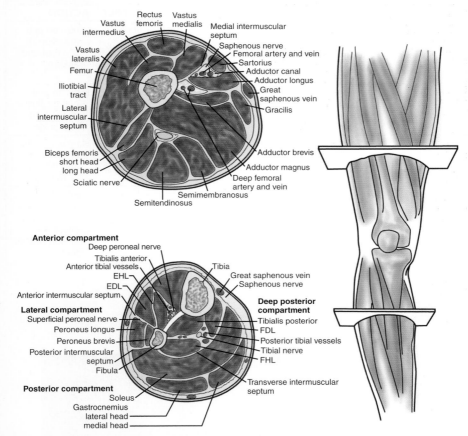

Figure 7-2. Cross-sectional anatomy of the thigh and leg. EDL, extensor digitorum longus; EHL, extensor hallucis longus; FDL, flexor digitorum longus; FHL, flexor hallucis longus. *(From Miller MD, Hart JA, MacKnight JM, editors:* Essential orthopaedics, *Philadelphia, 2010, Saunders.)*

Table 7-2. Muscle Compartments of the Thigh

COMPARTMENT	MUSCLES	INNERVATION	BLOOD SUPPLY	ACTION
Anterior	Vastus lateralis, vastus medialis obliquus, vastus intermedius, rectus femoris, sartorius	Femoral nerve	Superficial femoral artery	Extension of the knee
Medial	Adductors (longus, magnus, brevis) and gracilis	Obturator and sciatic nerves	Deep femoral artery	Adduction of the leg
Posterior	Semimembrano-sus, semitendi-nosus, biceps femoris	Sciatic nerve	Inferior gluteal and perforating branches of the femoral artery	Flexion of the knee and extension of the hip

Table 7-3. Muscle Compartments of the Lower Leg

COMPARTMENT	MUSCLES	INNERVATION	BLOOD SUPPLY	ACTION
Anterior	Tibialis anterior, extensor hallucis longus, extensor digitorum longus	Deep peroneal nerve	Anterior tibial artery	Extension and inversion of the foot and ankle
Lateral	Peroneus brevis, peroneus longus, peroneus tertius	Superficial peroneal nerve	Peroneal artery	Eversion and plantar flexion of the foot and ankle
Superficial posterior	Gastrocnemius, soleus, plantaris	Tibial nerve	Sural arteries	Plantar flexion of the foot and flexion of the knee
Deep posterior	Flexor hallucis longus, flexor digitorum longus, tibialis posterior, popliteus	Tibial nerve	Posterior tibial artery, popliteal artery (popliteus only)	Plantar flexion and inversion of the foot and ankle, flexion of the toes

Normal Radiographic Appearance: Figures 7-3 and 7-4

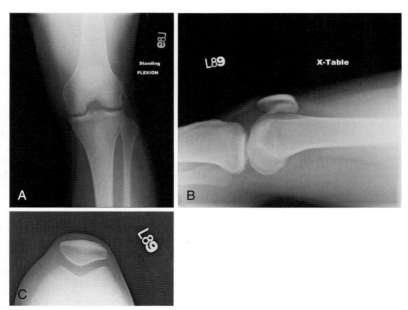

Figure 7-3. Normal knee radiographs. **A,** Standing flexion view. **B,** Lateral view. **C,** Sunrise view.

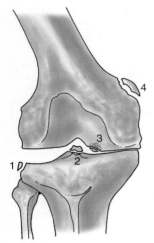

Figure 7-4. Illustration showing multiple radiographic findings. *1,* Segond fracture (lateral capsular sign); *2,* tibial eminence fracture; *3,* osteochondritis dissecans; *4,* Pellegrini-Stieda lesion. *(From Miller MD, Hart JA, MacKnight JM, editors:* Essential orthopaedics, *Philadelphia, 2010, Saunders.)*

PHYSICAL EXAMINATION

Observe: gait (antalgic, assistive devices), alignment (valgus, varus), and feet (pes planus or cavus), ecchymosis, abrasion, gross deformity, effusion, quadriceps atrophy, and leg length discrepancy

Palpate: quadriceps muscle and tendon, patella (all poles, tendon, and fat pads), medial collateral ligament (MCL) and medial joint line, lateral collateral ligament (LCL) and lateral joint line, bursa (prepatellar and infrapatellar, pes anserine), and popliteal fossa

Normal range of motion (ROM): up to 10 degrees of hyperextension and 130 degrees of flexion

Neurovascular examination (Table 7-4): assessment of sensation and motor function of the foot; palpation of dorsalis pedis, posterior tibial, and popliteal pulses; test of patellar reflex

Special Tests

Patella

■ **Patellar apprehension test:** The patient lies supine with the knee in 20 to 30 degrees of flexion and the quadriceps relaxed. Carefully glide the patella laterally. A positive test result is the presence of a reactive contraction of the quadriceps muscles by the patient in an attempt to avoid a recurrence of the dislocation or a sense of apprehension or fear that the patella will dislocate.

■ **Patellar grind test:** The patient lies supine with knee fully extended. Push the patella distally in the trochlear groove. Have the patient tighten the quadriceps against patella resistance. Pain with or without crepitus is considered a positive test result.

Ligament Examination: Table 7-5 and Figures 7-5 and 7-6

Meniscal Examination

■ **McMurray test:** With patient supine, take hold of the heel with one hand and flex the leg. Place the free hand on the knee with fingers along the medial joint line and the thumb and thenar eminence on the lateral joint line. Apply valgus force, and externally rotate the lower leg, and then maintain valgus force while internally

Table 7-4. Lower Extremity Neurologic Examination

NERVE	MOTOR FUNCTION	SENSORY DISTRIBUTION
Sural	Foot plantar flexion	Lateral heel
Saphenous	None	Medial leg and ankle
Superficial peroneal	Foot eversion	Dorsum of the foot
Deep peroneal	Great toe flexion	First web space
Tibial	Toe plantar flexion	Sole of the foot

209

Table 7-5. Special Tests to Assess for Ligament Injury

LIGAMENT OR STRUCTURE	SPECIAL TEST
Anterior cruciate ligament (ACL)	**Lachman test:** With the patient in the supine position with knee at 30 degrees of flexion (placing a pillow under the knee may help the patient relax), place one hand slightly superior to the knee to stabilize the thigh, and use the other hand to apply anterior pressure to the proximal tibia. Increased anterior translation compared with the unaffected side is a positive finding.
	Anterior drawer test: With the patient lying supine with the hip flexed to 45 degrees and the knee to 90 degrees, grasp the tibia just below the joint line. Place the thumbs on either side of the patellar tendon. Use the index fingers to palpate the hamstring tendons to ensure that the tendons are relaxed. Pull forward on the tibia. Increased anterior translation compared with the unaffected side is a positive finding.
	Pivot shift test: The patient is in the supine position, the knee is extended, and the foot is internally rotated. Apply valgus stress while flexing the knee. Pivoting of the tibia is a positive finding. It is easiest to perform this test while the patient is under anesthesia.
Posterior cruciate ligament (PCL)	**Posterior drawer test:** With the patient lying supine with the hip flexed to 45 degrees and the knee to 90 degrees, grasp the tibia just below the joint line. Place the thumbs on either side of the patellar tendon. Use the index fingers to palpate the hamstring tendons to ensure that they are relaxed. Apply posterior force on the tibia. Increased posterior translation compared with the unaffected side is a positive finding.
Medial collateral ligament (MCL)	**Valgus stress test:** With the patient supine with the knee flexed to 30 degrees, apply valgus force and assess for medial opening. Repeat in full extension. Medial opening and pain are positive findings; opening in full extension indicates possible concurrent ACL injury.
Lateral collateral ligament (LCL)	**Varus stress test:** With the patient supine with the knee flexed to 30 degrees, apply varus force and assess for lateral opening. Repeat in full extension. Lateral opening and pain are positive findings.
Posterolateral corner (PLC)	**Dial test (external rotation asymmetry):** With the patient prone with the knees flexed at 30 degrees, stabilize the knees and externally rotate the feet. Repeat at 90 degrees of flexion. Asymmetry of ≥15 degrees in 30 degrees of flexion indicates isolated PLC injury; asymmetry at 90 degrees indicates combined PCL and PLC injury.
Posteromedial corner (PMC)	**Slocum test:** An anterior drawer test is performed with the patient's foot in neutral position and with the foot externally rotated. Anterior displacement should be reduced in the externally rotated position unless there is a PMC injury.

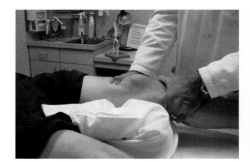

Figure 7-5. The Lachman examination. Note that the hand closest to the head of the patient grasps the thigh, and the opposite hand performs the examination with the thumb close to the joint line. A pillow can be placed under the knee to help the patient relax. *(From Miller MD, Hart JA, MacKnight JM, editors: Essential orthopaedics, Philadelphia, 2010, Saunders.)*

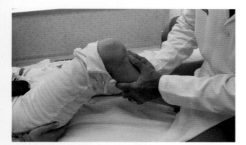

Figure 7-6. The posterior drawer examination. Note that the starting point is evaluated by palpating the medial tibial plateau in relation to the medial femoral condyle before a posteriorly directed force is applied. *(From Miller MD, Hart JA, MacKnight JM, editors: Essential orthopaedics, Philadelphia, 2010, Saunders.)*

Table 7-6. Differential Diagnosis Based on Location of Knee Pain

LOCATION	DIFFERENTIAL DIAGNOSES
Anterior	Patellofemoral chondromalacia, prepatellar bursitis, patellar tendinitis, patellar fracture, patellofemoral osteoarthritis
Medial	Meniscus tear, MCL injury, osteoarthritis, pes anserine bursitis
Lateral	Meniscus tear, LCL injury, osteoarthritis, iliotibial band syndrome
Posterior	Tear of posterior horn of medial or lateral meniscus, neurovascular injury (popliteal artery or nerve), PLC injury

LCL, lateral collateral ligament; MCL, medial collateral ligament; PLC, posterolateral corner.

rotating. A palpable or audible click is considered a positive finding.

Differential Diagnosis: Table 7-6
- The differential diagnosis for immediate effusion, in order of frequency, is as follows: anterior cruciate ligament (ACL) tear, patella dislocation, osteochondral fracture, and peripheral meniscus tear.

ANTERIOR CRUCIATE LIGAMENT INJURY
History
- The mechanism is typically a noncontact pivoting injury.
- The patient often reports feeling or hearing a "pop" at the time of injury.
- Immediate effusion is noted.
- The patient is typically unable to continue activity or complete a sporting event.
- Instability with pivoting and swelling after activity are seen in chronic ACL tears.

Physical Examination
- Observation: Note effusion, abrasion, and deformity.
- Palpation: Patellar ballottement is performed to assess for effusion. Joint line tenderness may be present secondary to concurrent meniscus tear.
- ROM: Decreased ROM may result from effusion. The lack of ability to extend the knee fully may occur with a concurrent displaced bucket handle meniscus tear.

 ORTHOPAEDIC WARNING

Loss of full extension may indicate a "locked knee," indicating a flipped bucket handle tear of the meniscus. This is an urgent finding and should prompt magnetic resonance imaging for possible early surgical meniscal repair if appropriate.

Special Tests
- Lachman, anterior drawer, and pivot shift tests
- Posterior drawer test to evaluate for posterior cruciate ligament (PCL) injury
- McMurray test to evaluate for meniscus tear
- Dial test to evaluate for posterolateral corner (PLC) injury
- Valgus and varus stress to evaluate the collateral ligaments

- Patella apprehension and patella glide tests to evaluate for possible patella dislocation

Imaging

- Radiographs
  - Obtain standing flexion, lateral, and sunrise views.
  - Findings are often unremarkable; however, lateral tibial avulsion (Segond fracture) is highly suggestive of an ACL tear.
- Magnetic resonance imaging (MRI) of the knee without contrast (Fig. 7-7)
  - Scans show disruption of the ACL and can also identify other ligamentous, osseous, or meniscal injuries.
  - Bony contusions of the lateral femoral condyle and posterior tibia are classic in ACL tears.

Classification

- ACL tears are classified by the amount of anterior translation noted with the Lachman test:
  Grade I: less than 5 mm
  Grade II: 5 to 10 mm
  Grade III: more than 10 mm

Initial Treatment

Patient Education

- Treatment options, as well as the risks and benefits of all options, should be thoroughly reviewed and discussed with the patient.
- Graft selection for surgical reconstruction is made based on a variety of factors. In most cases, it is preferable to use a patient's own tissue (autograft). Allograft (cadaveric tissue) is used when autograft is not available or to supplement inadequate autograft.
- The most common sources of autograft are the hamstring tendons (typically gracilis and semitendinosus) or a bone patella tendon bone (BPTB) graft (central third of the inferior patella, patella tendon, and a small portion of the tibial tuberosity).

First Treatment Steps

- Rest, ice, compression, and elevation are indicated.
- Aspiration may be performed to decrease effusion.
- Maintaining ROM is vital; do not place the patient in a knee immobilizer unless occult fracture is suspected.
- Crutches may be used if the patient cannot bear weight comfortably.

Treatment Options

Nonoperative Management

- Conservative management may be appropriate for patients with a low activity level and less than 5 mm of laxity compared with the unaffected side.

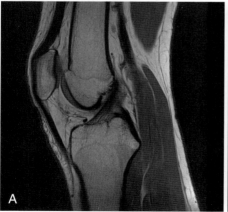 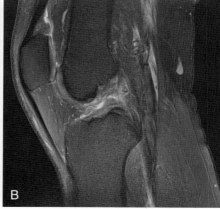

Figure 7-7. Magnetic resonance imaging demonstrating (**A**) intact and (**B**) ruptured anterior cruciate ligament.

- Physical therapy (PT) for ROM and quadriceps strengthening is indicated.
- Without surgery, the patient may have recurrent instability and be at increased risk for meniscus tears and chondral injury or degeneration.

Operative Management
Codes
ICD-9 code: 844.2 Anterior cruciate ligament tear
CPT code: 29888 Anterior cruciate ligament reconstruction

Operative Indications
- Most active patients with symptomatic instability who wish to continue with sports or significant physical activity require surgery to reconstruct the ACL.

Informed Consent and Counseling
- Possible complications include instrument breakage, aberrant tunnels, cartilage injury, hardware failure, loss of motion, residual laxity, paresthesia, effusion, deep vein thrombosis (DVT), and infection. Persistent anterior knee pain, patella tendon rupture, and patella fracture are potential complications if BPTB autograft is used.
- Anesthesia risks include paralysis, cardiac arrest, brain damage, and death.
- Postoperative PT is essential to regain motion and return to sports or physical activities.
- Return to sports is usually not expected until 6 months postoperatively.

Anesthesia
- General anesthesia with regional nerve block

Patient Positioning
- Supine with a knee holder or post, with a tourniquet

Surgical Procedures
Anterior Cruciate Ligament Reconstruction
- Prepare and drape the lower extremity in a sterile fashion.
- Diagnostic arthroscopy is used to visualize the ACL and confirm injury, as well as to evaluate and treat meniscus

tears, loose bodies, and chondral defects.
- Graft harvesting: Techniques vary based on graft choice. A midline incision is made for BPTB graft, and a small oscillating saw is used to cut bone plugs from the patella and tibial tubercle. A medial vertical incision approximately 5 cm below the joint line is made for harvest of a hamstring graft. The semitendinosus and gracilis are identified and harvested with a tendon stripper.
- Graft preparation: This varies based on the graft source. All grafts should be handled carefully and are prepared by a qualified assistant at area separate from the operative field.
- Débridement and notchplasty: Excess fibrous tissue and the ACL stump are débrided with a motorized shaver and bur to allow for better visualization of the back of the notch and to provide clearance for the graft.
- Tunnel placement: The technique for tibial and femoral tunnel placement is determined by the surgeon's preference. The goal is to recreate the normal anatomic position of the ACL.
- Graft passage: Sutures that are attached to both ends of the graft are passed through the tunnels.
- Graft fixation: If BPTB graft is used, the graft is fixed with interference screws. For hamstring graft, an implant designed for soft tissue fixation is used.
- Wound closure: Multilayer closure is augmented with Steri-Strips; then a sterile dressing and an elastic compression (ACE) wrap are applied.

Estimated Postoperative Course
- Postoperative day 0 to 6 weeks
  - The patient may remove the wound dressing the second day after surgery and replace it with self-adhesive bandages, gauze, and an elastic compression (ACE) wrap.
  - Ice, elevation, and pain medication as needed (PRN) are indicated for comfort.
  - The patient uses a cane or crutches for the first few days for comfort.

- Begin PT on postoperative day 1 or 2. Early-stage PT focuses on ROM, edema control, scar management, isometric quadriceps strengthening, and normalization of gait.
- A wound check, suture removal, and assessment of ROM and stability are performed at 10 to 14 days postoperatively.
■ Postoperative 6 weeks to 3 months
- Obtain radiographs to assess tunnels and the position of the graft fixation device.
- Evaluate healing of the surgical site, ROM, and stability of reconstruction.
- Advance PT.
■ Postoperative 3+ months
- Evaluate ROM and stability of reconstruction.
- The patient may begin straight ahead running at 3 months under the guidance of a physical therapist or a certified athletic trainer (ATC).
- The patient may return to sports at 6 months if able to pass functional testing with the ATC or the physical therapist.

Suggested Readings

Gianconi JC, Allen CR, Steinbach LS: Anterior cruciate ligament graft reconstruction, *Top Magn Reson Imaging* 20:129–150, 2009.

Michelic R, Jurdana H, Jotanovic Z, et al: Long-term results of anterior cruciate ligament reconstruction: a comparison with non-operative treatment with a follow-up of 17-20 years, *Int Orthop* 35:1093–1097, 2011.

Miller MD: Anterior cruciate ligament injury. In Miller MD, Hart JA, MacKnight JM, editors: *Essential orthopaedics*, Philadelphia, 2010, Saunders, pp 611–615.

Miller MD, Howard RF, Plancher KD: *Surgical atlas of sports medicine*, Philadelphia, 2003, Elsevier Science.

Neuman P, Kostogiannis I, Friden T, et al: Prevalence of tibiofemoral osteoarthritis 15 years after nonoperative treatment of anterior cruciate ligament injury, *Am J Sports Med* 36(9):1717–1725, 2008.

POSTERIOR CRUCIATE LIGAMENT INJURY

History

■ The mechanism of injury is typically a blow to the anterior tibia (i.e., dashboard injury) or a fall on a plantar flexed foot. Hyperextension or hyperflexion injuries also lead to PCL tear.
■ Effusion is noted.
■ Frank instability may or may not be present.
■ Anterior and medial knee pain may be reported in chronic injury.
■ Isolated PCL rupture is rare; it more commonly occurs in the multiligament knee injury.

Physical Examination

■ Observation: Note effusion, ecchymosis, abrasion, and obvious deformity.
■ Palpation: Patellar ballottement is performed to assess for effusion. Joint line tenderness may be present because of concurrent meniscus tear.
■ ROM: Decreased ROM may result from effusion.

Special Tests: Figures 7-8 and 7-9

■ Posterior drawer test: See the classification section.
■ Posterior sag test: With the knee and hip at 90 degrees of flexion, look for posterior sag of the tibia.
■ Dial test: This is used to assess the PLC.
■ Complete a thorough knee examination to rule out other ligamentous, meniscal, or patellar disorders.

Imaging

■ Radiographs: Standing flexion, lateral, and sunrise views are often unremarkable, but they may show a PCL avulsion fragment. Stress views are obtained by applying posterior force to the proximal tibia with a Telos device.

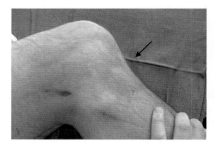

Figure 7-8. Positive posterior sag test. Note the position of the tibia *(arrow)*. *(From Miller MD, Hart JA, MacKnight JM, editors:* Essential orthopaedics, *Philadelphia, 2010, Saunders.)*

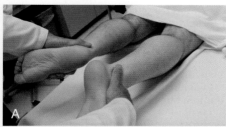
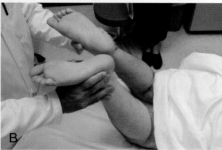

Figure 7-9. External rotation asymmetry. With the knees stabilized, both feet are passively externally rotated and the thigh-foot angle is measured. Asymmetry of 15 degrees or more implies injury to the posterolateral corner structures. The test is performed in both 30 degrees (**A**) and 90 degrees (**B**) of knee flexion. Asymmetry in both 30 and 90 degrees implies injury to both the posterolateral corner and the posterior cruciate ligament. *(From Miller MD, Hart JA, MacKnight JM, editors:* Essential orthopaedics, *Philadelphia, 2010, Saunders.)*

- MRI: Imaging helps to identify the degree of injury (partial versus complete tear) and associated ligament, meniscus, and chondral injuries.

Classification
- Classification is based in the degree of posterior subluxation of the tibia in relation to the femoral condyles:
  Grade I: partial tear; posterior drawer demonstrating posterior tibial displacement that is anterior to the anterior aspect of the femoral condyles
  Grade II: posterior drawer demonstrating posterior tibial displacement that is flush with the anterior aspect of the femoral condyles
  Grade III: complete tear; posterior drawer demonstrating posterior

tibial displacement posterior to the anterior aspect of the femoral condyles

Initial Treatment
Patient Education
- Unlike the ACL, the PCL has some healing potential.
- Not all PCL injuries require surgical reconstruction. Nonoperative management consists of intensive PT.
- Some research indicates an increased risk of developing degenerative changes in the PCL-deficient knee, especially in the patellofemoral compartment.

First Treatment Step
- Elevation, ice, and nonsteroidal antiinflammatory drugs (NSAIDs) to decrease pain and effusion

Treatment Options
Nonoperative Management
- Grade I and II injuries with no or small bone fragment can be managed with PT. The focus of PT is on quadriceps strengthening and ROM.
- Patients may return to sports when quadriceps strength is near normal, approximately 4 weeks after injury.

Operative Management
Codes
ICD-9 code: 844.2 Posterior cruciate ligament tear
CPT code: 29889 Posterior cruciate ligament reconstruction

Operative Indications
- Grade I or II injury with large bone fragment
- Grade III injury
- Chronic grade II or grade III injuries that do not respond to extensive (>6 months) PT.
- Multiligament injury

Informed Consent and Counseling
- Possible complications include residual laxity, instrument breakage, aberrant tunnels, avascular necrosis of the medial femoral condyle, cartilage injury, heterotopic ossification, hardware failure, loss of motion, neurovascular injury, paresthesia, effusion,

DVT, and infection. Anesthesia risks include paralysis, cardiac arrest, brain damage, and death.
- Postoperative PT is essential to regain full ROM, strengthen quadriceps, and return to sport or physical activities.
- Full recovery may take up to 1 year.

Anesthesia
- General with regional nerve block

Patient Positioning
- Supine with a knee holder or post or lateral decubitus, with a tourniquet

Surgical Procedure: Figure 7-10
- Autograft (patellar tendon, quadriceps tendon, or hamstring tendons) or allograft (patellar tendon, quadriceps tendon, Achilles tendon, and hamstring tendons) may be used.

Transtibial Single-Bundle Technique
- The extremity is prepared and draped in standard sterile fashion. The tibial tunnel is drilled at the anterolateral cortex of the proximal tibia. The knee is flexed to 110 degrees while the proximal tibia is pushed in posteriorly. A plastic sheath is placed in contact with the lateral femoral condyle, and then a femoral tunnel is created 2 to 3 mm proximal to the articular junction at the 1 o'clock position in the right knee

or the 11 o'clock position in the left. A fixation device (chosen based on surgeon preference) is attached to the graft with a whipstitch. The graft is passed through both tunnels and secured with interference screws. The incisions are irrigated, then closed, and a sterile dressing is applied.

Arthroscopic Tibial Inlay Technique (Single- or Double-Bundle)
- The extremity is prepared and draped in standard sterile fashion. Anterolateral and anteromedial portals are established. Diagnostic arthroscopy is performed; meniscal and cartilage disorders are addressed. Next, a posteromedial portal is established for instrument passage. The PCL stump is débrided, while preserving the anterior edge of the PCL footprint to serve as a reference point for the inlay. The tibial tunnel is prepared with the knee in flexion. An arthroscopic PCL guide is used to position a pin in the proximal aspect of the PCL footprint. A flip cutter is used to create the tibial socket in an inside-out fashion. A C-arm and the arthroscope are used for guidance. The femoral tunnels are created using a PCL guide centered over the medial femoral condyle at the border of the vastus medialis. For single-bundle reconstruction, the femoral tunnel is drilled at the 11 o'clock position; for double-bundle reconstruction, tunnels are drilled at

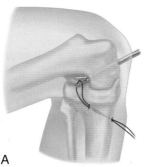
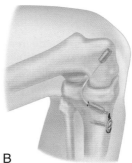

A   B

Figure 7-10. Posterior cruciate ligament reconstruction. **A,** The graft is passed from tibia to femur. **B,** Fixation is established with interference screws, and back-up fixation may be used if desired. (*From Miller MD, Hart JA, editors: SMART: sports medicine assessment and review textbook, Philadelphia, 2011, Saunders.*)

9 o'clock and 11 o'clock positions. Grafts are passed with the knee flexed at 90 degrees. The grafts are fixed (various fixation devices are available). The incisions are irrigated, then closed, and a sterile dressing is applied.

Estimated Postoperative Course

- Postoperative day 0 to 6 weeks
  - Hinged brace locked in full extension at all times for 6 weeks. 50% weight bearing in brace with crutches to assist with ambulation, prone passive ROM with PT.
  - Remove the dressing on the second day after surgery, and replace it with gauze or self-adhesive bandages and an elastic compression (ACE) wrap.
  - Ice, elevation, and PRN pain medications are used for comfort.
  - A wound check, suture removal, and assessment of ROM and stability are performed at 10 to 14 days postoperatively.
- Postoperative 6 weeks to 3 months
  - Obtain radiographs.
  - Assess ROM and stability at 3 months.
  - Wean the patient off crutches and discontinue the brace.
  - Advance PT.
- Postoperative 3+ months
  - Assess ROM and stability.
  - The patient may begin treadmill running and continue to advance PT.
  - The patient may return to recreation activities or sports at 9 to 12 months.

Suggested Readings

Keller T, Miller MD: Posterior cruciate ligament reconstruction: posterior inlay technique. In Scott WM, editor: *Insall and Scott surgery of the knee*, ed 5, Philadelphia, 2012, Churchill Livingstone, pp 538–547.

Kim S, Kin T, Jo S, et al: Comparison of the clinical results of three posterior cruciate ligament reconstruction techniques, *J Bone Joint Surg Am* 91:2543–2549, 2009.

Miller MD, Howard RF, Plancher KD: *Surgical atlas of sports medicine*, Philadelphia, 2003, Elsevier Science.

Patel DV, Answorth AA, Warren RF, et al: The nonoperative treatment of acute isolated (partial or complete) posterior cruciate ligament deficient knees: an intermediate-term follow-up study, *HSS J* 3:137–146, 2007.

Salata MJ, Wojtys EM, Sekiya JK: Posterior cruciate ligament injury. In Miller MD, Hart JA, MacKnight JM, editors: *Essential orthopaedics*, Philadelphia, 2010, Saunders, pp 616–619.

Voos JE, Mauro CS, Wente T, et al: Posterior cruciate ligament: anatomy, biomechanics, and outcomes, *Am J Sports Med* 40:221–231, 2012.

MEDIAL COLLATERAL LIGAMENT INJURY

History

- Acute injury
  - The mechanism of injury is typically valgus stress to the knee. It can result from contact or noncontact injury.
  - Medial knee pain is present.
  - The patient is typically able to bear weight.
  - The patient may report a sensation of instability with pivoting.
  - Effusion may or may not be noted; localized swelling is more common.

Physical Examination

- Observation: Note effusion, ecchymosis, deformity, abrasion or contusion, and gait.
- Palpation: Palpate the entire course of the MCL, from proximal to distal. Tenderness typically indicates some degree of MCL injury. Joint line tenderness is indicative of concomitant meniscus tear. Lateral tenderness of the distal femur and proximal tibia may result from bony contusion.
- ROM: This may be limited by effusion.

Special Tests: Figure 7-11

- Valgus stress testing with the knee in 30 degrees of flexion isolates the MCL and is the most sensitive test.
- Valgus stress testing should also be performed in full extension. Laxity in this position suggests grade III injury (complete rupture), as well as other ligamentous injury.
- The Slocum test is used to evaluate for posteromedial corner (PMC) laxity.
- Complete a through knee examination to rule out other ligamentous, meniscal, or patellar injury.

Imaging

- Radiographs
  - Standing flexion, lateral, and sunrise views are typically normal in acute injury unless bony avulsion

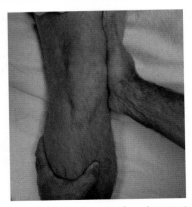

Figure 7-11. Varus stress testing. A varus stress is applied across the knee. This examination is done in both 30 degrees of knee flexion and full extension. Opening in full extension implies concurrent injury to the cruciate ligament. *(From Miller MD, Hart JA, MacKnight JM, editors:* Essential orthopaedics, *Philadelphia, 2010, Saunders.)*

is present. Stress radiographs may be helpful.
- Pellegrini-Stieda lesion: MCL calcification is seen on plain radiographs in chronic MCL injury.
▪ MRI (Fig. 7-12)
- MRI is not required to make the diagnosis, but it may be helpful to identify additional injuries.
- Coronal sequences are best for identifying MCL injury.

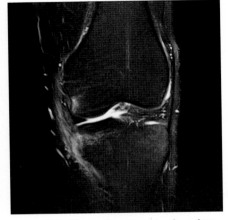

Figure 7-12. Magnetic resonance imaging demonstrating a medial collateral ligament tear.

- Bone bruises of the lateral femoral condyle and lateral tibial plateau may be seen.
- MRI allows for grading: grade I, periligamentous swelling and minor tearing; grade II, complete disruption of superficial layers, deep layers intact; grade III, complete disruption and fluid extravasation.

Classification
▪ Classification is based on the amount of opening noted with valgus stress test:
- Grade I: 1 to 4 mm of laxity with end point
- Grade II: 5 to 9 mm of laxity with end point
- Grade III: 10 to 15 mm of laxity with no firm end point
▪ MCL injury is also graded by MRI findings as previously described.

Initial Treatment
Patient Education
▪ The MCL is the most commonly injured ligament in the knee.
▪ Most MCL sprains will heal with bracing and activity modification.
▪ Persistent laxity may occur if the patient is noncompliant with brace wear.

First Treatment Step
▪ Rest, ice, compression, elevation, NSAIDs

Treatment Options
Nonoperative Management
▪ Playmaker brace: worn during weight-bearing activities until physical examination reveals pain-free motion and stability, typically for 6 to 8 weeks
▪ Typical return to play: grade I, 10 days; grade II, 20 days; grade 3, at least 4 weeks (typically recommend the use of the brace with sports activities for an additional 6 weeks)

Operative Management
Codes
ICD-9 code: 844.1 Medial collateral ligament tear
CPT codes: 27427 Medial collateral ligament reconstruction
27405 Medial collateral ligament primary repair

Operative Indications
- Surgical repair or reconstruction is indicated in patients with persistent laxity or rotatory instability following adequate bracing or in patients with acute multiligament injuries.

Informed Consent and Counseling
- Possible complications include loss of motion, bleeding, infection, DVT, neurovascular injury, residual laxity, instrument breakage, cartilage injury, hardware failure, and effusion. Anesthesia risks include cardiac arrest, paralysis, brain damage, and death.
- Postoperative PT is essential for full recovery and return to sports or physical activities.

Anesthesia
- General, with or without regional nerve block

Patient Positioning
- Supine
- Tourniquet used if needed

Surgical Procedures
Primary Repair
- A medial incision is made between the medial epicondyle and the adductor tubercle. Various suturing techniques are used to re-tension and repair the MCL and surrounding structures such as the posterior oblique ligament and semimembranosus. Suture, suture anchor, or screw with washer is used to repair MCL avulsions from the origin or insertion.
- Wound closure: Multilayer closure is augmented with Steri-Strips; then a sterile dressing and an elastic compression (ACE) wrap are applied.

Reconstruction
- Diagnostic arthroscopy is performed to evaluate and treat concurrent meniscus tear and to determine whether the MCL is torn from the femoral or tibial side.
- A 10- to 15-cm medial hockey stick incision is made. Primary repair is typically completed as described earlier and is then combined or reinforced with MCL reconstruction using

semitendinosus autograft or allograft. The graft tissue is used to reconstruct the superficial MCL anatomically. The graft is secured at the anatomic origin and insertion with screws and washers or sutures. The posteromedial capsule can be secured to the graft to eliminate laxity.
- Wound closure: Multilayer closure is augmented with Steri-Strips; then a sterile dressing and an elastic compression (ACE) wrap are applied

Estimated Postoperative Course
- Postoperative day 0 to 6 weeks
  - An integrated ROM (IROM) brace locked in full extension is worn at all times for the first 2 weeks, then at 0 to 90 degrees for weeks 2 to 6. The patient has 50% weight bearing with crutches.
  - The patient may remove the dressing on the second day after surgery and replace it with gauze or self-adhesive bandages and an elastic compression (ACE) wrap.
  - Ice, elevation, and PRN pain medications are used for comfort.
  - A wound check, suture removal, and assessment of ROM and stability are performed at 10 to 14 days postoperatively.
  - Begin PT 10 to 14 days postoperatively.
- Postoperative 6 weeks to 3 months
  - Full weight bearing is allowed as tolerated; the patient may be weaned off crutches. Discontinue the brace.
  - Obtain radiographs, evaluate healing of the surgical site, and assess ROM and stability of reconstruction.
  - PT: Advance to full ROM as soon as possible, facilitate gait normalization with treadmill walking, and continue quadriceps strengthening.
- Postoperative 3+ months
  - Evaluate ROM and stability of reconstruction.
  - PT: The patient may begin jogging on a treadmill.
  - The patient may initiate sport-specific activities under supervision of a physical therapist or an ATC at

4 months, with full return to sports at 6 months.

Suggested Readings

Fanelli GC, Harris, MD: Surgical treatment of acute medial collateral ligament and postero-medial corner injuries of the knee, *Sports Med Arthrosc Rev* 14:78–83, 2006.
Jacobson KE, Chi FS: Evaluation and treatment of medial collateral ligament and medial-sided injuries of the knee, *Sports Med Arthrosc Rev* 14:58–66, 2006.
Kurzweil RK, Kelley ST: Physical exam and imaging of the medial collateral ligament and posteromedial corner of the knee, *Sports Med Arthrosc Rev* 14:67–73, 2006.
Long JL, Carpenter JE: Medial collateral ligament injury. In Miller MD, Hart JA, MacKnight JM, editors: *Essential orthopaedics*, Philadelphia, 2010, Saunders, pp 620–623.

KNEE DISLOCATION

History
- The mechanism of injury is typically high-energy trauma such as a motor vehicle collision, but it can also occur in lower-velocity sports injuries. Knee dislocation can occur in obese patients with events that involve minimal trauma.
- Large effusion is noted.
- Pain is extreme.
- An obvious deformity may be present, but the knee may also spontaneously reduce before the patient seeks medical attention.

Physical Examination
- Observation
  - Effusion
  - Bruising and/or abrasions
  - Deformity

Special Tests
- Compartment syndrome evaluation
  - Remember the six Ps: pain, pressure, paresthesia, pulselessness, pallor, and paralysis.
  - Monitor compartment pressures.
  - Consider checking serum creatine kinase and urine myoglobin levels.
- Vascular examination
  - Serial examination must be performed.
  - Dorsalis pedis and posterior tibial pulses should be symmetric bilaterally.
  - Check the ankle-brachial index (ABI). An ABI greater than 0.9 is considered normal.
  - An abnormal ABI is an indication for an arteriogram with venous runoff.
  - Request a vascular surgery consultation if available.
- Neurologic examination
  - Evaluate motor function and sensation.
- Knee ligament examination (knee dislocation often causes multiligament injury)
  - ACL: Lachman, pivot shift, and anterior drawer tests
  - PCL: posterior drawer test
  - Collateral ligaments: valgus and varus stress tests
  - PLC: dial test

Pearl
Many knee dislocations are obvious on clinical examination because of joint deformity, but the clinician should be cautious because some dislocations spontaneously reduce before medical examination. *Always* complete a thorough neurovascular examination on a patient who presents with an acute traumatic knee injury.

 ORTHOPAEDIC WARNING

Neurovascular injury is exceedingly common with knee dislocation. Serial examination is key, and a high index of suspicion must be maintained when evaluating these injuries. Many centers recommend arteriograms and/or vascular consultations for all knee dislocations in the emergency department.

Imaging
- Radiographs (Fig. 7-13): Anteroposterior (AP) and lateral views help to identify associated osseous injuries such as tibial plateau fracture, proximal fibular fracture, avulsion of Gerdy tubercle, intercondylar spine fracture, fibular head avulsion, and Segond or PCL avulsion fragments. Stress views

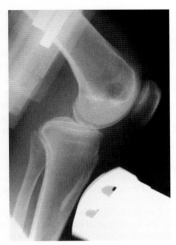

Figure 7-13. Stress radiograph demonstrating posterior translation secondary to posterior cruciate ligament rupture.

will help assess degree of laxity resulting from ligamentous injury.
- MRI is not needed on an emergency basis, but it is helpful for identifying the extent of ligament injury and preparing for surgical reconstruction.
- Arteriogram with venous runoff is used to assess for vascular injury.

Classification
- Open versus closed
- Reducible versus irreducible
- Types of dislocations also defined by the direction of displacement of the

tibia in respect to the femoral condyles: posterior, anterior, medial, lateral, and rotator (Fig. 7-14)

Initial Treatment
Patient Education
- Knee dislocation can result in multiligament injury.
- The peroneal nerve, which provides sensation to the dorsum of the foot and controls dorsiflexion of the ankle, is injured in up to 20% of knee dislocations.
- Popliteal artery injury occurs in approximately 19% of knee dislocations.
- The long-term risk of posttraumatic arthritis is approximately 50%.

First Treatment Steps
- Closed reduction should be performed as soon as possible. Once the dislocation is reduced, repeat a neurovascular examination. Apply a long-leg splint or knee immobilizer; then repeat the radiographs to ensure that reduction is maintained.
- Rapid identification and repair of vascular injuries are essential. Delay of 6 to 8 hours is associated with a high amputation rate.

Treatment Options
Nonoperative Management
- Nonoperative management is usually associated with significant instability and poor outcome.

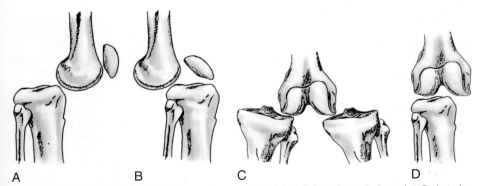

A   B   C   D

Figure 7-14. Descriptive classification system of knee joint dislocations. **A,** Posterior. **B,** Anterior. **C,** Medial or lateral. **D,** Rotatory. (From Bryant BJ, Musahl V, Harner CD: The dislocated knee. In Scott WN, editor: Insall and Scott surgery of the knee, ed 5, Philadelphia, 2012, Churchill Livingstone.)

Operative Management
- Emergency surgery may be necessary if the dislocation is not reducible or evidence indicates vascular injury.
- Surgical reconstruction will address multiligament injury. Timing often depends on the presence or absence of vascular injury. If vascular injury was previously repaired, consult a vascular surgeon for clearance before proceeding with ligament reconstruction.
- If initial surgery must be delayed because of other more urgent injuries, the use of an external fixator may be necessary until definitive treatment with ligament reconstruction can be safely performed.
- A combination of allograft and autograft is typically used for multiligament reconstruction.
- Ligament reconstruction is performed as described in previous sections.
- Later tendon transfer may be needed for patients with nerve injury.

Estimated Postoperative Course
- Postoperative day 0 to 6 weeks
  - An IROM brace locked in full extension is worn at all times for the first 2 weeks and then at 0 to 90 degrees for weeks 2 to 6. The patient is 50% weight bearing with crutches for 6 weeks.
  - Remove the dressing on the second day after surgery, and replace it with gauze or self-adhesive bandages and an elastic compression (ACE) wrap.
  - Ice, elevation, and PRN pain medications are indicated.
  - A wound check, suture removal, and assessment of ROM and stability are performed at 10 to 14 days postoperatively.
  - PT: Straight leg raises with brace locked in extension, ROM exercises in the prone position, scar management, and modalities are used. The patient may begin using the stationary bike at 2 weeks.
- Postoperative 6 weeks to 3 months
  - Full weight bearing is allowed as tolerated; the patient may be weaned off crutches. Discontinue the brace.
  - PT: Advance to full ROM as soon as possible, facilitate gait normalization

with treadmill walking, and continue quadriceps strengthening.
- Postoperative 3+ months
  - PT: The patient may begin jogging on a treadmill and doing isokinetic exercises.
  - The patient may initiate sport-specific activities under the supervision of a physical therapist or an ATC at 4 months, with full return to sports at 6 months.

Suggested Readings
Harner CD, Waltrip RL, Bennet CH: Surgical management of knee dislocations, *J Bone Joint Surg Am* 45:889, 2004.
Levy BA, Fanelli GC, Whelan DB, et al: Controversies on the treatment of knee dislocation and multiligament reconstruction, *J Am Orthop Surg* 17:197–206, 2009.
Mook WR, Miller MD, Diduch DR, et al: Multiple-ligament knee injuries: a systematic review of the timing of operative intervention and postoperative rehabilitation, *J Bone Joint Surg Am* 19:2946–2857, 2009.
Salata MJ, Wojtys EM, Sekiya JK: Knee dislocation. In Miller MD, Hart JA, MacKnight JM, editors: *Essential orthopaedics*, Philadelphia, 2010, Saunders, pp 628–632.

PATELLA CHONDROMALACIA
History
- Patients complain of anterior knee pain that is aggravated by running, squatting, ascending or descending stairs, walking on inclines, sitting with the knee bent for a prolonged period, and rising from a seated position.
- Pain is typically described as "achy," but it may be sharp at times.
- Patients may complain that the knee gives way. This pseudoinstability is the result of pain, which inhibits proper contraction of the quadriceps.
- "Popping" or "creaking" under the patella is a common complaint.
- The patient may complain of "catching" under the patella (pseudolocking); however, true locking is not typical of patellofemoral chondromalacia. Locking is an indication of other disorders such as a meniscus tear.

Physical Examination
- Observation: Gait, body habitus, knee alignment (valgus/varus), foot pronation,

pes planus/cavus, quadriceps atrophy, and effusion are noted.
- Palpation: Note patellar tenderness, tenderness of quadriceps or patellar tendon, tight lateral retinaculum, and crepitus.
- ROM should be normal. There may be anterior knee pain with the upper range of flexion.
  - Assess patellar mobility.

Special Tests
- Patellar grind and patellar apprehension tests (Fig. 7-15)

Imaging
- Radiographs (Fig. 7-16)
  - Obtain standing flexion, lateral, and sunrise views.
  - Radiographs are helpful in ruling out other causes of pain such as loose body, degenerative changes, bipartite patella, and fracture.
  - Patellar tilt may be seen on the sunrise view.
- MRI
  - This is warranted only in refractory cases to rule out other pathologic processes.

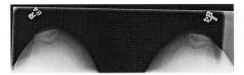

Figure 7-16. Lateral patellar tilt is seen on a radiograph in a patient with patellofemoral pain.

Initial Treatment
Patient Education
- Patellofemoral pain can almost always be managed nonoperatively with activity modification, PT, and a home exercise program.
- It may take an extended period for symptoms to improve; compliance with PT and a home exercise program is essential for recovery.
- Patients should be counseled on the importance of obtaining or maintaining a healthy body weight.

First Treatment Step
- Rest, ice, NSAIDs

Treatment Options
Nonoperative Management
- Initial treatment includes:
  - Activity modification: Patients must avoid activity that causes pain. Runners must decrease distance and frequency. Those with severe pain may have to stop running and cross train on a stationary bike or elliptical machine during the rehabilitation period.
  - NSAIDs: A short course (2 to 3 weeks) may help to decrease pain.
- PT for quadriceps strengthening with emphasis on the VMO, hip adductor strengthening, and stretching to increase quadriceps hamstring and iliotibial band (ITB) flexibility.
- Other modalities such as ice, electrical stimulation, iontophoresis. and ultrasound may be beneficial.
- Patellar taping or bracing is used.
- Custom orthotics may be used to address foot pronation and/or pes planus.
- Corticosteroid injection may be indicated.

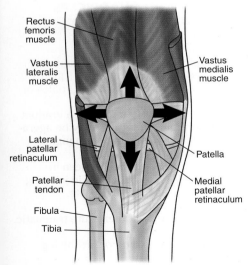

Rectus femoris muscle

Vastus lateralis muscle

Vastus medialis muscle

Lateral patellar retinaculum

Patella

Patellar tendon

Medial patellar retinaculum

Fibula

Tibia

Figure 7-15. The patella is stabilized by dynamic (muscles) and static (retinaculum and tendon) restraints. *(From Miller MD, Hart JA, MacKnight JM, editors:* Essential orthopaedics, *Philadelphia, 2010, Saunders.)*

Operative Management
Codes
ICD-9 code: 717.7 Patellofemoral chondromalacia
CPT code: 29877 Arthroscopic débridement and shaving chondroplasty

Operative Indications
- Arthroscopic débridement may be considered as a last resort when extensive conservative treatment has failed.

Informed Consent and Counseling
- Potential risks: bleeding, infection, DVT or pulmonary embolism (PE), loss of motion, cartilage injury, damage to nearby structures, and tourniquet complications
- Anesthesia complications: paralysis, cardiac arrest, brain damage, and death

Anesthesia
- General, and local anesthetic injected at portal sites after closure

Patient Positioning
- Supine with a leg holder or post and a tourniquet

Surgical Procedures
Arthroscopic Débridement and Chondroplasty
- Two small incisions are made medial and lateral to the patella tendon slightly above the joint line. An arthroscope is used to explore the suprapatellar pouch, patellofemoral joint, intercondylar notch, medial and lateral compartments, and medial and lateral gutters. A shaver is used to débride the patella and other areas of cartilage fraying.

Estimated Postoperative Course
- Postoperative day 0 to 6 weeks
  - Full weight bearing is allowed as tolerated, and crutches or a cane may be used if needed.
  - Ice, elevation, and PRN pain medications are indicated for comfort.
  - Remove the dressing 2 days after surgery, and replace it with a self-adhesive bandage or gauze.
  - Patients may begin using a stationary bicycle 2 to 3 days after surgery.

Start with low resistance for short periods and advance as tolerated. Swimming and use of an elliptical trainer may be started 1 week after surgery.
- Sutures are removed 10 to 14 days after surgery.
- Formal PT is indicated in patients with decreased ROM, persistent effusion, or quadriceps atrophy.
- Postoperative 6+ weeks
  - Full recovery is likely by this time. If the patient is still experiencing pain; continued PT should be recommended.

Suggested Readings
Collado H, Fredericson M: Patellofemoral pain syndrome, *Clin Sports Med* 29:379–398, 2010.
Fredericson M, Koon K: Physical examination and patellofemoral pain syndrome, *Am J Phys Med Rehabil* 85:234–243, 2006.
Parker RD: Patellofemoral pain syndrome. In Miller MD, Hart JA, MacKnight JM, editors: *Essential orthopaedics*, Philadelphia, 2010, Saunders, pp 660–662.
Prins MR, van der Wurff P: Females with patellofemoral pain syndrome have weak hip muscles: a systematic review, *Aust J Physiother* 55:5–15, 2009.

PATELLA AND QUADRICEPS TENDON DISORDERS
History
- Tendinitis
  - Typically, presentation is anterior knee pain at the superior (quadriceps) or inferior (patellar) poles of the patella.
  - The patient often reports a gradual onset, but symptoms may be aggravated by increasing or changing workouts.
  - This is most commonly seen in patients who participate in jumping, running, and kicking sports.
- Tendon rupture
  - Usually present after acute traumatic injury
  - Inability to extend or lift the leg
  - Severe pain
  - Immediate effusion
  - Possible history of knee pain or tendinitis before acute injury
  - Possible history of steroid injection or anabolic steroid use

- Patella tendon ruptures more common in patients less than 40 years of age, whereas quadriceps tendon ruptures more common in patients more than 40 years of age

Physical Examination
- Tendinitis
  - Observation: focal swelling of the affected tendon
  - Palpation: tenderness at the patellar poles and along the tendon
  - ROM: should be full; pain possible with the upper range of flexion

Tendon Rupture
- Observation: effusion, ecchymosis
- Palpation: palpable defect at the site of rupture
- ROM: complete loss of active extension
- Quadriceps tendon rupture: no movement of the patella with contraction of the quadriceps
- Patella tendon rupture: movement of the patella with contraction of the quadriceps

Imaging: Figure 7-17
- Radiographs: AP, lateral, and sunrise views are used to rule out fracture

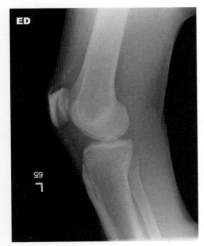

Figure 7-17. A bony fragment avulsed from the patella can be seen on this lateral radiograph of a patient following quadriceps tendon rupture.

(the patella may be "high" with patella tendon rupture and "low" with quadriceps tendon rupture).
- MRI is not typically needed to evaluate acute tendon rupture, but it may be helpful in chronic tendinitis to evaluate degree of tendinopathy and other disorders.

Classification
- Patellar tendinitis can be classified using the system developed by Blazina in 1973:
  Phase I: pain only after activity
  Phase II: pain or discomfort during activity, but no interference with participation
  Phase III: pain both during and after participation that interferes with competition
  Phase IV: complete tendon disruption

Initial Treatment
Patient Education
- Tendinitis is an overuse injury. Activity modification and rest are the mainstays of treatment.
- Tendinitis can progress to tendon rupture.
- Tendon rupture should be surgically repaired acutely to improve the chances of a good outcome.

First Treatment Steps
- Tendinitis: rest, ice, NSAIDs
- Tendon rupture: immobilization in extension, ice, elevation

Treatment Options
Nonoperative Management
- Tendinitis
  - Rest for 4 to 6 weeks followed by gradual return to the previous level of activity
  - PT: stretching (quadriceps, hamstring, and Achilles), core strengthening, endurance training
  - Therapeutic modalities: ice, ultrasound, electrical stimulation
  - Patella tendon strap or taping
- Tendon rupture
  - Immobilization in extension
  - Crutches with weight bearing as tolerated

Operative Management

Codes
ICD-9 codes: 726.64 Patellar tendinitis
844.8 Patella or quadriceps tendon
rupture
CPT codes: 27350 Tendon débridement
27380 Patella tendon repair
27385 Quadriceps tendon repair

Operative Indications
■ Tendinitis
  • Persistent symptoms after 3 to
    6 months of extensive nonoperative
    measures
■ Tendon rupture
  • Surgical repair: performed as soon
    as possible in all patients unless
    they are medically unstable

Informed Consent and Counseling
■ Potential risks include rerupture,
  extensor mechanism dysfunction, loss
  of motion, failure to restore normal
  patella height, bleeding, infection,
  wound complications, and DVT or PE.
■ Anesthesia risks include paralysis, cardiac arrest, brain damage, and death.
■ Postoperative PT is essential to regain
  function, strength, and to return to
  sports or physical activity.

Anesthesia
■ General, with or without regional block

Patient Positioning
■ Supine

Surgical Procedures

Tendon Débridement
■ The surgical site is prepared and draped
  in standard sterile fashion. A midline
  incision is made to expose the tendon.
  The diseased portion of the tendon is
  excised and débrided. A rongeur or
  small drill bit may be used on the patellar pole to create marrow stimulation
  and promote healing. The tendon, peritenon, and skin are closed in a multilayer
  fashion, and a sterile dressing is applied.

Tendon Repair
■ Patellar tendon
  • The surgical site is prepared and
    draped in standard sterile fashion.
    A midline incision is made to expose

the patella and ruptured tendon.
Degenerated or inflammatory tissue
is débrided. The distal pole of
patella is dissected with a curette
and rongeur; #5 Ethibond sutures
are woven into the patellar tendon.
Three longitudinal holes are drilled
from the distal pole to the proximal
pole of the patella. Ethibond sutures
are passed through the drill holes
with a suture passer. Sutures are tied
to complete an anatomic reconstruction. The wound is irrigated and
closed in a multilayer fashion, and
then a sterile dressing is applied.
■ Quadriceps tendon
  • The surgical site is prepared and
    draped in standard sterile fashion.
    A midline incision is made to expose
    the patella and ruptured tendon.
    The superior pole of the patella is dis-
    sected using a curette and rongeur.
    Using #5 FiberWire, three stitches are
    placed into the quadriceps tendon.
    Four longitudinal tunnels are drilled
    through the patella, and sutures are
    passed through the tunnels. Ana-
    tomic reconstruction is completed
    by securing knots at the distal end of
    the patella. The wound is irrigated
    and closed in a multilayer fashion,
    and then a sterile dressing is applied.

Estimated Postoperative Course
■ Postoperative day 0 to 6 weeks
  • A hinged knee brace locked in full
    extension is used for 4 weeks.
  • The patient is allowed full weight
    bearing in a brace.
  • Perform a wound check and
    suture removal at 10 to 14 days
    postoperatively.
  • Begin PT at 2 weeks postoperatively.
  • ROM can progress to 0 to 60 degrees
    at 4 weeks.
■ Postoperative 6 weeks to 3 months
  • Assess surgical site healing.
  • ROM is from 0 to 90 and advanced
    as tolerated.
  • Advance PT.
■ Postoperative 3+ months
  • Assess the surgical site, extensor
    mechanism, and ROM.
  • The patient may initiate jogging on
    a treadmill.

Suggested Readings

Blazina ME, Kerlan RK, Jobe FW, Carter VS, Carlson GJ: Jumper's Knee, *Orthop Clin North Am* 4(3):665–78.

Bolvig FU: Jumper's knee, *Scand J Med Sci Sports* 9:66–73, 1999.

Boublik M, Schlegel T, Koonce R, et al: Patellar tendon rupture in national football league players, *Am J Sports Med* 39:2436–2442, 2011.

Miller MD, Howard RF, Plancher KD: *Surgical atlas of sports medicine*, Philadelphia, 2003, Elsevier Science.

Parker RD: Extensor tendon rupture. In Miller MD, Hart JA, MacKnight JM, editors: *Essential orthopaedics*, Philadelphia, 2010, Saunders, p 677.

Parker RD: Quadriceps and patellar tendonitis. In Miller MD, Hart JA, MacKnight JM, editors: *Essential orthopaedics*, Philadelphia, 2010, Saunders, p 669.

Rees JD, Wilson AM, Wolman RL: Current concepts in the management of tendon disorders, *Rheumatology* 45:508–521, 2006.

PATELLA INSTABILITY

History

- The patient may present with acute traumatic dislocation or with a complaint of chronic dislocation or subluxation.
- Acute patellar dislocation is a common cause of hemarthrosis.
- The patella may have to be manually reduced or may spontaneously reduce.
- Patients with chronic instability often report anterior knee pain and a sensation that the knee is "giving way" or "going out."

Physical Examination

- Observation: gait, lower extremity alignment, effusion
- Palpation: tenderness along the medial border of the patella

Special Tests

- Patellar grind
- Patella apprehension
- J sign: The patella shifts laterally when the knee is extended (Fig. 7-18).
- Q angle: The angle is formed from a line drawn from the anterior superior iliac spine to the center of the kneecap and from the center of the kneecap to the tibial tubercle. Measure that angle, and subtract from 180 degrees to determine Q angle.
- Thorough knee examination to rule out ligamentous and meniscal injury

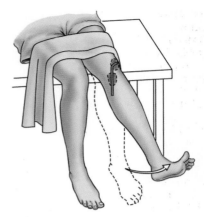

Figure 7-18. The J sign is positive when the patella suddenly shifts laterally when the knee is extended. *(From Miller MD, Hart JA, MacKnight JM, editors:* Essential orthopaedics, *Philadelphia, 2010, Saunders.)*

Imaging

- Radiographs: Standing flexion, lateral and sunrise views may show trochlear dysplasia, patella alta subluxation or tilt of the patella, and degenerative changes.
- MRI may show effusion, loose body, avulsion fracture, chondral injury, medial patellofemoral ligament (MPFL) tear, and subchondral edema (lateral femoral condyle and medial patella) (Fig. 7-19).

Classification

- A classification system was developed by Dejour et al:
  - Major patellar instability: more than one documented dislocation
  - Objective patellar instability: one dislocation with associated anatomic abnormality
  - Potential patellar instability: patellar pain with associated radiographic abnormalities
- Patellar instability is also classified as congenital, traumatic, obligatory, subluxation, or dislocation.

Initial Treatment

Patient Education

- The etiology of patellar instability is multifactorial. The following structural and functional factors can play a role

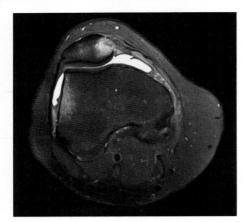

Figure 7-19. Magnetic resonance imaging demonstrating subchondral edema of the medial patella and lateral femoral condyle following patella dislocation.

in instability: patella alta, trochlear dysplasia or shallow groove, malalignment of the tibial tubercle, vastus medialis insufficiency, tight lateral structures, deficient MPFL, and joint laxity.
- The rate of recurrent dislocation can be as high as 60%.

First Treatment Step
- Reduction: Pain control and sedation may be required. Place the patient in the supine position with the hips flexed. Slowly extend the knee while applying medial pressure to the lateral aspect of the patella.

Treatment Options
Nonoperative Management
- Crutches may be needed initially to assist with ambulation.
- Rest, ice, elevation, and NSAIDs are indicated.
- Limit activities that cause pain.
- Aspiration may be indicated for a large effusion that interferes with ROM.
- PT is indicated for quadriceps strengthening with emphasis on the vastus medialis, strengthening of the hip abductors and flexors, edema control, and ROM.
- Patella taping or a patella stabilizing brace may provide symptomatic relief.

- Weight loss is recommended to reduce the patellofemoral load.

Operative Management
Codes
ICD-9 code: 718.86 Patella instability
CPT codes: 29873 Arthroscopic lateral release
27427 Medial patellofemoral ligament reconstruction
27418 Fulkerson osteotomy

Operative Indications
- Recurrent instability despite adequate PT

Informed Consent and Counseling
- Potential risks: loss of motion, infection, DVT or PE, wound complications, neurovascular injury, recurrent dislocation, and nonunion (Fulkerson osteotomy)
- Anesthesia risks: paralysis, cardiac arrest, brain damage, and death

Anesthesia
- General, with or without regional block

Patient Positioning
- Supine

Surgical Procedures
Proximal Repair and Realignment Procedures
- Primary repair of the MPFL: This procedure is indicated when instability is secondary to avulsion of the MPFL from the patellar or femoral attachment, rather than abnormal alignment. If the MPFL is disrupted at the patellar attachment, it is reattached to the patella with nonabsorbable sutures placed through drill holes in the patella. When the MPFL is torn from its femoral attachment, two suture anchors are placed into the femur at the MPFL origin, and mattress sutures are used to secure the MPFL.
- Reconstruction of the MPFL: This procedure is indicated when the MPFL is deficient or attenuated. Soft tissue autograft or allograft (semitendinosus tendon) is used. The graft can be fixed to the patella with an

EndoButton fixation device, interference screw, or biotenodesis screw. A screw and washer are used for femoral fixation.

■ Lateral retinaculum release: This procedure is most often performed in combination with the previously mentioned medial stabilization techniques. Lateral release is indicated only for patients with a tight retinaculum leading to patellar tilt. The lateral retinaculum is released proximal to the patellar pole; the vastus lateralis is left intact to reduce medial patellar subluxation.

Distal Realignment Procedure
■ This procedure is performed when instability results from malalignment.

Anterior Tibial Tubercle Transfer (Fulkerson Osteotomy): Figure 7-20
■ This procedure is indicated when the patella does not track properly because of an abnormal trochlea or high patella. The tibial tubercle is detached and then anteriorized, medialized, and secured with cortical screws. This procedure unloads the patellofemoral joint and corrects the Q angle.
■ Proximal and distal realignment procedures are often used in combination.

Estimated Postoperative Course
■ Postoperative day 0 to 6 weeks
  • Hinged brace locked in full extension
  • Crutches and toe touch weight bearing for 2 weeks for MPFL

reconstruction and 6 weeks for Fulkerson osteotomy
  • Removal by the patient of the surgical dressing the third day after surgery and replacement with gauze or self-adhesive bandages.
  • Wound check and suture removal 10 to 14 days postoperatively
  • Passive ROM 0 to 90 degrees for the first 6 weeks
■ Postoperative 6 weeks to 3 months
  • Discontinuation of brace
  • Radiographs after Fulkerson osteotomy; partial weight bearing and gait training begun for patients with adequate healing
  • ROM: 0 degrees to full
  • Exercise bicycle, closed chain kinetic exercises, and hamstring, adductor, abductor, quadriceps, and Achilles stretching begun
■ Postoperative 3+ months
  • Radiographs to assess bony union after Fulkerson osteotomy at 3 months.
  • Progressive quadriceps strengthening exercises; return to sports typically 3 to 5 months after MPFL repair and reconstruction and 8 to 12 months after Fulkerson osteotomy

Suggested Readings

Dejour H, Walch G, Nove-Josserand L, et al: Factors of patella instability: an anatomic radiographic study, *Knee Surg Sports Traumatol Arthrosc* 2:19–26, 1994.

Farr J, Schepsis AA: Reconstruction of the medial patellofemoral ligament for recurrent patellar instability, *J Knee Surg* 19:307–316, 2008.

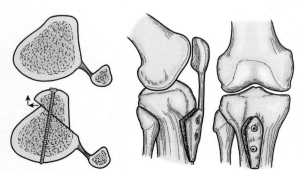

Figure 7-20. Fulkerson osteotomy. *(From Aglietti P, Buzzi R, Insall J: Disorders of the femoral joint. In Scott WN, editor: Insall and Scott surgery of the knee, ed 4, Philadelphia, 2006, Churchill Livingstone.)*

Parker RD: Patellar instability. In Miller MD, Hart JA, MacKnight JM, editors: *Essential orthopaedics*, Philadelphia, 2010, Saunders, pp 663–665.

Post WR, Fulkerson JP: Distal realignment of the patellofemoral joint: indications, effects, results and recommendations. In Scott WM, editor: *Insall and Scott surgery of the knee*, ed 5, Philadelphia, 2012, Churchill Livingstone, pp 624–639.

Redziniak DE, Diduch DR, Mihalko WM, et al: Patellar instability, *J Bone Joint Surg Am* 91: 2264–2265, 2009.

CARTILAGE INJURIES

History
- These injuries may occur along with acute injury to ACL, meniscus, collateral ligaments or patella dislocation.
- These injuries can occur secondary to high-energy trauma or dashboard injury when the patella is forced into the trochlea.
- Acute pain with or without effusion (possible hemarthrosis if subchondral bone is fractured) is noted.
- Pain is aggravated by weight bearing.
- Mechanical symptoms such as locking or catching may occur if there is a cartilage flap or loose body (cartilage displaced into the joint).
- Osteochondritis dissecans (OCD) is a condition that typically affects the pediatric population. This condition is characterized by separation of an osteochondral fragment with or without articular cartilage involvement. It manifests with the foregoing symptoms. The origin appears to be idiopathic.

Physical Examination
- Observation: gait, effusion, ecchymosis or abrasion, quadriceps atrophy
- Palpation
  - Tenderness of the femoral condyles or undersurface of the patella
  - Ballotable effusion
  - Palpable "clunk" with ROM an indication of a displaced cartilage flap
- ROM
  - Possibly decreased secondary to effusion
  - Possible blockage by loose body of full extension and/or flexion
  - Crepitus possible with large lesions

Special Tests
- No special test for cartilage injury is available, but a thorough examination should be completed to rule out ligamentous or meniscal injury.

Imaging
- Radiographs
  - Standing flexion, lateral, and sunrise views to rule out osteoarthritis (OA), fracture, or OCD
- MRI (Fig. 7-21)
  - Helps to identify location and size of lesion
  - May show bone edema indicating overloading of the affected area
  - Can identify or rule out other disorders
- Computed tomography (CT)
  - Identifies fractures and size of bone fragments

Classification: Tables 7-7 to 7-9
- Classification systems for articular cartilage defects are shown in Tables 7-8 and 7-9.

Initial Treatment
Patient Education
- Articular cartilage lesions have limited healing potential, and persistent defects may progress to secondary OA.

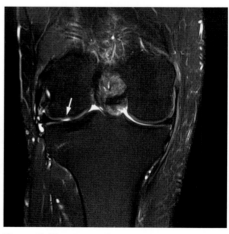

Figure 7-21. Magnetic resonance imaging demonstrating a chondral defect.

Table 7-7. Clanton and DeLee Classification System for Osteochondritis Dissecans Lesions

Type I	Depressed chondral fracture
Type II	Fragment attached by osseous bridge
Type III	Detached nondisplaced fragment
Type IV	Displaced fragment

Data from Clanton TO, DeLee JC: Osteochondritis dissecans. History, pathophysiology, and current treatment concepts, Clin Orthop Relat Res 167:50-64, 1982.

Table 7-8. Outerbridge Arthroscopic Grading System

Grade 0	Normal cartilage
Grade I	Softening and swelling
Grade II	Partial thickness defect, fissures <1.5 cm diameter
Grade III	Fissures down to subchondral bone, diameter >1.5 cm
Grade IV	Exposed subchondral bone

Data from Spahn G, Klinger HM, Hofmann GO: How valid is the arthroscopic diagnosis of cartilage lesions? Results od an opinion survey among highly experienced arthroscopic surgeons, Arch Orthop Trauma Surg 129:1117-1121, 2010.

Table 7-9. International Cartilage Repair Society Grading System

Grade 0	Normal
Grade 1	Nearly normal, superficial lesions
Grade 2	Abnormal, lesions extend <50% of cartilage depth
Grade 3	Severely abnormal, lesions extend >50% of cartilage depth
Grade 4	Lesions extend to subchondral bone

Data from Spahn G, Klinger HM, Hofmann GO: How valid is the arthroscopic diagnosis of cartilage lesions? Results od an opinion survey among highly experienced arthroscopic surgeons, Arch Orthop Trauma Surg 129:1117-1121, 2010.

- The goal of surgical intervention is to repair the defect or promote the formation of tissue with structure and durability similar to those of normal articular cartilage, thus leading to pain-free joint function.

First Treatment Step
- Rest, ice, compression, elevation, NSAIDs

Treatment Options
Nonoperative Management
- Rest, ice, elevation, NSAIDs, and compression for symptom management
- PT for quadriceps strengthening and to restore ROM
- An unloader brace possibly helpful if there is overloading in a single compartment
- Surgical intervention possibly required if no response to conservative measures
- Surgical options: arthroscopic chondroplasty and loose body removal, microfracture, cartilage transfer (autograft versus allograft)

Operative Management
Codes
ICD-9 code: 718.0 Articular cartilage defect of the knee
CPT codes: 29879 Microfracture
29877 Chondroplasty/débridement
29866 Osteochondral autograft, knee arthroscopic
27415 Osteochondral allograft, knee open

Operative Indications
- Operative management is indicated in symptomatic focal full-thickness cartilage lesions, without significant concomitant arthritis, that have not responded to nonoperative measures.

Informed Consent and Counseling
- Potential risks: bleeding, infection, wound complications, loss of motion, DVT or PE, and failure of the procedure to hold up over time
- Anesthesia complications: paralysis, cardiac arrest, brain damage, and death
- Postoperative PT and compliance with weight-bearing restrictions essential for full recovery

Anesthesia
- General, with or without regional block

Patient Positioning
- Supine, with tourniquet use

Surgical Procedures

Chondroplasty/Débridement
- Two small incisions are made medial and lateral to the patella tendon slightly above the joint line. An arthroscope is used to explore the suprapatellar pouch, patellofemoral joint, intercondylar notch, medial and lateral compartments, and medial and lateral gutters. A shaver is used to débride identified cartilage defects.

Fixation of Unstable Fragments
- This procedure can be performed if there is an osteochondral fragment and adequate subchondral bone. The defect is identified arthroscopically, and then underlying nonviable tissue is débrided with a shaver. Subchondral bone may be drilled or supplemented with bone graft, after which the osteochondral fragment is fixed with absorbable or nonabsorbable screws.

Microfracture
- This procedure is performed arthroscopically. The defect is identified and débrided to subchondral bone. An awl is used to make holes in the bone. This procedure stimulates the production of fibrocartilage, which will eventually fill the defect (Fig. 7-22).

Osteochondral Autograft Plug Transfer (OATS)
- This procedure may be performed open or arthroscopically. A cylindrical instrument is used to harvest plugs of cartilage and bone from a non–weight-bearing area. The cartilage defect is débrided and prepared, and then the plug is placed into the defect.

Osteochondral Allograft
- Two different techniques using osteochondral allograft exist. Very large defects can be "filled" using large osteochondral allograft plugs ("megaOATS") that are cut to size and press fit into the defect. Minced juvenile allograft cartilage has also gained popularity to fill smaller defects and is particularly useful for patella defects, in which traditional OATS procedures have been difficult. The cartilage defect is débrided and filled with juvenile cartilage cells and is then sealed with fibrin glue. Hyaline cartilage fills the defect and functions similar to normal articular cartilage.

Estimated Postoperative Course
- Postoperative day 0 to 6 weeks
  - The surgical dressing can be removed on the second day after surgery and replaced with adhesive bandages or gauze.
  - A wound check and suture removal are performed at 10 to 14 days postoperatively.
  - Microfracture: Crutches and 25% weight bearing are indicated for 6 weeks. No limits on ROM are necessary; advance as tolerated.

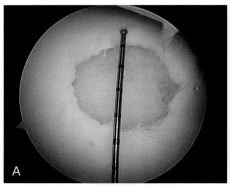
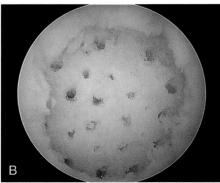

Figure 7-22. Arthroscopic images of a cartilage defect. **A,** Defect after débridement. **B,** Microfracture of the defect.

- OATS: A brace and 50% weight bearing are indicated for 6 weeks.
- A continuous passive motion (CPM) machine may be ordered after microfracture or OATS.
- Ice, elevation, and PRN pain medication indicated for comfort.
- Begin PT at 10 to 14 days postoperatively.
- Arthroscopic débridement and chondroplasty: Only one postoperative visit is typically needed. The patient may bear weight and progress activity as tolerated.
- Postoperative 6 weeks to 3 months
  - Assess surgical site healing and ROM.
  - Discontinue the brace and advance to full weight bearing.
  - Normalize gait mechanics and progress open and closed chain exercises as tolerated.
- Postoperative 3+ months
  - Begin sport-specific drills and plyometrics.
  - Return to sports typically occurs 5 to 6 months after microfracture or OATS; however, some surgeons may allow earlier return.

Suggested Readings

Cole BJ: Surgical management of articular cartilage defects in the knee, *J Bone Joint Surg Am* 91(7):1778–1790, 2009.

Magnussen RA, Dunn WR, Carey JL, et al: Treatment of focal articular cartilage defects in the knee: a systematic review, *Clin Orthop Relat Res* 466(4):952–962, 2008.

Marcu DM, Baer GS: Chondral injuries of the knee. In Miller MD, Hart JA, MacKnight JM, editors: *Essential orthopaedics*, Philadelphia, 2010, Saunders, pp 642–646.

Vanlauwe J, Saris BF, Victor J: Five-year outcome of characterized chondrocyte implantation versus microfracture for symptomatic cartilage defects of the knee: early treatment matters, *Am J Sports Med* 39(12):2566–2574, 2011.

KNEE OSTEOARTHRITIS

History

- Joint swelling
- Pain aggravated by weight bearing and relieved by rest
- Stiffness
- Periodic flares
- Night pain and pain at rest with severe OA

- Mechanical symptoms such as catching and locking possible secondary to loose bodies, cartilage flap, and concurrent meniscus tears
- Most common in older obese patients

Physical Examination

- Observation
  - Gait and use of assistive device
  - Alignment: valgus (medial compartment OA), varus (lateral compartment OA)
  - Quadriceps atrophy
  - Effusion
- Palpation
  - Effusion
  - Crepitus
  - Tenderness
- ROM
  - Often decreased; may lack full extension

Imaging

- Radiographs
  - Standing flexion weight-bearing, AP lateral, and sunrise views are obtained. Bilateral films are often helpful for comparison.
  - Common radiographic changes seen in OA include decreased joint space, osteophyte formation, subchondral sclerosis, cyst formation, and flattening of the femoral condyles (Fig. 7-23).
  - Full-length hip to ankle films are helpful to assess alignment if surgical intervention is indicated.

Classification

- Primary: Arthritis is not associated with a specific trauma, inflammatory, or metabolic condition.
- Secondary: Arthritis develops secondary to injury of the articular cartilage or other structures in the knee, such as intra-articular fracture, chondral defect, meniscus tear, or ligament rupture.

Initial Treatment

Patient Education

- OA is a common joint disease that can cause significant disability.
- It is caused by cartilage breakdown and subsequent changes to the underlying bone.

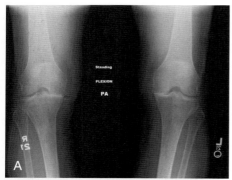

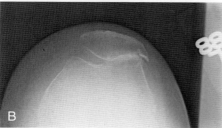

Figure 7-23. Radiographs demonstrating osteoarthritis (OA). **A,** Medial compartment OA. PA, posteroanterior. **B,** Patellofemoral OA.

■ Joint changes are irreversible, but lifestyle modification, such as weight loss, can help slow the progression.

First Treatment Step
■ Activity modification, ice or heat, acetaminophen or NSAIDs

Treatment Options
Nonoperative Management
■ Lifestyle modification includes low-impact exercise (stationary bicycle, elliptical trainer, swimming) and weight loss.
■ PT may help patients to develop an appropriate exercise routine.
■ Medications: Acetaminophen and NSAIDs are indicated. Narcotics are not recommended for long-term symptom management.
■ Topical NSAIDs are used.
■ Dietary supplements: Glucosamine (1500 mg) and chondroitin sulfate (1200 mg) are recommended.
■ Orthotics consist of a heel wedge and/ or unloader brace (if OA is isolated to a single compartment).

■ Intra-articular injections: Corticosteroid injections can be administered up to three times per year. Hyaluronic acid injections act as a lubricant, have few side effects, and may be helpful in patients in whom corticosteroid injection has failed.

Operative Management
Codes
ICD-9 code: 715.96 Knee osteoarthritis
CPT codes: 29877 Arthroscopic débridement and chondroplasty
  • 27457 High tibial osteotomy
  • 27446 Unicondylar arthroplasty
  • 27447 Total knee arthroplasty

Operative Indications
■ Surgical intervention is indicated in patients in whom extensive conservative measures fail and who have significant disability or decreased quality of life.
■ Arthroscopic débridement is typically used in patients with loose bodies or meniscus tears along with OA. It may help relieve mechanical symptoms (catching, locking).
■ High tibial osteotomy is indicated for young to middle-aged active patients with degenerative changes that are isolated to the medial or lateral compartment.
■ Unicondylar arthroplasty is indicated for isolated medial or lateral compartment OA in older, low-demand patients.
■ Total knee arthroplasty is indicated for older, low-demand patients with multicompartment OA.

Informed Consent and Counseling
■ Potential risks include DVT or PE, patella fracture, component loosening, peroneal nerve palsy, periprosthetic fracture, wound complications, infection, instability, popliteal artery injury, quadriceps and patellar tendon rupture, stiffness, fat embolism, collateral ligament injury, and need for revision.
■ Anesthesia complications include paralysis, cardiac arrest, brain damage, and death.
■ Research indicates that 10-year survivorship for unicompartmental arthroplasty is approximately 90%, and it drops to 85% at greater than 10 years.

- Research indicates that 5-year success rates for high tibial osteotomy range from 80% to 96%; the 10-year success rate ranges from 53% to 85%.
- Research indicates that 15-year survivorship for total knee arthroplasty may be as high as 94%.

Anesthesia
- General, with or without regional block

Patient Positioning
- Supine

Surgical Procedures
Arthroscopic Débridement
- The extremity is prepared and draped in standard sterile fashion. Two small incisions are made medial and lateral to the patella tendon slightly above the joint line. An arthroscope is used to explore the suprapatellar pouch, patellofemoral joint, intercondylar notch, medial and lateral compartments, and medial and lateral gutters. A shaver is used to débride identified cartilage defects. Loose bodies are identified and removed, and meniscus tears are débrided. Portals are closed, and a sterile dressing is applied.

High Tibial Osteotomy
- The extremity is prepared and draped in standard sterile fashion. A midline or lateral incision is made to expose the proximal tibia. An opening wedge or closing wedge osteotomy is performed to correct alignment and unload the affected compartment. During opening wedge osteotomy, a bone wedge is removed from the tibia, and a plate is applied and tensioned; bone graft is often used to fill the defect. During closing wedge osteotomy, a wedge of bone is removed from the tibia, and plate systems or staples are used for compression. Incisions are closed in a multilayer fashion, and a sterile dressing is applied.

Unicondylar Replacement
- The extremity is prepared and draped in standard sterile fashion. A short vertical incision is made from the top of the patella to the tibial tubercle.

The knee is positioned in 90 degrees of flexion. The collateral ligaments are retracted and protected throughout the case. Osteophytes are removed. Tibial resection is then performed with a saw, and tibial trial components are used to determine the appropriate component size. The flexion gap is measured and balanced using spacer blocks. A cutting block is used to prepare the femoral side, and the trial components are again used to determine the appropriate component size. Components are cemented in place, the wound is irrigated and closed in a multilayer fashion, and a sterile dressing is then applied.

Total Knee Replacement
- Various prostheses and surgical techniques are available. The extremity is prepared and draped in standard sterile fashion. A midline incision is made over the patella, and then subcutaneous tissue and peritenon are dissected. The patella is everted, and osteophytes are excised from all three compartments. Using a tibial intramedullary (IM) guide, a hole is drilled in line with tibial shaft, usually just lateral to insertion of the ACL. The MCL and LCL are retracted and protected. A transverse osteotomy of the proximal tibia is then performed. Then femoral component is sized, and the distal femoral cut is made with the assistance of an IM guide and cutting block. Next, the patella is measured, and holes are drilled for placement of the patellar component. All components are secured with cement. Multilayer closure is performed, and a sterile dressing is applied (Fig. 7-24).

Estimated Postoperative Course
Postoperative Day 0 to 6 Weeks
- High tibial osteotomy
  - Surgical dressing removal by the patient 2 to 3 days after the procedure
  - Ice, elevation, and PRN pain medication for comfort
  - No weight bearing, and use of a hinged brace for 6 to 8 weeks
  - Wound check and suture removal at 10 to 14 days

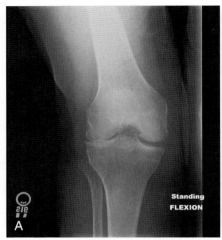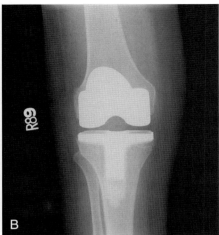

Figure 7-24. A, Radiograph before total knee replacement. **B,** Radiograph after total knee replacement.

- PT begun at 10 to 14 days postoperatively, with flexion limited to 120 degrees for 15 days and then gradually advanced
- Unicondylar arthroplasty
  - 1- to 2-day hospital stay
  - Ice, elevation, and PRN pain medication for comfort
  - Removal of the surgical dressing by the patient 2 to 3 days after the procedure
  - Weight bearing as tolerated and walking with an assistive device shortly after surgery
  - PT begun in the hospital, with transition to home health or outpatient therapy
  - Wound check and suture or staple removal at 10 to 14 days
- Total knee arthroplasty
  - 2- to 3-day hospital stay
  - CPM begun shortly after surgery 0 to 90 degrees initially and then advanced as tolerated; used for 8 hours daily
  - Ice, elevation, and PRN pain medication for comfort
  - Weight bearing as tolerated and ambulation with an assistive device
  - PT begun in the hospital, with transition to home health or outpatient therapy

Postoperative 6 Weeks to 3 Months
- High tibial osteotomy
  - Brace discontinued
  - Evaluation of surgical site healing and ROM
  - PT advanced
  - Radiographs obtained and reviewed
- Unicondylar arthroplasty
  - Evaluation of surgical site healing and ROM
  - PT advanced
  - Radiographs obtained and reviewed
- Total knee arthroplasty
  - Goal: full ROM at this point
  - Ambulation indoors possible without an assistive device

Postoperative 3+ Months
- High tibial osteotomy
  - Return to strenuous work at 3 months and sports at 6 months
- Unicondylar arthroplasty
  - Evaluation of ROM; repeat radiographs considered at 6 or 12 months
- Total knee arthroplasty
  - Ambulation with no assistive device
  - Radiographs obtained and reviewed

Suggested Readings
Fitz W, Scott RD: Unicompartmental knee arthroplasty. In Scott WM, editor: *Insall and Scott surgery of the knee*, ed 5, Philadelphia, 2012, Churchill Livingstone, pp 988–995.

Leone JM, Hanssen AD: Osteotomy about the knee: American perspective. In Scott WM, editor: *Insall and Scott surgery of the knee*, ed 5, Philadelphia, 2012, Churchill Livingstone, pp 910–925.

Marcu DM, Baer GS: Osteoarthritis of the knee. In Miller MD, Hart JA, MacKnight JM, editors: *Essential orthopaedics*, Philadelphia, 2010, Saunders, pp 651–656.

Micheal JW, Schuluter-Brust KU, Eysel P: The epidemiology, etiology, diagnosis and treatment of osteoarthritis of the knee, *Dtsch Arztebl Int* 107(9):152–162, 2010.

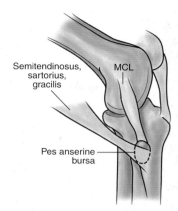

Figure 7-26. Location of the pes anserine bursa on the medial side of the knee. MCL, medial collateral ligament. *(From Miller MD, Hart JA, MacKnight JM, editors:* Essential orthopaedics, *Philadelphia, 2010, Saunders.)*

KNEE BURSITIS

History

■ Prepatellar bursitis (Fig. 7-25)
  • Anterior knee pain and swelling
  • Difficulty kneeling
  • Possible occupation requiring excessive kneeling
  • Possible history of trauma to the anterior knee
■ Pes anserine bursitis (Fig. 7-26)
  • Common causes: athletic overuse, medial knee acute trauma, and chronic mechanical or degenerative processes.
  • Pain in the medial knee, over the proximal tibia
  • Pain possibly particularly severe at night
  • Pain possibly aggravated by ascending or descending stairs and rising from a seated position

Physical Examination

■ Prepatellar bursitis
  • A ballotable collection of fluid is located just over the patella, with or without erythema and warmth.
  • Tenderness over the bursal sac is noted.
  • Crepitus may or may not be present.
  • Chronic bursitis is characterized by palpable subcutaneous cobblestone-like roughness.
■ Pes anserine bursitis
  • Examination should include observation and analysis of gait.
  • Palpate the tibial plateau to localize tenderness, and differentiate between tenderness of the MCL and that of the pes anserine bursa.
  • The patient may have pain with valgus stress, resisted internal rotation, and resisted flexion.

Imaging

■ Radiographs: Standing flexion, lateral, and sunrise views are obtained. Radiographs are not needed to make the diagnosis of bursitis, but they can rule out underlying fracture if the patient has a history of trauma and assess for

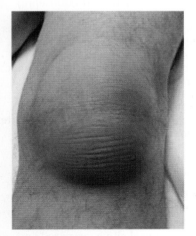

Figure 7-25. Patient with acute prepatellar bursitis. *(From Miller MD, Hart JA, MacKnight JM, editors:* Essential orthopaedics, *Philadelphia, 2010, Saunders.)*

concurrent arthritis. Typically, radiographs are unremarkable, except for soft tissue swelling of the anterior knee in prepatellar bursitis.

- MRI is not necessary, but it rules out other disorders. Fluid may be seen in the bursa.

Initial Treatment
Patient Education
- Prepatellar bursitis
  - It is most commonly caused by trauma, such as a fall onto the anterior knee, or direct pressure and friction caused by repetitive kneeling ("housemaid's knee").
  - It may become chronic in a small percentage of patients.
  - The prepatellar bursa may become infected (typically by *Staphylococcus aureus*) and can also be inflamed secondary to gout.
- Pes anserine bursitis
  - It commonly occurs along with medial compartment OA or results from overuse.
  - It can result from trauma, but abnormal gait is a more common cause. Increased friction on the bursa secondary to loss of normal mechanical relationships leads to inflammation.
- Knee bursitis typically responds well to nonoperative treatment.

First Treatment Step
- Symptom management: ice and NSAIDs

Treatment Options
Nonoperative Management
- Prepatellar bursitis
  - Avoid activities that put direct pressure on the bursa, such as squatting and crossing the legs.
  - Use knee pads.
  - Limit repetitious bending.
  - If infection of the prepatellar bursa is suspected, aspiration is recommended. Send fluid for cell counts, Gram stain, culture and sensitivity, and crystal analysis. Serum erythrocyte sedimentation rate and C-reactive protein determinations may be helpful as well. Treat septic bursitis with appropriate antibiotics.

- PT is indicated for stretching and strengthening, as well as treatment modalities such as ultrasound and electrical stimulation.
- If symptoms persist despite conservative measures, corticosteroid injection is indicated.
- Pes anserine bursitis
  - Activity modification, rest, and NSAIDs are recommended.
  - PT is indicated for stretching and strengthening, as well as treatment modalities such as ultrasound and electrical stimulation.
  - If symptoms persist despite conservative measures, corticosteroid injection is indicated.
  - It may be helpful to place a small cushion between the thighs while sleeping.

Operative Management
Codes
ICD-9 codes: 726.65 Prepatellar bursitis
726.61 Pes anserine bursitis
CPT codes: 27340 Prepatellar bursectomy
27599 Pes anserine bursectomy

Operative Indications
- Surgical bursectomy is rarely needed, but it is indicated for severe intractable bursitis.

Informed Consent and Counseling
- Possible complications: bleeding, infection, wound complication, loss of motion, and damage to nearby tissues, vessels, and nerves
- Anesthesia risks: paralysis, cardiac arrest, brain damage, and death

Anesthesia
- General, and local at portal site after closure

Patient Positioning
- Supine, with tourniquet

Surgical Procedures
Arthroscopic Prepatellar Bursectomy
- The surgical site is prepared and draped in standard sterile fashion. An anteromedial portal and an anterolateral portal are routinely used. The

bursal cavity and synovial thickening are visualized with the arthroscope. A motorized shaver is inserted, and total synovectomy (including the bursa) is performed. Portals are closed, and a sterile dressing is applied.

Pes Anserine Bursectomy
- The surgical site is prepared and draped in standard sterile fashion. A small incision is made over the pes anserine. Soft tissues are dissected so that the bursa can be visualized. The bursa and any bony exostosis are excised. The wound is irrigated and closed in a multilayer fashion.

Estimated Postoperative Course
- The surgical dressing can be removed on the second postoperative day.
- Sutures are removed at 10 to 14 days postoperatively.
- Prepatellar bursectomy: No vigorous physical activity is allowed for 2 weeks after surgery; return to normal physical activity occurs at 3 weeks postoperatively.
- Pes anserine bursectomy: The knee should be braced in extension or slight flexion for 2 weeks; then, advance ROM as tolerated.
- PRN follow-up occurs after the initial postoperative clinic appointment.

Suggested Readings
Huang Y, Yeh W: Endoscopic treatment of prepatellar bursitis, *Int Orthop* 35(3):355–358, 2011.
Parker RD: Pes anserine bursitis. In Miller MD, Hart JA, MacKnight JM, editors: *Essential orthopaedics*, Philadelphia, 2010, Saunders, pp 674–676.
Parker RD: Prepatellar bursitis. In Miller MD, Hart JA, MacKnight JM, editors: *Essential orthopaedics*, Philadelphia, 2010, Saunders, pp 671–673.
Rennie WJ, Saiffuddin A: Pes anserine bursitis: incidence in symptomatic knees and clinical presentation, *Skeletal Radiol* 34:395–398, 2005.

MENISCUS INJURY
History
- Acute injury
  - The mechanism of injury is typically twisting or hyperflexion.
  - Acute pain is present, with or without effusion.

- Pain is aggravated by squatting or pivoting.
- Mechanical symptoms such as locking and catching may be present.
- Chronic (degenerative) injury
  - This often occurs in older patients with OA.
  - It is frequently caused by an atraumatic mechanism.

Physical Examination
- Observation
  - Effusion
  - Antalgic gait
  - Ecchymosis or abrasion
- Palpation
  - Joint line tenderness: Assess the medial and lateral joint lines with the knee flexed.
  - Perform patella ballottement to evaluate for effusion.
  - Palpate the popliteal fossa for a Baker cyst.
- ROM
  - Lack of full extension, which is referred to as a locked knee, may be caused by a displaced bucket handle tear.
  - Decreased flexion may occur secondary to effusion.

Special Tests
- McMurray test: Pain with McMurray test is more common and is often considered a positive test result, but pain is less sensitive for a meniscus tear than a palpable click.
- The patella apprehension, Lachman, pivot shift, posterior drawer, and valgus and varus stress tests should also be performed to rule out concurrent injury.

Imaging
- Radiographs
  - Order standing flexion, lateral, and sunrise views.
  - Radiographs are often unremarkable in younger patients with acute tear; they may show effusion if present. Joint space narrowing is seen in patients with degenerative meniscus tears secondary to OA.
- MRI
  - No contrast is needed to evaluate for meniscus tears, but arthrogram

MRI is useful to evaluate healing or recurrent tear at the site of previous meniscal repair.

- MRI can determine location of the tear, tear pattern, and displacement.

Classification

- Meniscus tears are classified by location and tear pattern (Fig. 7-27).
- Discoid meniscus: Typically, this is a normal anatomic variant in which the meniscus is abnormally shaped, covering a larger portion of the tibial plateau than the normally shaped meniscus. This condition is classified into three types: incomplete, complete, and Wrisberg variant. Discoid meniscus is typically asymptomatic, but it may require meniscectomy or repair if it is torn or if snapping and popping develop.

Initial Treatment

Patient Education

- Meniscus tears may become less symptomatic over time, or symptoms may be intermittent and aggravated by physical activity.
- Peripheral meniscus tears can be repaired, but tears that involve the inner portion of the meniscus are débrided.

First Treatment Step

- Initial treatment is symptom based: rest, ice, compression, and elevation are helpful to relieve pain and swelling.

Treatment Options

Nonoperative Management

- Observation is indicated for small tears or in arthritic patients with no mechanical symptoms.
- PT may be beneficial to restore motion, reduce swelling, and increase quadriceps strength.

Operative Management

Codes

ICD-9 code: 836.0 Meniscus tear

CPT codes: 29881 Arthroscopic partial medial or lateral meniscectomy

29880 Arthroscopic partial medial and lateral meniscectomy

29882 Medial or lateral meniscus repair

29883 Medial and lateral meniscus repairs

Operative Indications

- Failure of nonoperative management, mechanical symptoms (catching, clicking, locking), and persistent pain or swelling that interferes with activity are operative indications.
- Vertical and longitudinal tears in the periphery of the meniscus (red-red/white zone) can be repaired. Meniscus tears that occur in the avascular region of the meniscus are treated with partial meniscectomy.
- Meniscus transplant is an option for younger patients with near total meniscectomy, particularly in the lateral meniscus.

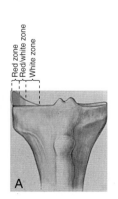
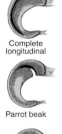

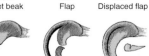

Figure 7-27. Classification of meniscal tears. **A,** Classification based on location. **B,** Classification based on appearance and orientation. *(From Miller MD: Review of orthopaedics, ed 5, Philadelphia, 2008, Saunders.)*

Red zone
Red/white zone
White zone

Complete longitudinal

Bucket handle

Displaced bucket handle

Parrot beak

Flap

Displaced flap

Radial

Double flap

Incomplete longitudinal

A   B

Informed Consent and Counseling
- Potential complications: damage to articular cartilage, hemarthrosis, neurovascular injury, tourniquet complications, fluid extravasation, DVT, loss of motion, and infection
- Anesthesia risks: paralysis, cardiac arrest, brain damage, and death

Anesthesia
- General, and local at portal sites after closure

Patient Positioning
- Supine with a leg holder or post, with a tourniquet

Surgical Procedures
Arthroscopic Partial Meniscectomy
- The extremity is prepared and draped in a sterile fashion. Two small incisions are made medial and lateral to the patella tendon slightly above the joint line. An arthroscope is used to explore the suprapatellar pouch, patellofemoral joint, intercondylar notch, medial and lateral compartments, and medial and lateral gutters. Shavers and biters are used to débride the meniscus tear back to a stable border. Any visualized loose bodies are removed, and areas of cartilage fraying can be débrided with a shaver. Portals are closed, and local anesthetic is injected. A sterile dressing and an elastic compression (ACE) wrap are applied.

Meniscus Repair: Figure 7-28
- The extremity is prepared and draped in a sterile fashion. Diagnostic arthroscopy is used to identify the meniscus tear, after which a 2- to 3-cm vertical incision (medial or lateral) is made to allow for tying of the sutures. Various techniques are available for meniscus repair. Placement of inside-out vertical mattress sutures is a commonly used technique and remains the gold standard. Tensionable all-inside devices have been developed and are most commonly used with concomitant ACL reconstruction, which provides the best environment for meniscal healing. Neurovascular structures must be identified and protected: the saphenous nerve and vein medially and the common peroneal nerve laterally. The incision is closed in a multilayer fashion. A sterile dressing and an elastic compression (ACE) wrap are applied.

Estimated Postoperative Course
Postoperative Day 0 to 6 Weeks
- Partial meniscectomy
  - The wound dressing can be removed and replaced with self-adhesive bandages after 2 days.
  - Sutures are removed at 10 to 14 days postoperatively.

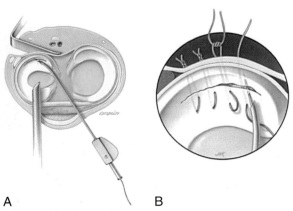

A   B

Figure 7-28. Inside-out meniscal repair technique. **A,** Passing the suture. **B,** Tying the knots and completing the repair. *(From Miller MD:* Review of orthopaedics, *ed 5, Philadelphia, 2008, Saunders.)*

- Weight bearing is allowed as tolerated, with crutches for assistance if needed.
- Use of a stationary bicycle and quadriceps strengthening exercise can be started several days after surgery, and activity is advanced as tolerated.
- Formal PT is not typically needed, but it may be beneficial for patients who have decreased ROM, quadriceps atrophy, or persistent edema.
- Return to sports typically occurs 3 to 4 weeks postoperatively.
- Follow-up PRN occurs after the initial postoperative visit.
- Meniscus repair
  - The wound dressing can be removed and replaced with self-adhesive bandages after 2 days.
  - Sutures are removed at 10 to 14 days postoperatively.
  - Toe touch weight bearing with crutches is allowed for 4 weeks, followed by 50% weight bearing.
  - ROM is from 0 to 90 degrees.
  - Begin PT at 10 to 14 days postoperatively.

Postoperative 6 Weeks to 3 Months
- Meniscus repair
  - Assess ROM and surgical site healing at the clinic visit.
  - Progress ROM as tolerated.
  - Continue to advance PT.

Postoperative 3+ Months
- Meniscus repair
  - The patient begins running on a treadmill and plyometrics at 3 months.
  - The patient returns to full sport at 5 months.

Suggested Readings
Kalliakmanis A, Zourntos S, Bousgas D, et al: Comparison of arthroscopic meniscus repair results using 3 different devices in anterior cruciate ligament reconstruction patients, *Arthroscopy* 24:810–816, 2008.

Marcu DM, Baer GS: Meniscus tears. In Miller MD, Hart JA, MacKnight JM, editors: *Essential orthopaedics*, Philadelphia, 2010, Saunders, pp 671–673.

Miller MD, Howard RF, Plancher KD: *Surgical atlas of sports medicine*, Philadelphia, 2003, Elsevier Science.

Noyes FR, Chen RC, Barber-Westin SD, et al: Greater than 10-year results of red-white longitudinal meniscal repairs in patients 20 years of age or younger, *Am J Sports Med* 39(5):1008–1016, 2011.

ILIOTIBIAL BAND SYNDROME
History
- Lateral knee pain worsens with activity (Fig. 7-29).
- Typically, the syndrome has an insidious onset.
- Patients can typically point to the exact area of involvement.

Physical Examination
- Observation: There may be swelling at the insertion of the ITB.
- Palpation: Minimal to no effusion is noted; tenderness to palpation at the insertion of the ITB is evident.
- ROM: Typically, full ROM may cause pain.

Special Tests
- Ober test: Have the patent lie on the unaffected side with the involved

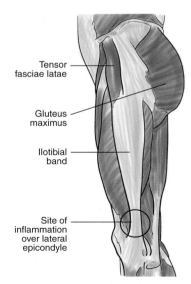

Figure 7-29. Anatomy of iliotibial band syndrome. Note the area of involvement over the lateral femoral epicondyle. *(From Miller MD, Hart JA, MacKnight JM, editors:* Essential orthopaedics, *Philadelphia, 2010, Saunders.)*

Tensor fasciae latae

Gluteus maximus

Ilotibial band

Site of inflammation over lateral epicondyle

extremity up. Extend and adduct the hip, and then flex and extend the knee. An inability to adduct the leg and pain with flexion or extension indicate a positive test result.
- Complete McMurray test, special tests for ligamentous injury, and patella examination to rule out other injury.
- Other tests: Injection of a local anesthetic (lidocaine or bupivacaine) may be diagnostic and therapeutic.

Imaging
- Radiographs and MRI are not indicated.

Initial Treatment
Patient Education
- The ITB is a superficial thickening of tissue that runs from the hip to just below the knee.
- The ITB rubs the lateral femoral epicondyle with flexion and extension.
- ITB syndrome primarily occurs secondary to overuse, particularly in cyclists, runners, and skiers.

First Treatment Step
- Ice, rest, activity modification

Treatment Options
Nonoperative Management
- Initial treatment involves the following conservative measures: rest, ice, PT (stretching and strengthening), orthotics, and cross training.
- Corticosteroid injection is performed at the point of maximal tenderness.

Operative Management
- If conservative measures fail and the patient is unwilling to change activity level, surgical interventions may be considered.
- Surgery typically involves open exploration of the area, débridement of the bursa, shaving of bony prominences, and excision or fenestration of the ITB over the lateral femoral condyle.

Codes
ICD-9 code: 728.89 Iliotibial band syndrome
CPT code: 27305 Open ITB fasciotomy/débridement

Operative Indications
- Intractable symptoms following extensive conservative treatment

Informed Consent and Counseling
- Possible complications: bleeding, infection, wound complication, stiffness and damage to nearby structures, loss of motion, and DVT or PE.
- Anesthesia risks: paralysis, cardiac arrest, brain damage and death

Anesthesia
- General

Patient Positioning
- Supine

Surgical Procedures
Iliotibial Band
- Prepare and drape the extremity in standard sterile fashion. A diagnostic arthroscopy may be performed to rule out concomitant meniscus tear or cartilage defect. A short longitudinal incision is made laterally over the later femoral condyle. Soft tissue is dissected. The synovium or bursa is débrided, and a small triangular piece of the ITB that contacts the lateral femoral epicondyle when the knee is flexed to 30 degrees is excised. The incision is closed in a multilayer fashion, and a sterile dressing is applied.

Estimated Postoperative Course
- A wound check and suture removal are performed at 10 to 14 days postoperatively.
- PT focuses on stretching, strengthening, and slow return to sports.
- The patient may return at 3 months for reevaluation or on a PRN basis.

Suggested Readings
Drogset JO, Rossvoli I, Grontvedt T: Surgical treatment of iliotibial band friction syndrome: a retrospective study of 49 patients, *Scand J Med Sci Sports* 9:296–298, 1999.

Hariri S, Savidge ET, Reinold MM, et al: Treatment of recalcitrant iliotibial band syndrome with open iliotibial band bursectomy: indications, technique, and clinical outcomes, *Am J Sports Med* 37:1417–1424, 2009.

Parker RD: Iliotibial band syndrome. In Miller MD, Hart JA, MacKnight JM, editors: *Essential orthopaedics*, Philadelphia, 2010, Saunders, pp 666–678.

CHRONIC EXERTIONAL COMPARTMENT SYNDROME

History
- Gradually increasing pain is noted in a specific muscle region during exertion.
- Symptoms typically occur at a specific and reproducible point of exercise, such as a particular distance or length of time.
- Pain is described as tightness, aching, squeezing, or cramping.
- The syndrome often occurs bilaterally.
- Neurologic symptoms such as paresthesia, weakness, and foot drop may be present.
- Pain typically resolves with rest, but some patients may report pain with daily activities and at rest.

Physical Examination: Table 7-10
- Findings are often unremarkable at rest; it may be helpful to examine the patient after exercise that is sufficient to elicit symptoms.
- Observation: Swelling may be noted.
- Palpation: Palpable fascial hernia may be present. Involved compartments may be tight and tender.

Imaging
- Radiographs, MRI, or CT may be used to identify concurrent stress fractures or to rule out other possible causes.

Compartment Pressure Measurement
- The definitive diagnosis of chronic exertional compartment syndrome (CECS) is made by measuring compartment pressures.
- Pressure measurements are obtained at rest and after exercise challenge.
- The diagnosis is made based on the presence of one or more of the following criteria:
  - Pre-exercise pressure 15 mm Hg or greater
  - 1-minute postexercise pressure 30 mm Hg or greater
  - 5-minute postexercise pressure 20 mm Hg or greater

Initial Treatment
Patient Education
- CECS is an overuse injury that most commonly occurs in young endurance athletes, particularly distance runners.
- Reversible ischemia is caused by increased pressure within the noncompliant fascial planes of a muscle compartment. It occurs during exercise as muscle volume expands in response to increased blood flow and edema.
- CECS occurs most commonly in the anterior compartment of the lower leg, followed by the deep posterior, lateral, and superficial posterior compartments. It may also occur in the foot, thigh, forearm, and hand.

First Treatment Step
- Rest, NSAIDs

Treatment Options
Nonoperative Management
- Limitation on or cessation of the activity that causes symptoms
- Cross training

Table 7-10. Physical Examination Findings Vary Based on Which Compartments Are Affected	
Anterior compartment	Numbness of the first web space or dorsum of foot, weakness of ankle dorsiflexion and toe extension, and possible foot drop
Deep posterior compartment	Weak toe flexion and foot inversion, as well as sensory changes on the plantar surface of the foot
Lateral compartment	Weak ankle eversion and numbness of the anterolateral leg
Superficial posterior compartment	Weak foot plantar flexion and numbness of the lateral foot

- NSAIDs
- Orthotics
- PT: massage, soft tissue mobilization, muscle stretching and strengthening

Operative Management
Codes
ICD-9 code: 729.9 Chronic exertional compartment syndrome
CPT codes: 27600 Anterior and lateral compartment release/fasciotomy
27603 Four compartment release/fasciotomy

Operative Indications
- Operative management is indicated in patients with intractable symptoms despite extensive conservative measures and documented increased compartment pressures.

Informed Consent and Counseling
- Possible complications: bleeding, wound infection, wound healing complications, nerve entrapment, nerve injury, swelling, arterial injury, hematoma, and DVT or PE
- Anesthesia risks: cardiac arrest, brain damage, paralysis, and death

Anesthesia
- General

Patient Positioning
- Supine, with or without a tourniquet

Surgical Procedures: Figure 7-30
Anterior and Lateral Compartment Release
- The lower extremity is prepared and draped in a sterile fashion. A 4- to 5-cm incision is made halfway between the fibular shaft and the tibia crest. A second more proximal incision may be made as needed. Skin edges are undermined, and a transverse incision is made in the fascia. The anterior intermuscular septum is identified; then Metzenbaum scissors and a fasciotome are used to release the fascia proximal and distal to the incision. Make sure the superficial peroneal nerve is identified and protected during the release.

Superficial Posterior and Deep Posterior Compartment Release
- The lower extremity is prepared and draped in a sterile fashion. A 4- to 5-cm incision is made 2 cm posterior to the posterior tibial margin. The saphenous nerve and vein are identified and protected. A transverse incision is made in the fascia, and the septum between the two compartments is identified; the superficial compartment is released first. The deep compartment is released distally and then proximally.

Wound Closure
- Deep tissues are closed with #3-0 Monocryl suture in an interrupted fashion, followed by #3-0 suture in a running fashion. Incisions are reinforced with Steri-Strips, and sterile dressings are applied. Posterior left splints are placed with the foot in neutral position.

Estimated Postoperative Course
- Postoperative day 0 to 6 weeks
  - At 10 to 14 days after surgery, splint removal, wound check, and suture removal are performed, and PT is begun.
  - Crutches and no weight bearing are indicated for the first 2 weeks, with gradual progression as tolerated.
  - Early PT focuses on edema control, scar management, and ROM (ankle and knee). PT may progress at approximately 4 weeks to include gentle stretching, ankle strengthening, balance and proprioception exercises, and gait training.
- Postoperative 6 weeks to 3 months
  - Check wound healing at the office visit.
  - PT: Progress from water walking (if wounds are well healed) to the elliptical trainer and then to light jogging at 6 to 8 weeks.
- Postoperative 3+ months
  - The patient may begin sport-specific training.

Suggested Readings
Schubert AG: Exertional compartment syndrome: review of the literature and proposed rehabilitation guidelines following surgical release, *Int J Sports Phys Ther* 6(2):126–141, 2011.

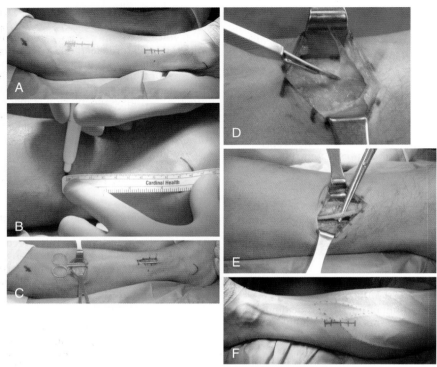

Figure 7-30. Surgical fasciotomy. A, Dual lateral incisions for release of the anterior and lateral compartments. **B,** The distal lateral incision is centered 10 to 12 cm proximal to the tip of the distal fibula, at the site where the superficial peroneal nerve penetrates the fascia. **C,** Blunt dissection produces subcutaneous connection of the incisions to allow adequate release of the compartments throughout their lengths. **D,** Anterior compartment fascial incision. The fascial incision is then extended proximally and distally under direct visualization. **E,** Superficial peroneal nerve after release of the anterior and lateral compartments. It is important to mobilize the nerve freely. **F,** Medial incision for release of the superficial and deep posterior compartments. *(From Miller MD, Hart JA, MacKnight JM, editors:* Essential orthopaedics, *Philadelphia, 2010, Saunders.)*

Tucker AK: Chronic exertional compartment syndrome, *Curr Rev Musculoskelet Med* 3: 32–37, 2010.
Wilder RP: Exertional compartment syndrome. In Miller MD, Hart JA, MacKnight JM, editors: *Essential orthopaedics*, Philadelphia, 2010, Saunders, pp 684–686.
Wilder RP, Sethi S: Overuse injuries: tendinopathies, stress fractures, compartment syndrome, and shin splints, *Clin Sports Med* 23: 55–81, 2004.

MEDIAL TIBIAL STRESS SYNDROME (SHIN SPLINTS)
History
- Vague diffuse pain occurs over the middle and/or distal tibia.

- Initially, pain is worse at the beginning of exercise, but it gradually resolves during exercise or shortly after cessation of activity.
- As the condition progresses, pain is more intense, persists throughout exercise, and may be present at rest and with ambulation.
- The patient has often had a change in a recent training regimen, such as increased activity, intensity, or duration.

Physical Examination
- Observation
  - Evaluation for biomechanical abnormalities: genu varus or valgus, pes

planus or pes cavus, hindfoot valgus, foot pronation, tibial torsion, femoral anteversion, and leg length discrepancy
- Muscle imbalance, tightness, or weakness of the gastrocnemius, soleus, and plantaris
- Shoe wear patterns
■ Palpation
- Diffuse tenderness over the medial ridge of the distal and middle tibia
- Tenderness possibly extending proximally with increasing severity
■ ROM
- Pain with passive ankle dorsiflexion, resisted plantar flexion, standing toe raises, or jumping

Imaging
■ Radiographs are usually not necessary for diagnosis, but they may show periosteal exostoses.
■ Bone scan can help determine whether medial tibial stress syndrome (MTSS) has progressed to stress fracture. Scans show diffuse uptake with MTSS; uptake is more focal in stress fracture.
■ MRI may help differentiate MTSS, stress fracture, and stress reaction. Scans can show periosteal edema, marrow involvement, and cortical stress fracture.

Initial Treatment
Patient Education
■ Shin splints are a common cause of exertional leg pain and most often occur in patients who run or participate in activities that require repetitive jumping.
■ Symptoms can worsen with continued activity; shin splints can progress to stress fracture without adequate rest and activity modification.

First Treatment Step
■ Rest, ice, activity modification

Treatment Options
Nonoperative Management
■ Acute phase: rest and ice
■ Activity modification: decreased intensity, frequency, and duration
■ Low-impact cross training

■ Gradual return to sport when pain free
■ Regular stretching and strengthening exercises of the gastrocnemius, soleus, ankle dorsiflexors and planter flexors, and foot invertors and evertors
■ Change of shoes in runners every 250 to 500 miles
■ Orthotics if indicated
■ Absolute rest possibly indicated if no response to conservative measures

Operative Management
Operative Indications
■ Failure of 6 to 12 months of conservative treatment is an indication for fasciotomy of the deep posterior compartment and periosteal stripping.

Surgical Procedure and Postoperative Course
The surgical procedure and postoperative course for fasciotomy are discussed in the CECS section earlier in this chapter.

Suggested Readings
Blackham J, Amendola N: Medial tibial stress syndrome (shin splints). In Miller MD, Hart JA, MacKnight JM, editors: *Essential orthopaedics*, Philadelphia, 2010, Saunders, pp 680–683.
Couture C, Karlson K: Tibial stress injuries: decisive diagnosis and treatment of "shin splints," *Phys Sportsmed* 30(6):29–36, 2002.
Galbraith RM, Lavallee ME: Medial tibial stress syndrome: conservative treatment options, *Curr Rev Musculoskelet Med* 2:127–133, 2009.
Wilder RP, Sethi S: Overuse injuries: tendinopathies, stress fractures, compartment syndrome, and shin splints, *Clin Sports Med* 23:55–81, 2004.

STRESS FRACTURE
History
■ Typically, patients present with progressively worsening activity-related pain. Pain may occur at rest as the injury progresses.
■ On occasion, the patient may present with a sudden increase in pain at a site where there has been a chronic low level discomfort; this finding indicates that a stressed bone has fractured.
■ This injury is common in athletes and military recruits.
■ It is more common in women than in men.
■ Female patients with eating disorders and amenorrhea are at increased risk.

Physical Examination

- Observation
  - Antalgic gait with walking or running
  - Localized swelling over the fracture site
- Palpation
  - Tenderness localized to a discrete area
  - Palpable bump resulting from periosteal edema

Special Tests

- Hop test: The result is positive if the patient is unable to hop on the affected leg for 10 repetitions.
- Tuning fork test: The result is positive if pain is elicited by placing a vibrating tuning fork over the fracture site.
- Percussion test: The result is positive if percussion of the bone at a site other than the fracture site causes pain.
- Neurovascular examination should be normal.

Imaging

- Radiographs: Obtain AP and lateral views of the tibia and fibula. Periosteal elevation, cortical thickening, sclerosis, and true fracture are positive findings. These findings are seen only in 20% to 30% of initial radiographs. Radiographs taken 3 to 4 weeks after diagnosis are more likely to show the previously mentioned changes. The "dreaded black line" seen on the lateral radiograph is a stress fracture of the midshaft anterior tibia, which is at high risk for delayed healing and nonunion (Fig. 7-31).
- Bone scan shows a focal area of uptake in stress fracture that helps differentiate stress fracture from MTSS, which has diffuse linear uptake.
- MRI can be particularly helpful in differentiating stress fracture from shin splints. MRI is also useful to differentiate intra-articular stress fracture from ligament, cartilage, or meniscal injury.
- CT may be helpful to determine whether the fracture has extended or developed into nonunion. It also defines fracture lines and shows evidence of healing with resolution

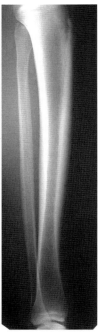

Figure 7-31. Radiograph showing the "dreaded black line" of an anterior tibia stress fracture with a thickened anterior cortex and a lucent line. *(From Miller MD, Hart JA, MacKnight JM, editors:* Essential orthopaedics, *Philadelphia, 2010, Saunders.)*

of lucency and development of sclerosis.

- Repeat imaging is not needed unless the patient fails to respond to treatment. Radiographic healing typically lags behind clinical healing; bone scan and MRI may remain positive for up to 1 year after the initial injury.

Initial Treatment

Patient Education

- The most common site of stress fracture is the tibia, followed by the fibula.
- Stress fractures are common in athletes, particularly runners. They also commonly occur in nonathletes who suddenly increase their activity level. Prolonged walking and jumping also increase the risk.
- Risk factors include excessive training, training on irregular or hard

terrain, poor foot wear, weak and inflexible calf muscles, leg length discrepancy, pes planus or pes cavus, and hormonal or nutritional imbalances that lead to bone demineralization.

First Treatment Step
- Rest and activity modification

Treatment Options
Nonoperative Management
- Diagnosis and treatment are often presumptive, based on history and physical examination because initial radiographic findings are often negative.
- NSAIDs, ice, and PT modalities can help alleviate pain.
- Calcium and vitamin D supplementation may be helpful.
- Treatment depends on the site of injury and the risk for delayed healing or nonunion.

High Risk: Anterior Tibia
- Avoidance of weight bearing: Use of crutches, casting, or bracing is indicated for 3 to 12 weeks; discontinue as symptoms allow.
- Activity can be gradually progressed as long as the patient is pain free.

Low Risk: Posteromedial Tibia or Fibula
- Treatment depends on the patient's goals and on whether pain interferes with performance.
- For athletes, if performance is not affected by pain and pain is not progressing, activity level may be continued without significant limitations.
- If performance is limited by pain, relative rest and cross training are recommended.
- If pain is present with walking, bracing or crutches and cross training should be implemented until the patient is pain free.

Operative Management
Operative Indications
- Operative management is indicated if there is a clear fracture line or conservative treatment has failed.

Codes
ICD-9 code: 733.93 Stress fracture of the tibia or fibula
CPT code: 27759 Tibial intramedullary nail

Surgical Procedure and Postoperative Course
The surgical procedure for tibial IM nail fixation and postoperative recovery are discussed in the tibial shaft fracture section later in this chapter.

Suggested Readings
Blackham J, Amendola N: Stress fractures of the tibia and fibula. In Miller MD, Hart JA, MacKnight JM, editors: *Essential orthopaedics*, Philadelphia, 2010, Saunders, pp 690–693.
Iwamoto J, Takeda T: Stress fractures in athletes: review of 196 cases, *J Orthop Sci* 8:273–278, 2008.
Kaeding CC, Yu JR, Wright R, et al: Management and return to play of stress fractures, *Clin J Sport Med* 15:442–447, 2005.
Ohta-Fukushima M, Mutoh Y, Takasugi S: Characteristics of stress fractures in young athletes under 20 years, *J Sports Med Phys Fitness* 42(2):198–206, 2002.

FRACTURES OF THE KNEE (PATELLA, DISTAL FEMUR, PROXIMAL TIBIA)
History
Patella Fracture
- Trauma: direct or indirect
- Pain and swelling
- Diminished or absent knee extension
- Difficulty bearing weight and ambulating

Distal Femur and Proximal Tibia Fractures
- Trauma: high or low energy
- Pain and swelling
- Inability to bear weight

Physical Examination
Patella Fracture
- Observation: effusion, visible patella deformity, skin abrasions or lacerations
- Palpation: palpable defect, effusion, tenderness
- ROM: active extension (intact, absent, extensors lag); flexion likely limited by effusion and pain
- Special tests
  - Saline load test: Sterile arthrocentesis is performed; then 60 mL of sterile saline with or without methylene

blue is injected into the joint. Extravasation confirms open fracture. The remaining fluid is aspirated.

Distal Femur and Proximal Tibia Fractures

- Observation: effusion, deformity, abrasion, laceration, fracture blisters
- Palpation: tenderness over fracture site, crepitus
- Neurovascular examination: assessment of sensory and motor function of the lower extremity and palpation of pulses
- Special tests
  - Complete a thorough knee examination to evaluate for ligamentous and/or meniscal injury.
  - Measure compartment pressures if indicated.
  - If vascular injury is suspected, measure the ABI.

Imaging
Patella Fracture

- Radiographs: AP, lateral, and sunrise (if patient is able to flex the knee) views are obtained. They help evaluate the fracture pattern and displacement.
- MRI is not typically needed to diagnose patella fracture, but it may identify osteochondral or ligament injuries.

Distal Femur and Proximal Tibia Fractures

- Radiographs: AP, lateral, and 45-degree oblique views are indicated. Obtain radiographs of the joint above and the joint below.
- CT characterizes intra-articular extension and depression and is helpful for surgical planning.
- MRI may be ordered to evaluate for ligamentous or meniscal disorders.

Classification
Patella Fracture

- Classified as open or closed and by fracture pattern (Fig. 7-32)

Distal Femur Fracture

- Open versus closed
- Supracondylar versus intercondylar
- Type A, extra-articular; type B, unicondylar (partial articular, portion of articular surface remains in continuity with shaft); type C, intra-articular (articular fragment separated from shaft)

Proximal Tibia Fracture

- Classified by the Schatzker grading system (Fig. 7-33)

Initial Treatment
Patient Education

- Counsel patients on weight-bearing and ROM restrictions.
- Patients should be informed to call or return to the clinic or emergency department if they experience the following symptoms: increased pain, swelling, or neurovascular changes.

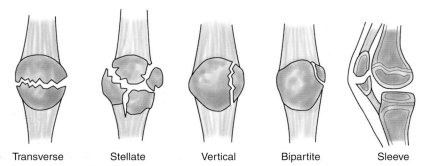

Transverse   Stellate   Vertical   Bipartite   Sleeve

Figure 7-32. Patella fracture classification. Adult fracture patterns include transverse, stellate or comminuted, and vertical. The bipartite patella is frequently confused with a patella fracture. (From Miller MD, Hart JA, MacKnight JM, editors: Essential orthopaedics, Philadelphia, 2010, Saunders.)

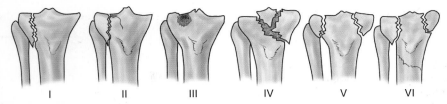

Figure 7-33. Schatzker classification of the tibial plateau fractures. I, lateral split; II, lateral split depression; III, lateral isolated depression; IV, medial; V, bicondylar; VI, bicondylar with metadiaphyseal dissociation. *(From Miller MD, Hart JA, MacKnight JM, editors:* Essential orthopaedics, *Philadelphia, 2010, Saunders.)*

First Treatment Steps

Patella Fracture

- A long-leg splint, immobilizer, or IROM brace locked in extension is used.
- For open fracture, apply a sterile dressing, and administer appropriate antibiotics and tetanus prophylaxis.

Distal Femur and Proximal Tibia Fractures

- Reduce the fracture, and apply a long-leg splint for closed fractures.
- For open fracture, apply a sterile dressing, and administer appropriate antibiotics and tetanus prophylaxis.

Treatment Options

Nonoperative Management

Patella Fracture

- Conservative management is indicated for minimally or nondisplaced fractures with an extensor mechanism that is intact.
- Immobilize the joint in full extension as discussed earlier.
- Patient may bear weight as tolerated with crutches or a walker.

Distal Femur and Proximal Tibia Fractures

- Nonoperative treatment is indicated in the following situations:
  - Isolated lateral tibial plateau fracture with less than 3 mm of articular step off and less than 10 degrees of valgus or varus instability
  - Isolated, nondisplaced, extra-articular distal femur fracture
- Place a locked hinged knee brace for 6 to 12 weeks.

- Begin gentle knee ROM under the guidance of a physical therapist at 2 to 4 weeks.
- Obtain serial radiographs to ensure proper alignment.

Operative Management

Codes

ICD-9 codes: 821.23 Closed supracondylar fracture of the femur
  821.33 Open supracondylar fracture of the femur
  832.00 Closed tibial condyle fracture
  823.10 Open tibial condyle fracture
  822.00 Patella fracture
CPT codes: 27524 Patella ORIF
  27535 ORIF of unicondylar tibial plateau fracture
  27536 ORIF of bicondylar tibial plateau fracture
  27506 Open treatment of femoral fracture

Operative Indications

- Patella fracture: Fixation is recommended for fractures that disrupt the extensor mechanism or demonstrate more than 2 to 3 mm of step-off and more than 1 to 4 mm of displacement.
- Distal femur fracture: Surgical fixation is indicated for any distal femur fracture other than isolated, nondisplaced, or extra-articular fractures.
- Proximal tibia fracture: Surgical fixation is indicated for open fracture, compartment syndrome, vascular injury, displaced bicondylar fracture, displaced medial condyle fracture, lateral plateau fracture with joint instability, more than 2 mm of articular

depression, and more than 10 degrees of varus or valgus instability.

Informed Consent and Counseling
- Possible risks: infection, nonunion, malunion, loss of fixation, painful hardware, DVT or PE, incomplete relief of pain, and incomplete return of function
- Anesthesia risks: cardiac arrest, brain damage, paralysis, and death

Anesthesia
- General, with or without regional block

Patient Positioning
- Supine, with all bony prominences well padded
- Tourniquet on thigh

Surgical Procedures

Patella Open Reduction, Internal Fixation
- The extremity is prepared and draped in standard sterile fashion. A vertical midline incision is made to expose the fracture site, as well as the medial and lateral retinaculum. The fracture is reduced with reduction forceps; reduction is confirmed by palpation of articular surface and/or C-arm images. Fixation can be obtained with a variety of methods, depending on the fracture pattern and the surgeon's preference (Fig. 7-34). The medial retinaculum and lateral retinaculum are repaired if indicated. Irrigate the wound, and close it in a multilayer fashion.

Tibial Plateau Open Reduction, Internal Fixation
- The extremity is prepared and draped in standard sterile fashion. Arthroscopy is performed to evacuate hematoma and evaluate the articular surface and for associated injury. Arthroscopy is not useful for type IV to VI fractures because of the loss of capsular integrity leading to extravasation. The fracture is reduced; reduction is maintained with Kirschner wires (K-wires), which can be exchanged for cannulated screws. Fluoroscopy is

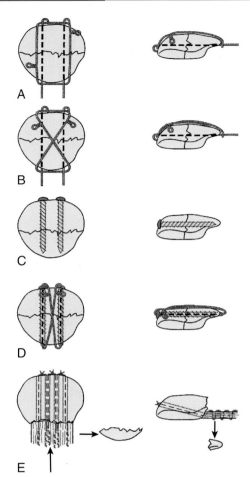

Figure 7-34. Techniques of patellar fracture fixation. **A,** Modified tension band with circular wire. **B,** Modified tension wire with figure-of-eight technique. **C,** Lag screw fixation. **D,** Combined cannulated lag screw and tension band wiring. **E,** Partial patellectomy. *(From Brinker MR: Review of orthopaedic trauma, Philadelphia, 2001, Saunders.)*

used to verify anatomic reduction (length, rotation, varus, valgus, and recurvatum). An appropriate plate is inserted, and proper alignment is verified in the AP and lateral planes. Locking screws are inserted in each fragment. Voids may be filled with bone graft. The wound is irrigated and then closed in a multilayer fashion, and a sterile dressing is applied.

Distal Femur Retrograde Intramedullary Nail Fixation

- The extremity is prepared and draped in standard sterile fashion. A midline incision from the patella to the tibial tubercle is made. Then the patellar tendon is split, and the fat pad is excised as needed. A guide pin is placed 1 cm anterior to the PCL origin; placement is verified with fluoroscopy. An entry hole is drilled. Longitudinal traction is used to reduce the fracture. A guidewire is passed across the fracture site under fluoroscopic guidance. The site is reamed and measured to determine nail length width. The nail is placed and locked distally, and then leg length and alignment are evaluated. After necessary adjustments are made, the nail is locked proximally. The wound is irrigated and then closed is a multilayer fashion, and a sterile dressing is applied.

Distal Femur Open Reduction, Internal Fixation

- The extremity is prepared and draped in standard sterile fashion. A medial or lateral incision is made; skin and soft tissues are dissected so the fracture site can be visualized. The fracture is reduced, and then reduction is maintained with K-wires, which can be exchanged for cannulated screws. Fluoroscopy is used to verify anatomic reduction (length, rotation, varus, valgus, and recurvatum). An appropriate plate is inserted, and alignment is verified in the AP and lateral planes. Locking screws are inserted in each fragment. Voids may be filled with bone graft. The wound is irrigated, the incision is closed in a multilayer fashion, and a sterile dressing is applied.

Estimated Postoperative Course

Postoperative Day 0 to 6 Weeks

- Patella open reduction, internal fixation (ORIF)
  - The knee brace is locked in extension, and weight bearing is allowed as tolerated in the brace.
  - Confirm reduction on radiographs at the initial postoperative visit.
  - Perform a wound check and suture removal at 10 to 14 days postoperatively.
  - Consider allowing knee ROM to some degree based on the stability of fixation at surgery.
- Tibial plateau ORIF and distal femur ORIF
  - Place a hinged knee brace; the patient is non–weight bearing for 6 weeks.
  - Confirm reduction on radiographs at the initial postoperative visit.
  - Perform a wound check and suture removal at 10 to 14 days postoperatively.
- Distal femur retrograde nail
  - Toe touch weight bearing is allowed, depending on the fracture configuration. Consider weight bearing as tolerated for short oblique or transverse fractures with 100% cortical contact.
  - Confirm reduction on radiographs at the initial postoperative visit.
  - Perform a wound check and suture removal at 10 to 14 days postoperatively.

Postoperative 6 Weeks to 3 Months

- Patella ORIF
  - Obtain radiographs to evaluate for union.
  - Advance ROM.
- Tibial plateau ORIF and distal femur ORIF
  - Obtain radiographs at 6 weeks; the patient may progress to toe touch weight bearing if adequate callus formation is seen.
- Distal femur retrograde nail
  - Obtain radiographs at 6 weeks; the patient may advance to full weight bearing when bridging callus is visible on radiographs.
  - Evaluate knee ROM.

Postoperative 3+ Months

- Patella ORIF
  - Progress with ROM and strengthening.
  - Permit full sport and activity at 5 to 6 months.

- Tibial plateau ORIF and distal femur ORIF
  - Obtain radiographs at 12 weeks; the patient may progress to full weight bearing if adequate callus formation is seen.

Suggested Readings

Gurkan V, Orhun H, Doganay M: Retrograde intramedullary interlocking nailing in fractures of the distal femur, *Acta Orthop Traumatol Turc* 43(3):199–205, 2009.

Melvin JS, Mehta S: Patellar fractures in adults, *J Am Acad Orthop Surg* 19:198–207, 2011.

Okike K, Bhattacharyya T: Trends in the management of open fractures: a critical analysis, *J Bone Joint Surg Am* 88:2739–2748, 2006.

Shuler FD, Beimesch CF: Distal femur and proximal tibia fractures. In Miller MD, Hart JA, MacKnight JM, editors: *Essential orthopaedics*, Philadelphia, 2010, Saunders, pp 694–698.

Shuler FD, Davis BC: Patella fractures. In Miller MD, Hart JA, MacKnight JM, editors: *Essential orthopaedics*, Philadelphia, 2010, Saunders, pp 699–702.

Zlowodzki M, Bhandari M, Marek DJ, et al: Operative treatment of acute distal femur fractures: systematic review of 2 comparative studies and 45 case series, *J Orthop Trauma* 5:366–371, 2006.

TIBIAL AND FIBULAR SHAFT FRACTURES

History

- Typically, patients present after acute injury; fractures may result from low- or high-energy trauma or penetrating injury such as a gunshot wound.
- The patient has leg pain and an inability to bear weight.

Physical Examination

- Observation: deformity, abrasion, laceration, fracture blisters, skin discoloration, capillary refill
- Palpation: crepitus, tenderness
- ROM: assessment of knee and ankle ROM after the fracture is stabilized
- Neurovascular examination:
  - Vascular examination: palpation of dorsalis pedis and posterior tibial pulses to ensure that they are present and equal to those in the uninjured extremity
  - Neurologic examination: evaluation of motor and sensory function
- Compartment syndrome evaluation
  - Manual compression of compartments to assessed firmness compared with the unaffected extremity
  - Compartment pressures obtained if indicated

Imaging

- Radiographs: AP and lateral views of the tibia a fibula identify fracture and help characterize the fracture pattern. Repeat radiography after reduction. Obtain radiographs of the knee and ankle as well, to assess for concomitant injuries.

Classification

- Open versus closed: Open fractures are further classified as follows: Grade I: less than 1 cm skin opening Grade II: 1 to 10 cm skin opening Grade III: A, 10 cm; B, 10 cm requiring soft tissue coverage; C, vascular injury requiring repair
- Location: proximal, middle, distal
- Pattern: transverse, oblique, spiral, segmental, comminuted
- Amount of shortening (cm) and degree of angulation and rotation

Initial Treatment

Patient Education

- Counsel patients on weight-bearing and ROM restrictions.
- Patients should be informed to call or return to the clinic or emergency department if they experience the following symptoms: increased pain, swelling, or neurovascular changes.

First Treatment Steps

- Tibial shaft: Reduce closed fractures and apply a long-leg splint. Apply a sterile dressing to an open fracture, and administer antibiotics and tetanus prophylaxis.
- Fibular shaft: Immobilize the leg in a short-leg splint.

Treatment Options

Nonoperative Management:
Figure 7-35

- Tibial shaft fracture with less than 1 cm of shortening, less than 5 degrees

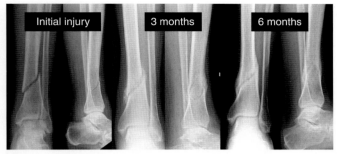

Figure 7-35. Nonoperative management: anteroposterior and lateral radiographs. Callus formation is noted in the 3-month radiograph, with healed fracture and acceptable alignment demonstrated 6 months after injury. *(From Miller MD, Hart JA, MacKnight JM, editors:* Essential orthopaedics, *Philadelphia, 2010, Saunders.)*

of angulation, less than 5 degrees of rotation, and competent soft tissues
- A long-leg splint is placed until swelling resolves (1 to 2 weeks); then it is converted to a long-leg cast.
- Non–weight bearing is indicated for 6 weeks. Begin protected weight bearing in a brace or cast if radiographs look favorable at 6 weeks.

Operative Management
Codes
ICD-9 code: 823.22 Tibial shaft fracture
CPT codes: 27759 Intramedullary nail fixation of the tibia
20690 Tibial shaft fracture external fixation

Operative Indications
- Tibial shaft
  - IM nail: unstable pattern (>1 cm of shortening, >5 degrees of angulation, >5 degrees of rotation) and incompetent soft tissues
  - External fixation: severe soft tissue injury and an unstable patient

Informed Consent and Counseling
- Possible complications: nonunion, infection, neurovascular injury, painful hardware, compartment syndrome, and DVT or PE
- Anesthesia risks: cardiac arrest, brain damage, paralysis, and death

Anesthesia
- General, with or without regional block

Patient Positioning
- Supine on a fracture table with all bony prominences well padded

Surgical Procedures
Tibial Shaft Fracture
- IM nail fixation (Fig. 7-36): The extremity is prepared and draped in standard sterile fashion. The fracture is reduced. A 2- to 3-cm longitudinal or transverse incision is made. The soft tissues medial to the patellar tendon are dissected. An awl is used to make a starting point, and then a guidewire is placed across the fracture site. The site is reamed in 0.5-cm increments to 1.5 mm greater than the selected nail size. Nail length is measured off the guidewire. The nail and distal locking screws are placed. The fracture site is compressed to eliminate any distraction that occurred during nail placement. Proximal locking screws are placed. Proximal and distal nail placement is evaluated using a C-arm. The wound is irrigated. The incision is closed in a multilayer fashion, and a sterile dressing is applied.
- External fixation: The extremity is prepared and draped in standard sterile fashion. A 1-cm incision is made over the preplanned pin site on the anteromedial border of tibia. Soft tissue is incised to bone. A tissue protector is used to predrill, and then half-pins are placed. Fluoroscopy is used to ensure proper pin placement. A frame is applied according to the manufacturer's

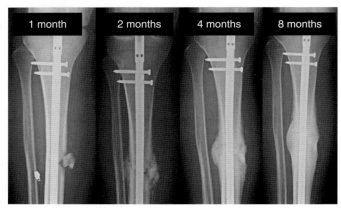

| 1 month | 2 months | 4 months | 8 months |

Figure 7-36. Operative management with intramedullary fixation: anteroposterior radiographs. Callus formation is noted in the 2-month postoperative radiograph. Note that surgery does not change the overall time required for fracture healing. *(From Miller MD, Hart JA, MacKnight JM, editors: Essential orthopaedics, Philadelphia, 2010, Saunders.)*

recommendations or the preoperative plan. Skin encroachment around the fixator pins is released, and pins are dressed with petrolatum gauze (Xeroform) and 4 × 4 gauze pads.

Estimated Postoperative Course
Postoperative Day 0 to 6 Weeks
- Tibial IM nail
  - At 10 to 14 days postoperatively, remove the splint and sutures, and obtain radiographs to evaluate alignment.
  - Allow weight bearing as tolerated.
  - Begin PT of knee and ankle mobilization if the fracture is stable.
- Tibial external fixator
  - At 10 to 14 days postoperatively, evaluate for pin site infection, and obtain radiographs to evaluate alignment,
  - Continue pin site care.
  - Convert to an IM nail at 2 weeks, if possible, to decrease the infection risk.

Postoperative 6 Weeks to 3 Months
- Tibial IM nail
  - Check radiographs at 6 weeks, and advance PT.
- Tibial external fixator
  - Evaluate for pin site infection and continue pin care.

- Obtain radiographs at 6 weeks to evaluate alignment. Advance weight bearing when callus is seen on radiographs.
- The frame may be removed, and a straight-leg cast may be placed at 8 weeks if adequate callous formation is seen.

Postoperative 3+ Months
- Tibial IM nail
  - Check radiographs. Begin sport-specific PT. The patient returns to full activity at 6 months.
- Tibial external fixator
  - Review radiographs.
  - Transition to a controlled ankle motion (CAM) walker or a fracture brace.
  - The patient returns to full activity at 6 months.

Suggested Readings
Beardi J, Hessman M, Hansen M, et al: Operative treatment of tibial shaft fractures: a comparison of different methods for primary stabilization, *Arch Orthop Trauma Surg* 128:709–715, 2008.

Dell Rocca GJ, Crist B: External fixation versus conversion to intramedullary nailing for definitive management of closed fractures of the femoral and tibial shaft, *J Am Acad Orthop Surg* 14:S131–S135, 2006.

Melvin JS, Domdroski DG, Torbert JT, et al: Open tibial shaft fractures: I. Evaluation and initial wound management. *J Am Acad Orthop Surg* 18:10–19, 2010.

Shuler FD, Dietz MJ: Tibial and fibular shaft fractures. In Miller MD, Hart JA, MacKnight JM, editors: *Essential orthopaedics*, Philadelphia, 2010, Saunders, pp 703–707.

White TO, Howell GE, Will EM, et al: Elevated intramuscular compartment pressures do not influence outcomes after tibial fracture, *J Trauma* 55:1133–1138, 2003.

ORTHOPAEDIC PROCEDURES
Knee Aspiration and/or Injection
Code
CPT code: 20610 Arthrocentesis, aspiration and/or injection; major joint or bursa

Indications
- Aspiration
  - Knee effusion or hemarthrosis
  - Suspected joint infection
- Injection with or without aspiration
  - OA of the knee
  - Gout or pseudogout of the knee
  - Rheumatoid arthritis of the knee
  - Patella chondromalacia

Contraindications
- Coagulopathy: severe or uncontrolled
- Suspected joint infection (may aspirate, do not inject steroid)
- Cellulitis or dermatitis of the overlying skin
- Adjacent osteomyelitis
- Impending knee surgery
- Bacteremia

Equipment and Supplies Needed
- Ethyl chloride
- Topical cleansing agent (e.g., povidone-iodine [Betadine])
- Sterile gloves and tray
- Needles: 25-gauge for injection of local anesthetic, 16- to 18-gauge for aspiration, 21-gauge for injection of steroid
- Hemostat
- Syringes: injection syringe (5- to 10-mL), aspiration syringe (30-mL)
- Sterile cup and appropriate laboratory tubes if fluid will be sent for analysis
- Injectate: steroid (1 mL) or other agent (e.g., triamcinolone [Kenalog],

40 mg/mL, hyaluronic acid) and 3 mL lidocaine, 1% without epinephrine
- Aspiration: 5 mL lidocaine, 1% without epinephrine anesthetize before aspiration
- Elastic compression (ACE) wrap, sterile dressing, or self-adhesive bandage

Procedure
1) Place the patient in the supine position on the examination table with the knee extended.
2) Palpate the superior pole of the patella, and locate the "soft spot," which is typically one fingerbreadth above and one fingerbreadth lateral to the superior pole. Mark this site with a pen or marker.
3) Apply ethyl chloride to the injection site. Put on sterile gloves. Prepare the skin with topical cleansing solution (Figs. 7-37 and 7-38).

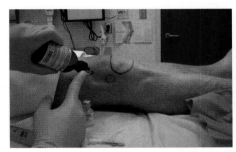

Figure 7-37. Ethyl chloride is applied to the injection site. *(From Miller MD, Hart JA, MacKnight JM, editors:* Essential orthopaedics, *Philadelphia, 2010, Saunders.)*

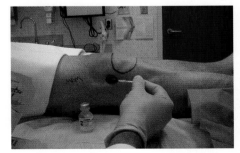

Figure 7-38. The skin is sterilized. *(From Miller MD, Hart JA, MacKnight JM, editors:* Essential orthopaedics, *Philadelphia, 2010, Saunders.)*

4) If aspiration is planned:
- Use a 25-gauge needle attached to a 5- to 10-mL syringe to infiltrate the skin with local anesthetic before inserting the larger aspiration needle (Fig. 7-39).
- Insert the larger-bore needle tilted at a 45-degree angle into the injection site (Fig. 7-40).
- Once the needle has been inserted, apply gentle pressure to the plunger to aspirate the fluid. Using the nondominant hand to compress the opposite side of the joint or the patella may be helpful (Fig. 7-41).
- When the syringe is full, place a hemostat on the hub of the needle to stabilize it; then the syringe can be disconnected and emptied into the sterile cup or tubes for laboratory studies. Reconnect the syringe,

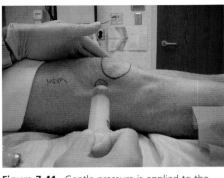

Figure 7-41. Gentle pressure is applied to the plunger to aspirate the fluid. Use of the nondominant hand to compress the opposite side of the joint or the patella may be helpful. *(From Miller MD, Hart JA, MacKnight JM, editors: Essential orthopaedics, Philadelphia, 2010, Saunders.)*

and continue aspiration if more fluid remains. If corticosteroid injection is indicated, attach the syringe with corticosteroid mixed with local anesthetic and then inject it into the joint. Hyaluronic acid injection can be performed in a similar manner.

5) Injection only: Identify the "soft spot," and prepare the injection site as described earlier. Insert the needle at a 45-degree angle, and inject the steroid-local anesthetic mixture or hyaluronic acid (Fig. 7-42).

6) Apply a sterile dressing or self-adhesive bandage to the injection site, and apply an elastic compression (ACE) wrap for compression.

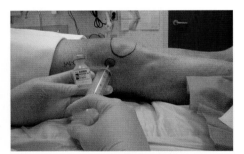

Figure 7-39. Local anesthetic is injected. *(From Miller MD, Hart JA, MacKnight JM, editors: Essential orthopaedics, Philadelphia, 2010, Saunders.)*

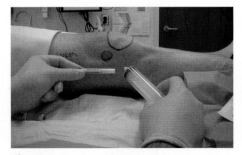

Figure 7-40. A large-bore needle tilted at a 45-degree angle is injected into the injection site. *(From Miller MD, Hart JA, MacKnight JM, editors: Essential orthopaedics, Philadelphia, 2010, Saunders.)*

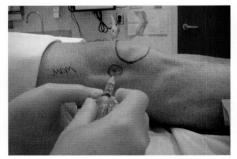

Figure 7-42. A steroid-local anesthetic mixture or hyaluronic acid is injected. *(From Miller MD, Hart JA, MacKnight JM, editors: Essential orthopaedics, Philadelphia, 2010, Saunders.)*

Aftercare Instructions

1) Remove the dressing the day following the injection.
2) Use ice for local discomfort at the injection site.
3) Diabetic patients may need to monitor blood glucose more closely because of the risk for transient increase in blood glucose level.
4) Possible side effects after the injection:
   • Pain or discomfort at the injection site may occur, but it typically subsides within 24 to 48 hours. This pain can be treated with ice and NSAIDs.
5) Contact your medical provider if any of the following symptoms develop: difficulty breathing, fever, chills, rash, or erythema and warmth at the injection site because they may be a sign of an adverse or allergic reaction.

PREPATELLAR BURSA ASPIRATION AND/OR INJECTION

Code
CPT code: 20610 (Arthrocentesis, aspiration and/or injection; major joint or bursa)

Indications
■ Acute or chronic prepatellar bursitis

Contraindications
■ Cellulitis or dermatitis of the skin overlying the injection site is a contraindication.
■ Do not inject steroid if septic bursitis is suspected.

Equipment and Supplies Needed
■ Ethyl chloride
■ Topical cleansing agent (e.g., povidone-iodine [Betadine])
■ Sterile gloves and tray
■ Needles (1- to 1.5-inch): 21-gauge needle for injection of local anesthetic, 16- to 18-gauge needle for aspiration
■ Syringes: injection syringe (5- to 10-mL), aspiration syringe (30-mL)
■ Injectate: 1 mL steroid (e.g., triamcinolone [Kenalog], 40 mg/mL) and 1 mL 1% lidocaine without epinephrine
■ Local anesthetic: lidocaine (1% without epinephrine) 5 mL to anesthetize the skin

■ Elastic compression (ACE) wrap and sterile dressing or self-adhesive bandage

Procedure
1) The patient should be in the supine position. A small pillow may be placed under the knee for comfort (Fig. 7-43).
2) Palpate the area over the patella for fluctuance (Fig. 7-44).
3) Use ethyl chloride to anesthetize the skin, and then prepare it with a topical cleansing agent (Figs. 7-45 and 7-46).
4) If aspirating the bursa, use the 21-gauge needle to inject local

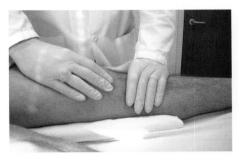

Figure 7-43. The patient is in the supine position. A small pillow may be placed under the knee for comfort. *(From Miller MD, Hart JA, MacKnight JM, editors:* Essential orthopaedics, *Philadelphia, 2010, Saunders.)*

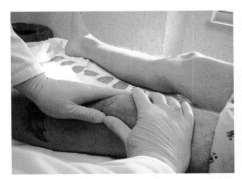

Figure 7-44. The area over the patella is palpated for fluctuance. *(From Miller MD, Hart JA, MacKnight JM, editors:* Essential orthopaedics, *Philadelphia, 2010, Saunders.)*

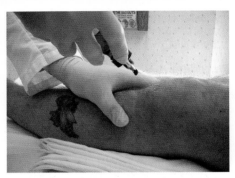

Figure 7-45. Ethyl chloride is used to anesthetize the skin site. *(From Miller MD, Hart JA, MacKnight JM, editors:* Essential orthopaedics, *Philadelphia, 2010, Saunders.)*

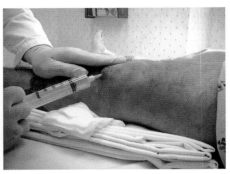

Figure 7-47. A 25-gauge needle and a 30-mL syringe are used to aspirate the bursa. *(From Miller MD, Hart JA, MacKnight JM, editors:* Essential orthopaedics, *Philadelphia, 2010, Saunders.)*

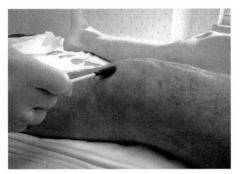

Figure 7-46. The skin site is prepared with a topical cleansing agent. *(From Miller MD, Hart JA, MacKnight JM, editors:* Essential orthopaedics, *Philadelphia, 2010, Saunders.)*

Aftercare Instructions
1) Remove the dressing the day after the injection.
2) Possible side effects after the injection:
   * Pain or discomfort at the injection site may occur, but it typically subsides within 24 to 48 hours. This pain can be treated with ice and NSAIDs.
3) Contact your medical provider if any of the following symptoms develop: difficulty breathing, fever, chills, rash, or erythema and warmth at the injection site because they may be a sign of an adverse or allergic reaction.

Pes Anserine Bursa Injection
Code
CPT code: 20610

Indications
▪ Pes anserine bursitis

Contraindications
▪ Cellulitis/dermatitis of the skin overlying the injection site

Equipment and Supplies Needed
▪ Ethyl chloride
▪ Topical cleansing agent (e.g., povidone-iodine [Betadine])
▪ Sterile gloves and tray
▪ 21-gauge needle
▪ 5- to 10-mL syringe
▪ Injectate: 1 mL steroid (e.g., triamcinolone [Kenalog], 40 mg/mL) and 1 mL

anesthetic before inserting the larger aspiration needle. From the lateral side, place the needle directly into the fluid-filled bursa.
5) Use the 25-gauge needle and the 30-mL syringe to aspirate the bursa (Fig. 7-47).
6) If steroid injection is planned, leave the needle in place. Use a hemostat to hold the needle while removing the aspiration syringe, and then connect the injection syringe and inject the steroid.
7) Apply a self-adhesive bandage or gauze and an elastic compression (ACE) wrap for compression.

local anesthetic (e.g., lidocaine 1% without epinephrine)
■ Elastic compression (ACE) wrap, sterile dressing, or self-adhesive bandage

Procedure

1) Place the patient in the supine position, and slightly flex the knee.
2) Identify the pes anserine bursa; it is located along the medial aspect of the knee approximately 2 cm below the joint line.
3) Apply ethyl chloride to the injection site, put on sterile gloves, and then prepare the skin with the topical cleansing agent (Fig. 7-48).
4) Insert the needle into the point of maximal tenderness, and gently advance it to bone. Retract the needle 2 to 3 mm, and then inject the mixture of the local anesthetic and steroid (Fig. 7-49).
5) Apply an elastic compression (ACE) wrap, sterile dressing, or self-adhesive bandage.

Aftercare Instructions

1) Remove the dressing the day after the injection.
2) Possible side effects after the injection:
   • Pain or discomfort at the injection site may occur, but it typically subsides within 24 to 48 hours. This pain can be treated with ice and NSAIDs.

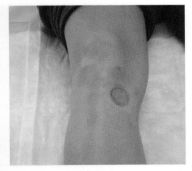

Figure 7-48. The skin site has been anesthetized with ethyl chloride and prepared with a topical cleansing agent. *(From Miller MD, Hart JA, MacKnight JM, editors: Essential orthopaedics, Philadelphia, 2010, Saunders.)*

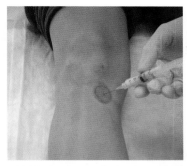

Figure 7-49. A mixture of a local anesthetic and steroid is injected. *(From Miller MD, Hart JA, MacKnight JM, editors: Essential orthopaedics, Philadelphia, 2010, Saunders.)*

3) Contact your medical provider if any of the following symptoms develop: difficulty breathing, fever, chills, rash, or erythema and warmth at the injection site because they may be a sign of an adverse or allergic reaction.

Iliotibial Band Injection

Code
CPT code: 20610

Indications
■ ITB syndrome

Contraindications
■ Cellulitis or dermatitis of the skin overlying the injection site

Equipment and Supplies Needed
■ Ethyl chloride
■ Topical cleansing agent for sterile preparation (e.g., povidone-iodine [Betadine])
■ Sterile gloves and tray
■ Injectate: 1 mL steroid (e.g., triamcinolone [Kenalog], 40 mg/mL) and 1 mL lidocaine (1% without epinephrine)
■ 21-gauge needle
■ 5- to 10-mL syringe
■ Sterile dressing or self-adhesive bandage

Procedure
1) Place the patient in the lateral decubitus position with the affected extremity up. Flex the knee 20 to 30 degrees (Fig. 7-50).

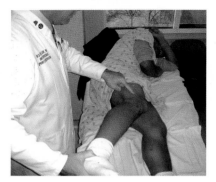

Figure 7-50. The patient is placed in the lateral decubitus position with the affected extremity up and the knee flexed 20 to 30 degrees. *(From Miller MD, Hart JA, MacKnight JM, editors: Essential orthopaedics, Philadelphia, 2010, Saunders.)*

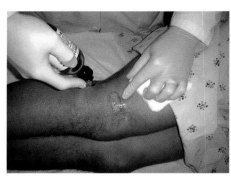

Figure 7-52. Ethyl chloride is applied to the injection site. *(From Miller MD, Hart JA, MacKnight JM, editors: Essential orthopaedics, Philadelphia, 2010, Saunders.)*

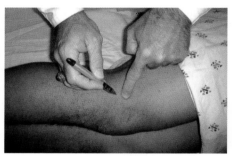

Figure 7-51. The point of maximal tenderness is identified. *(From Miller MD, Hart JA, MacKnight JM, editors: Essential orthopaedics, Philadelphia, 2010, Saunders.)*

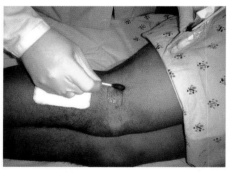

Figure 7-53. The skin is prepared with a topical cleansing agent. *(From Miller MD, Hart JA, MacKnight JM, editors: Essential orthopaedics, Philadelphia, 2010, Saunders.)*

2) Palpate the ITB, and identify its insertion site on the proximal tibia (Gerdy tubercle), and then identify the point of maximal tenderness (Fig. 7-51).
3) Apply ethyl chloride to the injection site, put on sterile gloves, and prepare the skin with the topical cleansing agent (Figs. 7-52 and 7-53).
4) Insert the needle into the point of maximal tenderness, and inject the combined steroid and lidocaine (Fig. 7-54).
5) Apply an elastic compression (ACE) wrap, sterile dressing, or self-adhesive bandage.

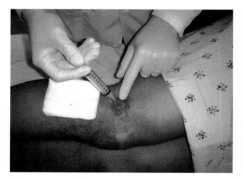

Figure 7-54. The needle is inserted into the point of maximal tenderness, and a combination of steroid and lidocaine is injected. *(From Miller MD, Hart JA, MacKnight JM, editors: Essential orthopaedics, Philadelphia, 2010, Saunders.)*

Aftercare Instructions

1) Remove the dressing the day after the injection.
2) Possible side effects after the injection:
   - Pain or discomfort at the injection site may occur, but it typically subsides within 24 to 48 hours. This pain can be treated with ice and NSAIDs.
3) Contact your medical provider if any of the following symptoms develop: difficulty breathing, fever, chills, rash, or erythema and warmth at the injection site because they may be a sign of an adverse or allergic reaction.

8 Foot and Ankle
Suzanne Eiss and Margaret Schick

ANATOMY
Bones: Figure 8-1

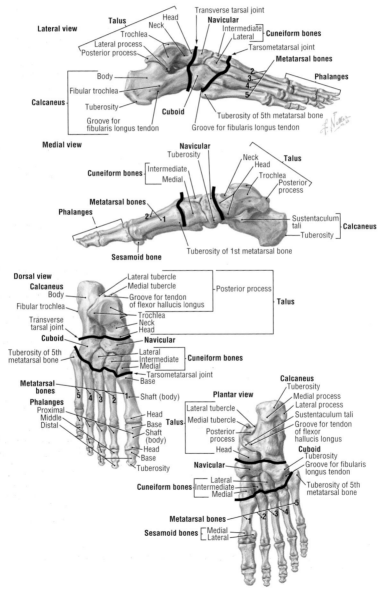

Figure 8-1. Bones of the foot. *(From Netter illustration from www.netterimages.com. Copyright Elsevier Inc. All rights reserved.)*

Ligaments: Figure 8-2

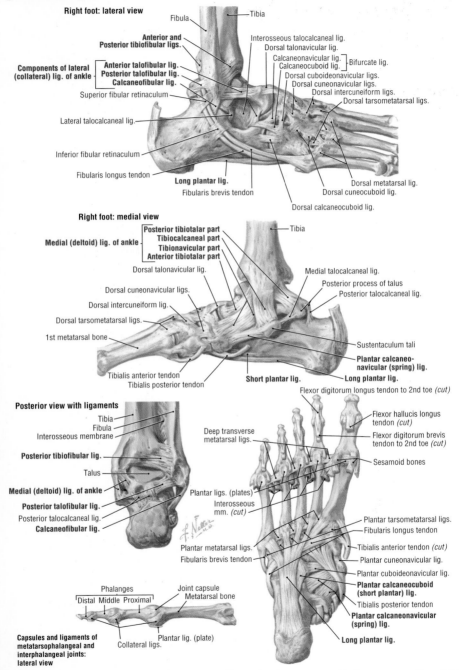

Right foot: lateral view

Fibula

Tibia

Anterior and
Posterior tibiofibular ligs.

Interosseous talocalcaneal lig.
Dorsal talonavicular lig.

Components of lateral
(collateral) lig. of ankle

Anterior talofibular lig.
Posterior talofibular lig.
Calcaneofibular lig.

Calcaneonavicular lig.
Calcaneocuboid lig.
Bifurcate lig.
Dorsal cuboideonavicular ligs.
Dorsal cuneonavicular ligs.
Dorsal intercuneiform ligs.
Dorsal tarsometatarsal ligs.

Superior fibular retinaculum

Lateral talocalcaneal lig.

Inferior fibular retinaculum

Fibularis longus tendon

Long plantar lig.
Fibularis brevis tendon

Dorsal metatarsal lig.
Dorsal cuneocuboid lig.
Dorsal calcaneocuboid lig.

Right foot: medial view

Medial (deltoid) lig. of ankle

Posterior tibiotalar part
Tibiocalcaneal part
Tibionavicular part
Anterior tibiotalar part

Tibia

Dorsal talonavicular lig.

Medial talocalcaneal lig.
Posterior process of talus
Posterior talocalcaneal lig.

Dorsal cuneonavicular ligs.

Dorsal intercuneiform lig.

Dorsal tarsometatarsal ligs.

1st metatarsal bone

Sustentaculum tali

Plantar calcaneo-
navicular (spring) lig.

Tibialis anterior tendon
Tibialis posterior tendon

Short plantar lig.

Long plantar lig.
Flexor digitorum longus tendon to 2nd toe (cut)

Posterior view with ligaments

Tibia
Fibula
Interosseous membrane

Deep transverse
metatarsal ligs.

Flexor hallucis longus
tendon (cut)

Flexor digitorum brevis
tendon to 2nd toe (cut)

Posterior tibiofibular lig.

Sesamoid bones

Talus

Medial (deltoid) lig. of ankle

Plantar ligs. (plates)
Interosseous
mm. (cut)

Posterior talofibular lig.

Posterior talocalcaneal lig.
Calcaneofibular lig.

Plantar tarsometatarsal ligs.
Fibularis longus tendon

Plantar metatarsal ligs.
Fibularis brevis tendon

Tibialis anterior tendon (cut)
Plantar cuneonavicular lig.
Plantar cuboideonavicular lig.
**Plantar calcaneocuboid
(short plantar) lig.**
Tibialis posterior tendon
**Plantar calcaneonavicular
(spring) lig.**

Phalanges
Distal Middle Proximal

Joint capsule
Metatarsal bone

Long plantar lig.

**Capsules and ligaments of
metatarsophalangeal and
interphalangeal joints:
lateral view**

Plantar lig. (plate)
Collateral ligs.

Figure 8-2. Ligaments of the foot. *(From Netter illustration from www.netterimages.com. Copyright Elsevier Inc. All rights reserved.)*

Muscles, Nerves, Arteries:
Figures 8-3, 8-4AB, **and** 8-5A-C

Superficial dissection

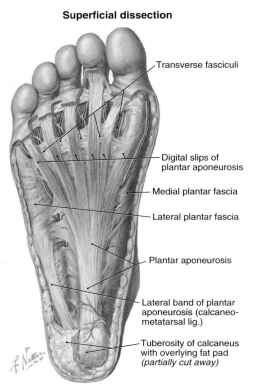

Transverse fasciculi

Digital slips of
plantar aponeurosis

Medial plantar fascia

Lateral plantar fascia

Plantar aponeurosis

Lateral band of plantar
aponeurosis (calcaneo-
metatarsal lig.)

Tuberosity of calcaneus
with overlying fat pad
(*partially cut away*)

Figure 8-3. Dorsal view of the foot sole. *(From Netter illustration from www.netterimages.com.*
Copyright Elsevier Inc. All rights reserved.)

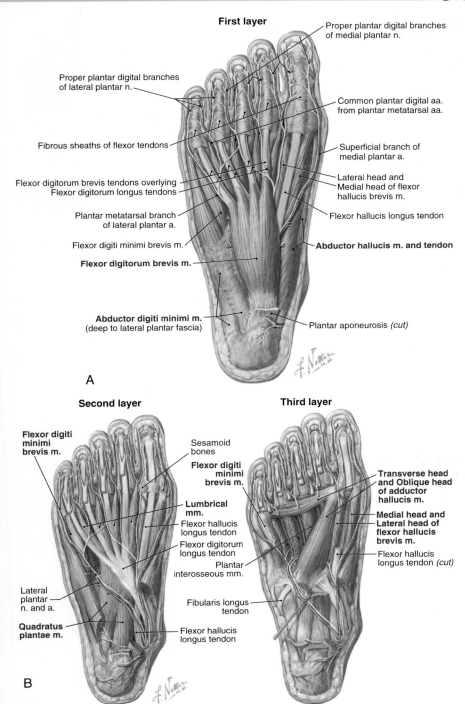

Figure 8-4A-B. Plantar views of the foot muscles. *(From Netter illustration from www.netterimages. com. Copyright Elsevier Inc. All rights reserved.)*

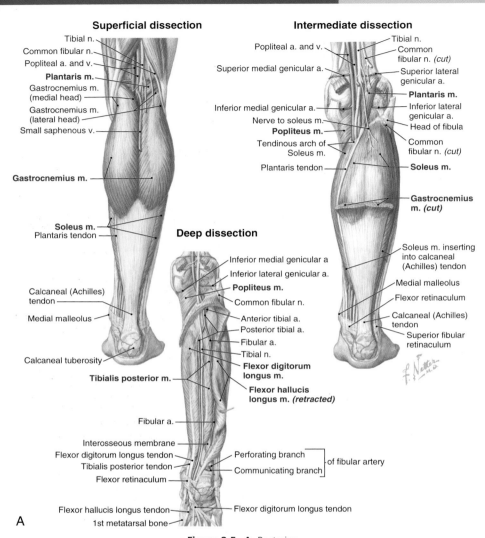

Superficial dissection

Tibial n.
Common fibular n.
Popliteal a. and v.
Plantaris m.
Gastrocnemius m. (medial head)
Gastrocnemius m. (lateral head)
Small saphenous v.

Gastrocnemius m.

Soleus m.
Plantaris tendon

Calcaneal (Achilles) tendon
Medial malleolus

Calcaneal tuberosity
Tibialis posterior m.

Fibular a.
Interosseous membrane
Flexor digitorum longus tendon
Tibialis posterior tendon
Flexor retinaculum

Flexor hallucis longus tendon
1st metatarsal bone

Intermediate dissection

Tibial n.
Popliteal a. and v.
Common fibular n. *(cut)*
Superior medial genicular a.
Superior lateral genicular a.
Plantaris m.
Inferior medial genicular a.
Inferior lateral genicular a.
Nerve to soleus m.
Head of fibula
Popliteus m.
Common fibular n. *(cut)*
Tendinous arch of Soleus m.
Soleus m.
Plantaris tendon
Gastrocnemius m. (cut)

Soleus m. inserting into calcaneal (Achilles) tendon
Medial malleolus
Flexor retinaculum
Calcaneal (Achilles) tendon
Superior fibular retinaculum

Deep dissection

Inferior medial genicular a
Inferior lateral genicular a.
Popliteus m.
Common fibular n.
Anterior tibial a.
Posterior tibial a.
Fibular a.
Tibial n.
Flexor digitorum longus m.
Flexor hallucis longus m. *(retracted)*

Perforating branch — of fibular artery
Communicating branch

Flexor digitorum longus tendon

A

Figure 8-5. A, Posterior,

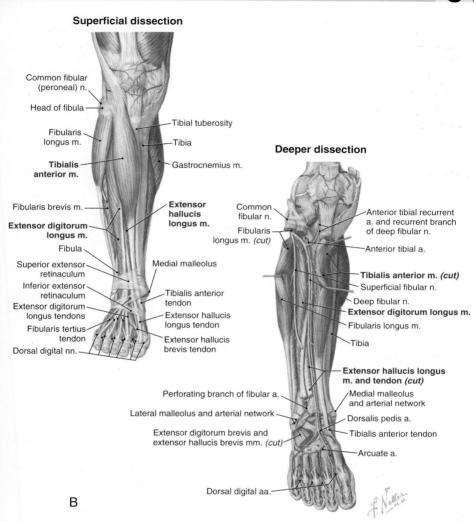

Superficial dissection

Common fibular (peroneal) n.

Head of fibula

Fibularis longus m.

Tibialis anterior m.

Fibularis brevis m.

Extensor digitorum longus m.

Fibula

Superior extensor retinaculum

Inferior extensor retinaculum

Extensor digitorum longus tendons

Fibularis tertius tendon

Dorsal digital nn.

Tibial tuberosity

Tibia

Gastrocnemius m.

Extensor hallucis longus m.

Medial malleolus

Tibialis anterior tendon

Extensor hallucis longus tendon

Extensor hallucis brevis tendon

Deeper dissection

Common fibular n.

Fibularis longus m. (cut)

Anterior tibial recurrent a. and recurrent branch of deep fibular n.

Anterior tibial a.

Tibialis anterior m. (cut)

Superficial fibular n.

Deep fibular n.

Extensor digitorum longus m.

Fibularis longus m.

Tibia

Extensor hallucis longus m. and tendon (cut)

Medial malleolus and arterial network

Dorsalis pedis a.

Tibialis anterior tendon

Arcuate a.

Perforating branch of fibular a.

Lateral malleolus and arterial network

Extensor digitorum brevis and extensor hallucis brevis mm. (cut)

Dorsal digital aa.

B

Figure 8-5, cont'd. B, anterior, and

Continued

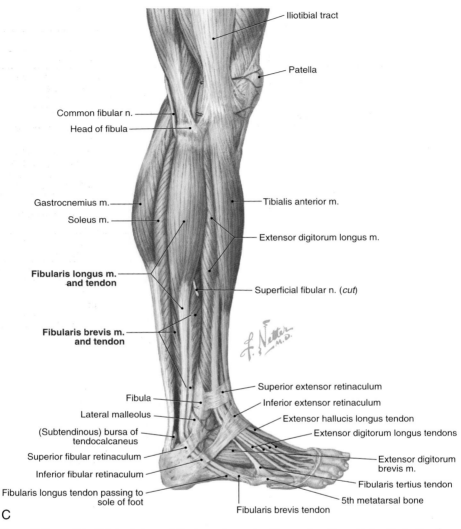

Iliotibial tract

Patella

Common fibular n.

Head of fibula

Gastrocnemius m.

Soleus m.

Fibularis longus m. and tendon

Fibularis brevis m. and tendon

Tibialis anterior m.

Extensor digitorum longus m.

Superficial fibular n. (*cut*)

Fibula

Lateral malleolus

(Subtendinous) bursa of tendocalcaneus

Superior fibular retinaculum

Inferior fibular retinaculum

Fibularis longus tendon passing to sole of foot

Superior extensor retinaculum

Inferior extensor retinaculum

Extensor hallucis longus tendon

Extensor digitorum longus tendons

Extensor digitorum brevis m.

Fibularis tertius tendon

5th metatarsal bone

Fibularis brevis tendon

C

Figure 8-5, cont'd. C, lateral views of the lower leg and ankle muscles. *(From Netter illustration from www.netterimages.com. Copyright Elsevier Inc. All rights reserved.)*

Nerve Function: Table 8-1

Table 8-1. Nerve Function

NERVE	BRANCHES	MOTOR	TESTING	SENSORY
Fibular (Peroneal)	Deep	Tibialis anterior, EHL, EDL, EDB, EHB	Ankle and great toe dorsiflexion, toe extension	Webspace between great toe and second toe
	Superficial	Peroneus longus and brevis	Ankle/subtalar eversion	Distal one third of anterior lower leg, dorsum of foot (except webspace between great toe and second toe and distal portion toes)
Saphenous		None		Medial portion of lower leg, medial foot
Sural		None		Posterior lower leg, lateral foot
Tibial		Gastrocnemius, soleus, plantaris, tibialis posterior, FHL, FDL	Ankle and great toe plantarflexion, Achilles reflex	Plantar surface of foot and toes, dorsal aspect of distal portion of toes

EDB, Extensor digitorum brevis; EDL, extensor digitorum longus; EHL, extensor hallucis longus; FDL, flexor digitorum longus; FHL, flexor hallicus longus.

Surface Anatomy: Figure 8-6

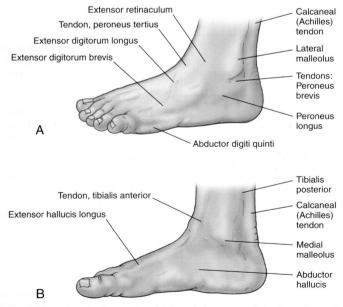

Figure 8-6. Surface anatomy of (**A**) lateral and (**B**) medial aspects of the foot. *(From O'Neal LW: Surgical pathology of the foot and clinicopathologic correlations. In Bowker JH, Pfeifer M (eds):* Levin and O'Neal's the diabetic foot, *ed 7, Philadelphia, 2008, Mosby.)*

PHYSICAL EXAMINATION
- Inspect for edema, erythema, ecchymosis, deformity, callus formation, ulceration, and hairlessness. On standing examination, note hindfoot alignment. Assess gait pattern.
- Palpate to evaluate clinical complaint:
  - Anterior ankle joint line
  - Fibula, both distally and proximally
  - Medial malleolus
  - Peroneal tendons
  - Posterior tibial tendon
  - Sinus tarsi
  - Achilles tendon
  - Anterior tibial tendon
  - Metatarsals
  - Insertion of plantar fascia

Normal Range of Motion:
Table 8-2
Neurovascular Examination:
Table 8-3

Table 8-2. Normal Ankle/Foot Range of Motion

Ankle dorsiflexion	10-23 degrees
Ankle plantarflexion	23-48 degrees
Inversion	5-35 degrees
Eversion	5-25 degrees
First metatarsophalangeal dorsiflexion	45-90 degrees
First metatarsophalangeal plantarflexion	10-40 degrees

Table 8-3. Neurovascular Examination

NERVE	LOCATION OF TEST	TESTS
SPN	Dorsum of foot	Tinel
DPN	1st/2nd MTP webspace	Tinel
Sural	Lateral border foot	Tinel
Saphenous	Medial border foot	Tinel
Tibial	Plantar foot	Tinel
Post tibialis artery	Posterior to medial malleolus	
Dorsalis pedis artery	Dorsum of midfoot	

DPN, Deep peroneal nerve; SPN, superficial peroneal nerve.

Table 8-4. Differential Diagnosis

Anterior ankle pain	Ankle arthritis, osteochondral dessicans talus
Medial ankle pain	Posterior tibial tendinopathy, medial malleolar injury
Lateral ankle pain	Peroneal tendinopathy, ankle sprain
Posterior ankle pain	Achilles tendinopathy or rupture, os trigonum, posterior impingement
Midfoot	Lisfranc injury, midfoot arthritis
Forefoot	Metatarsal fracture, stress fracture, metatarsalgia
Heel pain	Plantar fasciitis, calcaneal stress fracture, insertional Achilles tendinopathy
Great toe	Hallux rigidus, hallux valgus
Lesser toes	Toe fracture, hammertoe deformity, Morton neuroma

Differential Diagnosis: Table 8-4

ANKLE ARTHRITIS
History
- Ankle arthritis may affect tibiotalar or subtalar joints.
- Usually the patient has unilateral ankle pain, stiffness, swelling, ± history of injury. Pain worsens with weight-bearing activity.
- Post-traumatic most common etiology. Other causes include inflammatory arthritis, neuropathic arthropathy, and primary osteoarthritis (rare).

Physical Examination
- Standing evaluation may reveal varus/valgus deformity.
- Patient often experiences decreased motion in plantarflexion, dorsiflexion, or both.
- Tenderness occurs on palpation of the anterior tibiotalar joint line.

Imaging
- Radiographs: Weight-bearing anteroposterior (AP), mortise, lateral
  - May reveal joint space narrowing of the tibiotalar joint, osteophytes,

subchondral sclerosis and cysts, flattening of talus, loose bodies. Erosive changes are noted in inflammatory arthropathy. Neuropathic arthropathy joint collapse and significant bony deformity (Fig. 8-7)

Initial Treatment
Patient Education
- Ankle arthritis occurs when the cartilage between the tibia and talus wears out. It is most commonly the result of a previous injury. Arthritis is a progressive condition and worsens over time.

Treatment Options
Nonoperative Management
- First treatment steps include activity modification, weight loss if indicated, lace-up ankle brace, and nonsteroidal anti-inflammatory drugs (NSAIDs).
- Intra-articular corticosteroid injection (see ankle injection procedure, page 309). Risks include local skin reaction (depigmentation or subcutaneous fat atrophy) and infection.
- Bracing/shoe modification options are a lace-up ankle brace, an ankle-foot orthotic (AFO), an Arizona brace, and a rocker-bottom sole.

Operative Management
Codes
ICD-9 code:
  716.97 ankle arthritis

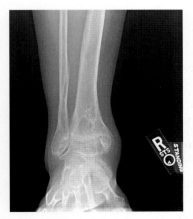

Figure 8-7. Severe post-traumatic ankle arthritis with complete loss of tibiotalar joint space.

CPT code:
  27625 Ankle arthrotomy with debridement/loose body removal
  27870 Ankle arthrodesis
  27702 Total ankle arthroplasty

Operative Indications
- **Ankle arthrotomy with debridement/loose body removal**
  - Generally has limited value and indicated only in mild arthritis without significant joint space narrowing
- **Ankle arthrodesis:**
  - Indications: painful tibiotalar arthritis not responsive to nonoperative treatment, failed arthroplasty
  - Contraindications: acute infection, acute neuropathic arthropathy, severe vascular disease
- **Total ankle arthroplasty:**
  - Indications: tibiotalar arthritis not responsive to nonoperative management, low demand patients older than age 50-55 years, weight < 200 lb, maintained range of motion, normal/near normal alignment, no preexisting subtalar arthritis.
  - Contraindications: acute infection, significantly diminished bone stock, neuropathy, severe vascular disease. Relative contraindications include deformity greater than 5 degrees and talar avascular necrosis.

Informed Consent and Counseling
- **Arthrodesis:**
  - Major risks include nonunion (<10%), wound complications, nerve injury, infection, deep vein thrombosis (DVT), hardware loosening/failure, and development of arthritis in hindfoot/subtalar joint. A risk of amputation exists in cases of severe complication (≤5%).
  - The complication rate increases with nicotine use, neuropathy, and vascular disease.
- **Total ankle arthroplasty:**
  - Informed consent and counseling: Risks are similar to arthrodesis (infection, wound complications, DVT, hardware loosening). Recent studies report 10% to 30% reoperation rate and survival rates of 77% to 90% at 5- and 10-year follow-up.

If surgery fails, consider conversion to arthrodesis (contraindicated in infection). Limited revision options are available.

Anesthesia
- General anesthesia with or without peripheral nerve block

Patient Positioning
- Positioning: supine with toes pointing directly toward ceiling. A small bump can be placed under the ipsilateral hip to internally rotate leg. A thigh tourniquet should be placed.

Surgical Procedures
Ankle arthrodesis (Fig. 8-8AB)
- Many implants for fixation are available, the most common being an anterior plate with cross-screws. An intraoperative radiograph is used to confirm appropriate placement.
- Open anterior approach is most common. An incision is made over the ankle between anterior tibial tendon and extensor hallucis longus (EHL).
- Structures at risk include superficial peroneal nerve and neurovascular bundle (posterior to EHL).

- The neurovascular bundle is mobilized, and the tibial osteophytes are removed to visualize joint. The joint is prepared by removing any remaining articular cartilage, and microfracturing and/or drilling the subchondral bone. A lamina spreader can be helpful for visualization.
- Align neutral dorsiflexion/plantarflexion, 0 to 5 degrees hindfoot valgus, 5 degrees external rotation. An intraoperative radiograph is used to determine correct alignment for fixation.
- A sugar tong splint is applied in the operating room after closure. The patient remains non–weight bearing.

Estimated Postoperative Course
- Postoperative 2 weeks:
  - Sutures are removed and radiographs are obtained. A non–weight-bearing cast is applied for 4 weeks.
- Postoperative 6 weeks:
  - Radiographs reviewed. The patient is transitioned to a weight-bearing cast for an additional 6 weeks.
- Postoperative 3 months:
  - Remove cast. Obtain radiographs to evaluate for healing.
  - Physical therapy is generally not indicated, but some patients may need some therapy for gait training.

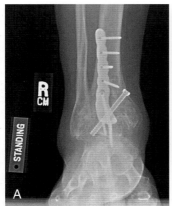 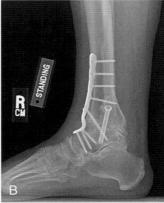

Figure 8-8. Postoperative anteroposterior (**A**) and lateral (**B**) views following ankle arthrodesis using anterior plate.

Total ankle arthroplasty (Fig. 8-9AB)

- Second- and third-generation implants are now available, but there are still limited data on longevity. First-generation implants have a high failure rate.
- Both 2 and 3 component implants are available, primarily depending on surgeon preference.
- An open anterior approach is used as described in ankle arthrodesis. Major structures at risk include the superficial peroneal nerve and neurovascular bundle.

Estimated Postoperative Course

- Postoperative 2 weeks: non–weight-bearing splint for 1 to 2 weeks. Remove sutures about 2 weeks after surgery and apply a non–weight-bearing cast.
- Postoperative 4 to 6 weeks: transition to weight bearing in a boot. Remove boot multiple times daily for gentle range of motion in plantarflexion and dorsiflexion.
- Postoperative 3 months: Formal physical therapy may be initiated about 3 months postoperatively if the patient has significant stiffness or weakness.
  - After recovery, radiographs may be obtained every 1 to 2 years.

SUBTALAR ARTHRITIS

History

- Post-traumatic most common etiology (calcaneal fracture or subtalar dislocation). Also common site for rheumatoid arthritis and Charcot arthropathy.
- Pain lateral aspect hindfoot, worse with walking on uneven ground

Physical Examination

- Tenderness over sinus tarsi, limited subtalar motion (inversion/eversion), pain and possible crepitus with subtalar motion

Imaging

- Radiographs: weight-bearing foot AP, lateral, oblique and weight-bearing ankle AP, mortise, lateral
  - Lateral views are best to evaluate subtalar joint (Fig. 8-10)
- Magnetic resonance imaging/computed tomography (MRI/CT) scan: not necessary for diagnosis. CT will show joint in more detail (osteophytes, subchondral cysts, and loose bodies)

Treatment Options

Nonoperative Management

Initial treatment should be nonoperative. NSAIDs, lace-up ankle brace, weight loss if indicated, activity modification (limit uneven surfaces), and corticosteroid injections

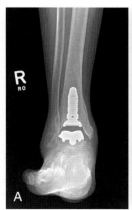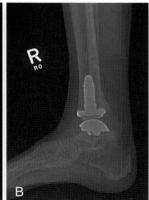

Figure 8-9. Postoperative anteroposterior (**A**) and lateral (**B**) views following ankle arthroplasty using Wright Medical INBONE prosthesis.

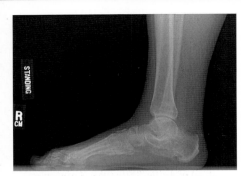

Figure 8-10. Post-traumatic subtalar arthritis on lateral radiograph. There is evidence of prior calcaneal fracture with collapse of subtalar joint.

Operative Management
Codes
ICD-9 Code
  716.97 Subtalar arthritis

CPT Codes
  29904 Arthroscopic subtalar joint
    debridement
  28725 Subtalar arthrodesis

Operative Indications
- **Arthroscopic subtalar joint debridement.**
  - Arthroscopy difficult due to joint space narrowing. Open debridement of osteophytes. Synovectomy is occasionally performed in mild/ moderate arthritis not responsive to nonoperative treatment. Generally limited value for long-term pain relief
- **Subtalar arthrodesis:**
  - Indication: Isolated subtalar degenerative disease unresponsive to nonoperative treatment
  - Contraindications: same as ankle arthrodesis

Informed Consent and Counseling
- Risks include infection, wound complications, arthritis in surrounding joints, nonunion (reported rates 0.5%), DVT, symptomatic hardware (especially if screw heads are prominent posteriorly). Some patients feel instability on uneven ground. At-risk structures: superficial peroneal and sural nerves, peroneal tendons

Anesthesia
- General anesthesia with or without peripheral nerve block

Patient Positioning
- Positioning for arthrodesis: supine with toes pointing directly toward ceiling. A small bump can be placed under ipsilateral hip to internally rotate leg. Thigh tourniquet placed.

Surgical Procedure
- *Subtalar arthrodesis*
  - Lateral incision is made about 2 cm distal to lateral malleolus, extending to the base fourth metatarsal. Extensor digitorum brevis is reflected to expose subtalar joint. Peroneal tendons are elevated from lateral calcaneous and retracted.
  - Any remaining cartilage is removed, and the joint is debrided to cancellous bone.
  - Fusion is performed at 5 degrees valgus. Two cannulated screws are placed from the non–weight-bearing portion of calcaneus toward the anterior margin posterior facet into the talus. Divergent screws have improved compression forces compared with parallel screws or a single screw. Intraoperative radiographs and guidewires are used to ensure appropriate placement of screws (Fig. 8-11).

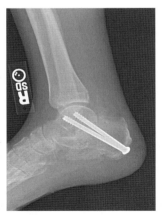

Figure 8-11. Lateral radiograph status post subtalar arthrodesis using two divergent cannulated screws.

- The patient may require bone grafting or bone block if bone loss is present from previous trauma/ calcaneal fracture.
- A posterior splint is applied in the operating room after closure. The patient remains non–weight bearing for 2 weeks.

Estimated Postoperative Course
- Postoperative 2 weeks: sutures removed. Non–weight bearing in a boot. Remove boot multiple times daily for ankle motion to prevent stiffness.
- Postoperative 6 weeks: radiograph reviewed. Start weight bearing in boot from weeks 6 to 12.
- Postoperative 3 months: Transition to regular shoes at 12 weeks if fusion is radiographically healed.

Suggested Readings

Coughlin MJ: *Surgery of the Foot and Ankle*, ed 8, Philadelphia, 2007, Mosby.
DiGiovanni CW, Greisberg J: *Foot and ankle: core knowledge in orthopaedics*, Philadelphia, 2007, Mosby.
Easley ME, Trnka HJ, Schon LC, Myerson MS: Isolated subtalar arthrodesis, *J Bone Joint Surg Am* 82(5):613–624, 2000.
Park JS, Mroczek KJ: Total ankle arthroplasty, *Bull NYU Hosp Jt Dis* 69(1):27–35, 2011.
Thomas RH, Daniels TR: Current concepts review: ankle arthritis, *J Bone Joint Surg Am* 85-A(5): 923–935, 2003.

ANKLE FRACTURES

History
- Trauma, low-energy twisting injuries to high-energy injuries (motor vehicle accidents or fall from height)
- Pain (worse with weight bearing), swelling, ecchymosis, ± deformity. Patient may report "pop" at the time of injury

Physical Examination
- Edema, ecchymosis, tenderness over fracture site. Medial tenderness without medial malleolus fracture suggests deltoid ligament injury; does not necessarily signify unstable ankle joint
- Fracture blisters with severe edema and soft tissue trauma
- Visual deformity present if ankle dislocated or severe displacement of fracture

- Complete neurovascular examination required. If ankle reduction performed, neurovascular examination should be repeated after reduction
- Evaluation for syndesmotic injury: palpation of proximal fibula (tenderness suggests syndesmotic injury), calf compression test, external rotation test
  - **Calf compression test:** medial-lateral compression at mid-calf. Pain at ankle joint suggests syndesmotic injury
  - **External rotation test:** external rotation of the ankle with the knee at 90 degrees of flexion. Pain at syndesmosis suggests injury

Imaging
- Radiographs:
  - Weight-bearing ankle AP, mortise, lateral. Assess fracture, alignment, displacement.
  - Weight bearing foot AP, oblique, lateral. Assess for fracture or malalignment.
  - Stress radiographs of the ankle should be performed for isolated fibular fractures at the level of the ankle joint. To perform, gravity stress or external rotation and/or abduction stress is applied in a non–weight-bearing mortise view. Medial clear space greater than 4 to 5 mm indicates deltoid ligament injury and ankle instability (Fig. 8-12).
  - Compare with contralateral ankle (mortise view is best). A 2-mm side-to-side difference in medial clear space indicates instability.
  - CT scans are helpful to evaluate comminution and subtle displacement. Scan should be performed of bilateral ankles to compare syndesmosis and medial clear space.
  - MRIs are usually not necessary but can be useful to evaluate the deltoid ligament and help determine ankle stability.

Classification Systems
- Danis-Weber classification is based on the location of the fibular fracture and does not address the medial structures.
  - Type A: Transverse fracture at the level of or distal to the tibial plafond

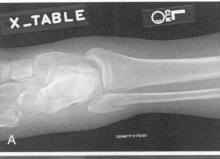

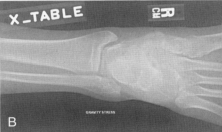

Figure 8-12AB. Gravity stress views of the injured (**A**) and uninjured (**B**) ankles. Medial clear space is obvious, and operative intervention is recommended for this fracture.

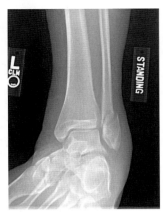

Figure 8-13. Mortise view of Weber B fracture, fracture line at the level of the ankle joint.

- Type B: Spiral, oblique fracture at the level of distal tibiofibular joint and extends proximally. Associated with possible disruption of syndesmosis (Fig. 8-13).
- Type C: Fracture proximal to distal tibiofibular joint. Syndesmosis completely disrupted; anterior and posterior tibiofibular ligaments and interosseous membrane ruptured (Fig. 8-14)
- Lauge-Hansen classification: Fracture types are described by two terms that describe the fracture mechanism. The first term is supination or pronation, and the second term is adduction or external rotation. Additional subtypes exist within each classification.

Initial Treatment
- Immobilization in sugar tong splint, non–weight bearing, and elevation. Refer to an orthopaedic surgeon to be seen within 7 to 10 days.

Patient Education
- Unstable fractures require surgical fixation. Fractures that heal in nonanatomic alignment result in pain and increased risk of post-traumatic arthritis.

Treatment Options
Nonoperative Management
- Weber A fractures: Nearly all can be treated nonoperatively, even with mild displacement.
  - Immobilization in cast or walking boot, weight bearing as tolerated. Most fractures heal in 6 weeks.
- Weber B: Isolated Weber B fractures require thorough evaluation to determine stability. If stable, consider nonoperative treatment. Unstable fractures require open reduction, internal fixation (ORIF).
  - Consider nonoperative management when medial clear space is less than 4 to 5 mm and less than 2 mm greater than contralateral side on stress and static radiographs.
  - Immobilization in cast or walking boot for 6 weeks. Weight bearing is progressed as tolerated.
  - Frequent follow-up with radiographs (weekly for first 2 to 3 weeks). Surgical fixation is recommended if there is a change in stability or alignment.

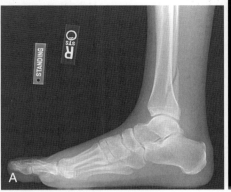
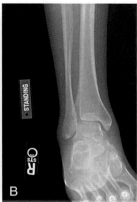

Figure 8-14. Lateral (**A**) and mortise (**B**) views of Weber C fracture. Medial clear space widening noted with fracture line above the ankle joint line.

- After 6 weeks of immobilization, transition to brace. Physical therapy may be helpful to regain motion and strength.
- ▪ Weber C: Nonoperative management is not recommended.
  - Medial malleolus fractures: Only small avulsion fractures can be treated nonoperatively if isolated and minimally displaced. Treatment includes short leg cast or cast boot for 6 weeks.

Operative Management
Codes
ICD-9
    824.0 Closed medial malleolus fracture
    824.2 Closed lateral malleolus fracture
    824.4 Closed bimalleolar ankle fracture
    824.6 Closed trimalleolar fracture
    824.8 Closed ankle fracture
CPT
    27792 ORIF lateral malleolus
    27814 ORIF bimalleolar fracture
    27823 ORIF trimalleolar fracture (with posterior malleolus ORIF)

Operative Indications
- ▪ Instability of ankle or syndesmosis, significant fracture displacement
- ▪ Open fractures require immediate surgical debridement and antibiotic therapy. Staged treatment is often used in open fractures. External fixator is initially placed to stabilize the fracture/joint followed by delayed ORIF once soft tissues allow.
- ▪ Bimalleolar and trimalleolar fractures result in instability of mortise and surgical fixation necessary to stabilize ankle.
- ▪ Medial malleolar fractures are often associated with injury to the deltoid ligament and most require ORIF.

Informed Consent and Counseling
- ▪ Risks include wound complications, infection, nonunion, and DVT. The rate of complication is significantly higher in diabetics, nicotine users, and patients with peripheral vascular disease. Post-traumatic arthritis may still occur despite proper stabilization. Major structures at risk are the superficial peroneal nerve (crosses fibula approximately 4 to 5 cm proximal to joint) and saphenous vein (for medial incisions).

Anesthesia
- ▪ General with ankle or popliteal block

Patient Positioning
- ▪ Supine with toes pointing directly toward ceiling. A small bump can be placed under the ipsilateral hip to internally rotate the leg. Place a thigh tourniquet.

Surgical Procedure
Open Reduction, Internal Fixation
- Hardware:
  - Distal fibular fractures—Multiple hardware options are available including locking and nonlocking plates and screws. Locking plates should be used when bone quality is poor or a patient is at high risk for nonunion (diabetes, osteoporosis).
  - Medial malleolus fractures— Fixation devices include lag, partially threaded, or cannulated screws; Kirshner wires; tension bands; and buttress plate (used only for vertical sheer fractures to prevent proximal migration of fracture fragment).
- Use a lateral approach for fixation of distal fibula, syndesmosis, and possibly posterior malleolus. Longitudinal incision is made directly over the distal fibula. Fibular fracture is reduced and stabilized, restoring proper length and rotation. Intraoperative radiograph is used for reduction, to confirm proper screw length, and to determine stability. After ORIF fibula, a radiograph is taken to evaluate medial clear space. If widening is present after ORIF fibula, a syndesmotic screw is placed (Fig. 8-15).
- Use a medial approach for fixation of medial malleolar fracture or deltoid ligament repair. A longitudinal incision is made over medial malleolus. The saphenous vein is identified and carefully retracted.
- Many fractures require both medial and lateral approaches.
- A sugar tong splint is applied before leaving the operating room, and the patient remains non–weight bearing on the affected extremity.

Estimated Postoperative Course
- Postoperative 2 to 3 weeks: Sutures removed. Radiographs are obtained at each postoperative visit until complete healing is noted.
- In general, the patient should be non–weight bearing with immobilization in a sugar tong splint, cast, or boot for 6 weeks postoperative. Gentle range of motion and partial weight bearing can begin 2 to 4 weeks postoperative when there is good bone quality and stable fixation. Strict immobilization and no weight bearing should be followed for full 6 weeks if there is poor bone quality, ligamentous instability, or less stable fixation.
- Postoperative 6 weeks: Progress to full weight bearing in boot. Remove boot daily for range of motion.
- Postoperative 8 to 10 weeks: Discontinue boot and progress to shoe with ankle brace.
- Syndesmotic screw removal should be performed no sooner than 3 to 4 months postoperative. No definitive evidence exists to show a difference in clinical outcome whether a syndesmotic screw is removed or left in place.

Suggested Readings
Clare MP: A rational approach to ankle fractures, *Foot Ankle Clin* 13:593–610, 2008.
Gumann G: *Fractures of the foot and ankle*, Philadelphia, 2004, Saunders.
Michel P, van den Bekeron J, Lamme B, et al: Which ankle fractures require syndesmotic stabilization? *J Foot Ankle Surg* 46(6):456–463, 2007.
Scott AM. Diagnosis and treatment of ankle fractures, *Radiol Technol* 81(5):457–475, 2010.

PLANTAR FASCIITIS (PF)
History
- PF is the most common cause of plantar heel pain.

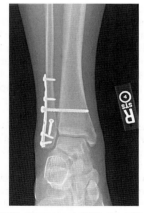

Figure 8-15. Status post ORIF distal fibular fracture (Weber B) requiring syndesmotic screw.

- Plantar heel pain at the distal plantar fascia (medial calcaneal tuberosity) may extend into midsubstance plantar fascia.
- Start-up pain is characteristic of PF. Pain is greatest with the first steps in the morning or after prolonged sitting. Symptoms improve or resolve with non–weight bearing.

Physical Examination
- Tenderness occurs on palpation of plantar fascia, most pronounced at insertion on plantar medial calcaneus.
- Patients often have a tight gastrocnemius and/or Achilles.
- Edema and ecchymosis are not present.

Imaging
- Radiograph: Weight-bearing foot AP, lateral, oblique. Presence of plantar calcaneal enthesophyte has no clinical relevance to PF
- MRI/Ultrasound: Usually not necessary, may reveal thickening of plantar fascia

Initial Treatment
Patient Education
- PF is a self-limiting process with 80-90% resolution within 10 months.

First Treatment Step
- Stretching program to include Achilles, gastrocnemius, and plantar fascia–specific stretches; ice, massage, heel cups

Treatment Options
Nonoperative Management
- Stretching should be done at minimum three times per day.
- Dorsiflexion splints worn at night keep the ankle at neutral position to prevent calf and plantar fascia contracture. Most improvement is noted in morning symptoms.
- Silicone heel cups, arch supports, custom orthotics, or over-the-counter (OTC) orthotics may be helpful. Custom inserts have no proven advantage over prefabricated inserts.
- Physical therapy and iontophoresis may provide symptomatic improvement, but symptoms return within 1 month of discontinuing treatment.

- Corticosteroid injections (see orthopaedic procedures, plantar fascia injection, page 310) provide focused delivery of anti-inflammatory medication. Risks include fascial rupture and fat pad atrophy. Improvement of symptoms generally lasts less than 3 months.

Operative Management
Codes
ICD-9:
   728.71 Plantar fasciitis
CPT:
   28060 Partial plantar fascia fasciectomy
- Rarely performed. Limited long-term outcome studies. Risks: arch collapse, persistent pain, injury to posterior tibial nerve

Suggested Readings
DiGiovanni B, Nawoczenski D, Malay D, et al: Plantar fascia-specific stretching exercise improves outcomes in patients with chronic plantar fasciitis, *J Bone Joint Surg Am* 88(8):1775–1781, 2006.
League A: Current concepts review: plantar fasciitis, *Foot Ankle Int* 29(3):358–366, 2008.
Thomas JL, Christensen JC, Kravitz SR, et al. The diagnosis and treatment of heel pain: a clinical practice guideline revision 2010, *J Foot Ankle Surg* 49(3 Suppl): S1–S19, 2010.

MORTON'S (INTERMETATARSAL) NEUROMA
History
- Compression neuropathy of common digital nerve: most common is third intermetatarsal space. Others are less common.
- Incidence in females is greater than males.
- Burning and/or radiating pain, and numbness/tingling exist, usually in plantar aspect of intermetatarsal space but can radiate to toes.
- Symptoms improve when barefoot.

Physical Examination
- Tenderness to palpation of intermetatarsal space. Pain is not reproduced with palpation of metatarsal heads or metatarsal-phalangeal (MTP) joints.
- **Mulder's sign:** Squeeze forefoot medial to lateral and apply dorsal pressure over affected web space. Positive test is audible or palpable click that causes pain.

- Edema, erythema, and ecchymosis are not present, and there is ± sensory deficit at affected web space/toes and ± divergence of toes.

Imaging
- Radiographs: Weight-bearing foot AP, lateral, oblique. Neuromas are not visible.
- Ultrasound and MRI: Can be used for atypical presentations, but usually not necessary. Neuroma appears as an ovoid/dumbbell-shaped plantar mass between metatarsal heads.
- Ultrasound: A hypoechoic signal is present, but not all neuromas are visible.
- MRI: Best identified on T1 images, low intensity signal. Contrast MRI can differentiate from other masses.
- Gold standard for diagnosis is surgical visualization.

Treatment Options
Nonoperative Management
- The goals are to alleviate pressure and decrease irritation of the nerve.
- Shoes with wide toe boxes are best. Avoid high heels.
- Metatarsal pads placed proximal to metatarsal heads spread apart the metatarsal heads and decrease pressure on nerve.
- Corticosteroid injections (see orthopaedic procedures, Morton's neuroma injection, page 311) have variable results. Multiple injections have higher success rates (reported resolution of symptoms 11% to 47%). Risks of injections include atrophy of plantar fat pad and MTP joint subluxation.

Operative Management
Codes
ICD-9:
  355.6 Lesion of plantar nerve
CPT Code:
  28080 Excision of Interdigital Neuroma

Operative Indications
- Persistent symptoms following nonoperative treatment

Informed Consent and Counseling
- Risks include infection, wound complication (greater for plantar approach), hematoma, stump neuroma formation, and chronic pain. Recurrent neuromas may require additional surgery. Major structures at risk are the digital artery and vein.

Anesthesia
- Ankle block with or without sedation or general anesthesia; ankle tourniquet

Patient Positioning
- Supine, toes toward ceiling; ipsilateral bump under the hip if necessary

Surgical Procedure
Interdigital Neuroma Excision
- Dorsal approach: A longitudinal incision is made over the involved web space. The dorsal interosseous fascia is split and retracted. Interosseous muscle is partially detached, metatarsal heads are retracted, and the intermetatarsal ligament is cut. The neuroma is exposed by retracting the digital artery and lumbrical muscle.
- Plantar approach: This is generally reserved for revision procedures. A longitudinal incision is made between the metatarsal heads. The plantar fascia is split and retracted to expose the neuroma.
- Once neuroma is exposed, it is dissected proximally and cut. The proximal stump retracts into the intrinsic muscles.
- Evaluate vascular status after excision to ensure digital artery intact and functioning.

Estimated Postoperative Course
- Dorsal approach: weight bearing as tolerated in hard-soled post-operative shoe. Progress to normal shoe wear and activities as tolerated once incision healed, usually between 2 and 3 weeks postoperative.
- The plantar approach requires greater protection with a splint or cast boot and more limited weight bearing to prevent wound complications. Sutures are removed 2 to 3 weeks postoperative. Progress to normal shoe wear and activities as tolerated once the wound has completely healed. This may be 3 to 4 weeks postoperative.

Suggested Readings

Thomas J, Blitch E, Martin Chaney D, et al: Diagnosis and treatment of forefoot disorders. Section 3. Morton's intermetatarsal neuroma, *J Foot Ankle Surg* 48(2):251–256, 2009.

Womack J, Richardson D, Murphy A, et al: Long-term evaluation of interdigital neuroma treated by surgical excision, *Foot Ankle Int* 29(6):574–577, 2008.

Wu K. Morton's interdigital neuroma: a clinical review of its etiology, treatment, and results, *J Foot Ankle Surg* 35(2):112–119, 1996.

DIABETIC FOOT AND CHARCOT ARTHROPATHY

History

- Diabetics with neuropathy are at high risk for developing ulcers and infections.
- Symptoms of neuropathy are numbness, paresthesias or dysesthesias, slow wound healing, and no pain after injury.
- Charcot arthropathy is a destructive disease of bones and joints that occurs in sensory neuropathy. It is noninfectious and progressive. Unilateral involvement occurs at initial presentation.
- Charcot arthropathy can develop in patients with diabetic neuropathy. The average duration of diabetes at onset is 20 to 24 years for type I and 5 to 9 years for type II.
- Risk factors for ulcers are peripheral neuropathy; absent pedal pulses; claudication; trophic skin changes (decreased hair growth, skin discoloration or atrophy); history of ulcer; and hospitalization for foot infection, bony deformity, or peripheral edema.
- The risk of osteomyelitis is high.

Physical Examination

- Visual deformities: Claw-toe deformities are common from loss of intrinsic muscle tone. Rocker-bottom midfoot deformity is often present in Charcot arthropathy of midfoot.
- Skin:
  - Inspect for presence of corns or calluses, open wounds, swelling, trophic changes, dependent rubor (arterial insufficiency), and bony prominences.
  - Ulcers often develop at sites of callus formation or as a result of microtrauma.

- Increased warmth compared with the contralateral side can indicate Charcot arthropathy, venous insufficiency, or infection.
- Sensory examination: Conduct monofilament testing (Semmes-Weinstein) for loss of protective sensation. The threshold for peripheral neuropathy is 10 grams. Generalized neuropathy with diminished sensation in "stocking" distribution is characteristic of diabetic neuropathy.
- Vascular: Decreased or absent pedal pulses indicate peripheral vascular disease. Delayed capillary refill indicates ischemic disease.

Imaging

- Radiograph: weight-bearing AP, lateral, oblique of foot and AP, lateral, mortise of ankle
  - May be normal in early disease processes
  - Difficult to differentiate Charcot arthropathy from osteomyelitis
  - Charcot arthropathy: disorganization of bony structure, bony erosion, intra-articular loose bodies, may have subluxation or dislocation of joints (Fig. 8-16)
- Nuclear medicine: Bone scan with indium labeled leukocyte scintigraphy useful to diagnosis osteomyelitis; 93% to 100% sensitivity, 80% specificity
- MRI:
  - Less specific than indium labeled scintigraphy. Difficult to differentiate acute Charcot arthropathy from osteomyelitis
  - Presence of sinus tract or abscess helpful in confirming osteomyelitis

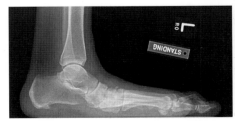

Figure 8-16. Charcot arthropathy of the midfoot. Joint debris and collapse of the midfoot are noted.

- Subchondral cysts and intra-articular loose bodies/debris suggest Charcot

Classification Systems

- Multiple classification systems for diabetic foot ulcers, and Charcot arthropathy
- Pinzer "risk factor" system to guide treatment of diabetic patients
  - Risk Category 0: Normal appearance and sensation, mild to no deformity
  - Risk Category 1: Normal appearance, insensate, no deformity
  - Risk Category 2: Insensate foot with deformity, no history of prior ulcer
  - Risk Category 3: Insensate foot with deformity and history of prior ulcer
- Classification system of Charcot arthropathy:
  - Stage 0: Clinical examination findings of erythema and edema. Radiographs are normal.
  - Stage I: Fragmentation or dissolution phase. Radiographs demonstrate periarticular fragmentation, subluxation, or dislocation of joint. On examination, foot is warm, edematous, and erythematous.
  - Stage II: Coalescence period, early healing phase. Radiographs show early sclerosis, fusion of bony fragments, and absorption of debris. On examination, there is less erythema and warmth than stage I.
  - Stage III: Reconstruction phase. Radiographs reveal subchondral sclerosis, osteophytes, and narrow or absent joint spaces. On examination, visual deformity is present and there is no acute inflammation.

Initial Treatment

Patient Education

Education is especially important for diabetic patients. Stress importance of regular foot examinations and proper shoe wear (wide and tall toe box, supportive insoles).

- Patients with neuropathy should not walk around barefoot or use corn or callous removers. Inspect feet daily and notify clinician if redness, ulceration, or blistering is present.

Treatment Options

Nonoperative Management

- **At-risk patients without Charcot arthropathy: based on Pinzur classification**
  - Risk Category 0: education, normal footwear, yearly clinical examination
  - Risk Category 1: education, daily foot self-examination, protective over-the-counter insoles, appropriate footwear, biannual clinical examination
  - Risk Category 2: education, daily foot self-examination, custom pressure-dissipating accommodative orthoses, inlay depth soft-leather shoes, clinical examination every 4 months
  - Risk Category 3: education, daily foot self-examination, custom pressure-dissipating orthoses, inlay depth soft-leather shoes, clinical examination every 2 months
- **Charcot arthropathy: based on stage**
  - Stage I: immobilization using total contact casting, which reduces total load on the foot by one third. Length of immobilization depends on progression of disease/collapse, often 2 to 4 months.
  - Stage II: ankle-foot orthosis or Charcot restraint orthotic walker (CROW) boot.
  - Stage III: accommodative shoe and custom insole to decrease pressure on bony prominences

Operative Management

Codes

ICD-9 Code
  713.5 Charcot foot
CPT Codes
  28124 Exostectomy CPT for ostectomy of toe. Multiple CPT codes exist and vary depending on which bone is involved. Options also include amputation or arthrodesis.

Operative Indications

- Exostectomy: Significant bony deformity not controlled by orthosis. May have osteomyelitis.

Informed Consent and Counseling
- Exostectomy: Recurrence requiring revision surgery is common (up to 25%). Patients are at high risk of wound complications. Due to decreased vascular and immune function, diabetics may require prolonged antibiotic use postoperatively.

Anesthesia
- General. Blocks are often not necessary in diabetics with peripheral neuropathy.

Patient Positioning
- Supine, toes toward the ceiling (ipsilateral bump under the hip may be necessary)

Surgical Procedures
- *Amputation:* Level of amputation and surgical techniques vary, depending on disease involvement.
- *Arthrodesis:* As described in earlier sections of the chapter

Exostectomy
- Procedure: Longitudinal incision is made at the border of plantar and dorsal skin. Careful dissection to prominent exostosis and prominent bone is excised using an osteotome or saw. Edges of bone are then smoothed, and precise closure is completed.
- *Estimated postoperative course*
  - A well-padded sugar tong splint is applied in the operating room, and the patient must not bear weight for 2 weeks. At 2 weeks, the patient is transitioned to a diabetic shoe if no ulcer is present. If an ulcer is present, a total contact cast or CROW boot is used until the ulcer heals.

Suggested Readings
Besse J, Leemrijse T, Deleu P: Diabetic foot: the orthopedic surgery angle, *Orthop Traumatol Surg Res* 97:314–329, 2011.

Kolker D, Weinfeld S: Diabetic foot disorders. In DiGiovanni C, Greisberg J: *First edition core knowledge in orthopaedics*—foot and ankle, Philadelphia, 2007, Elsevier.

Pinzur M, Slovenkai M, Trepman E, Shields N: Guidelines for diabetic foot care: recommendations endorsed by the Diabetes Committee of the American Orthopaedic Foot and Ankle Society, *Foot Ankle Int* 26:113–118, 2005.

Van der Ven A, Chapman C, Bowker J: Charcot neuroarthropathy of the foot and ankle, *J Am Acad Orthop Surg* 17:562–571, 2009.

Zgonis T: *Surgical reconstruction of the diabetic foot and ankle*, Philadelphia, 2009, Lippincott Williams & Wilkins.

METATARSAL FRACTURES (INCLUDING JONES FRACTURE)
History
- One of the most common foot injuries. Most have minimal or no displacement.
- Common mechanisms are inversion injuries or falls from heights. Symptoms include pain with weight bearing, swelling, and bruising.
- Multiple metatarsal (MT) fractures are common.

Physical Examination
- Edema, ecchymosis, and tenderness at fracture site(s) can exist.
- Inspect skin for evidence of open fracture.
- Displaced fractures may result in visual deformity or abnormal angulation of metatarsal.

Imaging
- Radiograph: Weight-bearing AP, lateral, oblique foot (Fig. 8-17).

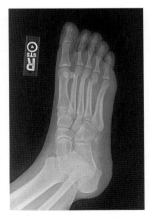

Figure 8-17. Second, third, and fourth metatarsal fractures. The fourth metatarsal fracture is displaced greater than 3 to 4 mm, so open reduction, internal fixation should be considered.

- MRI is generally not indicated but can be used to evaluate ligamentous structures if there is concern for injury.
- CT is often used when there is concern for occult fracture or to evaluate Lis Franc injury.

Classification System
- Fifth metatarsal fractures are classified on the basis of location. Treatment recommendations are based on this classification system.
  - Zone 1 (avulsion): Fifth metatarsal tuberosity fracture. Most common type (>90%). Often extends from insertion of peroneal brevis to involve the tarsometatarsal joint.
  - Zone 2 (Jones fracture): Distal to the tuberosity at metaphyseal-diaphyseal junction. Fracture extends to fourth to fifth intermetatarsal joint. Mechanism is adduction or inversion of the forefoot (Fig. 8-18).
  - Zone 3: Proximal diaphyseal shaft fracture. Rare, less than 3% of fifth MT fractures. Frequently a stress injury and patients may report prodromal pain.

Initial Treatment
- Immobilization in a sugar tong splint, short leg cast, or cast boot, non–weight bearing.
- Treatment is determined by fracture location and level of displacement.

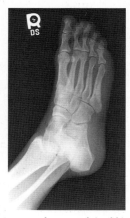

Figure 8-18. Jones fracture of the fifth metatarsal.

Treatment Options
Nonoperative Management
- First MT fractures nondisplaced, stable: immobilization (short leg cast or cast boot) for 6 weeks, weight bearing as tolerated.
- Lesser MT fractures nondisplaced or mild displacement (<4 mm translation, ≤10-degree sagittal angulation): hard-sole shoe for 4 to 6 weeks, weight bearing as tolerated.
- Fifth MT fractures:
- Zone 1: hard-soled shoe or short cast boot for 4 to 6 weeks, weight bearing as tolerated. Consider ORIF for significantly displaced fractures.
- Zone 2: short leg cast immobilization for 6 to 8 weeks, non–weight bearing.
- Concern for nonunion with nonoperative treatment exists, especially in noncompliant patients. ORIF is recommended for high-level athletes.
- Zone 3: high risk of nonunion, most surgeons recommend ORIF. If nonoperative treatment used, short leg cast immobilization with protected weight bearing for up to 3 months.

Operative Management
Codes
- ICD-9: 825.25 Metatarsal fracture
- CPT: 28485 ORIF 5th MT fracture, Zone 2 or Jones fracture

Operative Indications
- Significantly displaced fracture or fracture in Zone 2 or 3. Treatment of Zone 2 fractures is controversial and can be treated operatively or nonoperatively.
- ORIF or percutaneous pinning is recommended for fractures with significant displacement. Approach and exact procedure depend on location and fracture type.

Informed Consent and Counseling
- Risks include nonunion, surgical site infection, hardware irritation, and nerve or vascular injury. Nonunions are often associated with early return to weight-bearing activity. Structures at risk during fifth MT ORIF include cutaneous branches of sural nerve and peroneal tendons.

Anesthesia
- General, may use peripheral nerve block (ankle)

Patient Positioning
- Supine, a bump under the ipsilateral hip can help to internally rotate leg and allow for easier access to lateral foot

Surgical Procedure
ORIF Fifth Metatarsal Fracture
- Procedure: Screw fixation of fifth metatarsal fracture Zone 2 (Jones fracture)
  - Longitudinal incision is made proximal to base of the metatarsal just dorsal to the border of the dorsal and plantar skin. Dissection performed down to bone.
  - A guidewire is used to access the intramedullary canal from dorsal and medial position, under guidance of an intraoperative radiograph. Screw length is determined, and a 5.5-mm screw is placed across the fracture. The screw should be long enough for half of the threads to cross the fracture site. The screw is countersunk to decrease the risk of soft tissue irritation postoperatively. Due to the bend of the fifth MT, a screw with excess length can increase varus stress and result in a nonunion (Fig. 8-19).

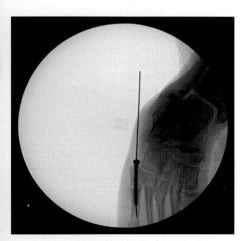

Figure 8-19. Intraoperative radiograph demonstrating guidewire and screw placement for fixation of fifth metatarsal fracture.

- A sugar tong splint is applied before leaving the operating room, and the patient is non–weight bearing for 2 weeks.

Estimated Postoperative Course
- Postoperative 2 weeks: sutures removed and patient transitioned to a cast boot, bearing weight as tolerated
- Postoperative 6 to 12 weeks: return to athletics depending on clinical and x-ray healing

Suggested Readings
Hatch R, Alsobrook J, Clugston J: Diagnosis and management of metatarsal fractures, *Am Fam Physician* 76:817–827, 2007.
Portland G, Kelikian A, Kodros S. Acute surgical management of Jones' fractures, *Foot Ankle Int* 24:829–833, 2003.
Schenck RC, Heckman JD: Fractures and dislocations of the forefoot: operative and non-operative treatment, *J Am Acad Orthop Surg* 3:70–78, 1995.

LISFRANC FRACTURE/INJURY (TARSOMETATARSAL JOINT COMPLEX INJURY)
History
- The Lisfranc ligament is a strong, interosseous attachment between the medial cuneiform and second metatarsal. A Lisfranc fracture describes an injury to the base of the metatarsal(s) at the attachment to the distal tarsal bones and Lisfranc ligament.
- Mechanism is trauma. About two thirds of injuries result from high-energy trauma (motor vehicle crash [MVC], fall from height), and one third result from lower-energy mechanisms (e.g., athletics).
- Symptoms include pain, inability to weight bear on affected foot, swelling, and bruising.
- Most injuries are subtle, and many are missed on first evaluation and radiograph.

Physical Examination
- Edema of midfoot and forefoot, tenderness midfoot/tarsometatarsal joints, and plantar ecchymosis are present.
- The neurovascular examination is usually normal, but severe dislocation of the second MT can compromise blood

flow, resulting in decreased or absent dorsalis pedis pulse.

Imaging

- Radiograph: weight-bearing AP, lateral, oblique of the foot. Include weight-bearing AP with both feet on same film for comparison.
  - Most common finding in Lisfranc injury is lateral step-off at second tarsometatarsal (TMT) joint.
  - Normal/uninjured foot: Medial border of second MT and medial border of middle cuneiform align on AP view. Oblique view demonstrates alignment of medial border fourth MT and medial border of cuboid (Fig. 8-20).
  - If radiographs appear normal, but high suspicion for Lisfranc injury, evaluate with CT scan or MRI.
- CT scan: can be used to evaluate subtle or occult fractures. CT scans allow for more precise evaluation of fractures including comminution and intra-articular extension (Fig. 8-21).
- MRI: can be used to evaluate soft tissues including Lisfranc ligament. MRI is used less frequently than CT scan to evaluate Lisfranc injuries.

Initial Treatment

- When Lisfranc injury is suspected, initialize immobilization in a sugar

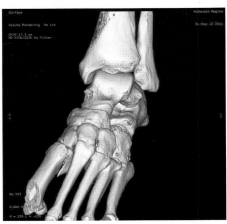

Figure 8-21. Computed tomography scan three-dimensional reconstruction demonstrating Lisfranc injury with fracture at the base of the second metatarsal.

tong splint or cast boot and instruct patient to not bear weight. Refer to an orthopaedic surgeon.

Patient Education

- Unstable fractures that are not appropriately managed lead to post-traumatic arthritis of the midfoot. Post-traumatic arthritis can develop quickly.

Treatment Options

Nonoperative Management

- Consider nonoperative management for stable injuries (no subluxation on radiograph or CT, no ligament tear on MRI, and negative stress examination under anesthesia).
- Immobilize in cast boot for 6 to 10 weeks, and bear weight as tolerated.
- Repeat weight-bearing radiographs 2 weeks postinjury. If there is a change in alignment, consider ORIF.
- After 6 to 10 weeks of immobilization, physical therapy may be indicated for gait training, balance, and functional strengthening. Full recovery occurs approximately 4 months postinjury.
- If pain is persistent in the future, midfoot arthrodesis can be performed.
- Nonoperative treatment is recommended for low-demand patients

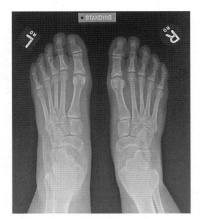

Figure 8-20. On the right (uninjured foot), there is good alignment of the medial borders of the second metatarsal (MT) and middle cuneiform. On the left, a subtle fracture is noted at the base of the second MT.

(little ambulation or nonambulatory), preexisting inflammatory arthritis, or insensate foot.

Operative Management
Codes
ICD-9
838.03 Closed dislocation of tarso-metatarsal joint (Lisfranc injury)
838.13 Open dislocation of tarsometa-tarsal joint
CPT
28615 Open reduction, internal fixation of tarsometatarsal fracture

Operative Indications
- Unstable injury (subluxation on radiograph or CT scan, ligament tear on MRI, or positive stress radiograph under anesthesia)

Informed Consent and Counseling
- If unstable injury is left untreated, significant post-traumatic arthritis develops resulting in persistent pain. Major structures at risk include dorsalis pedis artery and sensory branch of deep peroneal nerve. A second procedure is necessary 3 to 4 months after fixation to remove hardware.

Anesthesia
- General, with or without ankle block

Patient Positioning
- Supine with toes toward ceiling

Surgical Procedure
Open Reduction Internal Fixation
- Dorsal incision is made over the involved joint of midfoot. Many fixation techniques can be used, and multiple devices are available. Common techniques include screw fixation, dorsal plating, and Kirschner wires (most common for fourth or fifth TMT injuries).
- Fractures are reduced, alignment of TMT joints is corrected, and hardware is placed. Intraoperative radiograph is used to determine alignment and correct placement of hardware (Fig. 8-22).
- A sugar tong splint is applied before leaving the operating room, and the patient is non–weight bearing.

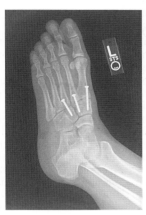

Figure 8-22. Postoperative oblique view of open reduction, internal fixation first, second, and third tarsometatarsal joints.

Estimated Postoperative Course
- Postoperative 2 weeks: Sutures are removed at about 2 weeks, and the patient is transitioned to a short leg cast
- Postoperative 4 to 6 weeks: Apply walking boot and begin partial weight bearing. K-wires are removed at about 6 weeks postoperative if present.
- Postoperative 8 weeks: Progress to full weight bearing in a cast boot. Continue boot for 3 to 4 months postoperative.
- Hardware removal performed about 4 months postoperative. Use walking boot, and bear weight as tolerated for 2 to 4 weeks after hardware removal. Progress to normal shoe full weight bearing.

Suggested Readings
Bellabarba C, Barei DP, Sanders RW: Dislocations of the foot. In Coughlin MJ, Mann RA, Saltzman CL: *Coughlin: surgery of the foot and ankle*, ed 8, Philadelphia, 2007, Mosby.

Coetzee JC: Making sense of Lisfranc injuries, *Foot Ankle Clin* 13:695–704, 2008.

Thompson M, Mormino M: Injury to the tarsometatarsal joint complex, *J Am Acad Orthop Surg* 11:260–268, 2003.

Watson T, Shurnas P, Denker J. Treatment of Lisfranc joint injury: current concepts, *J Am Acad Orthop Surg* 18:718–728, Dec 2010.

PHALANGEAL FRACTURES
History
- Common mechanisms include stubbing a toe or a direct blow from a falling object.
- Symptoms include pain, swelling, bruising, and difficulty walking or wearing a shoe.
- Sesamoid fractures are caused by overuse or avulsion forces or direct trauma. Patients report pain directly under the first MTP joint with weight bearing. The medial (tibial) sesamoid is more commonly injured than the lateral (fibular).

Physical Examination
- The affected area is edematous, tender to palpation, and ecchymotic.
- Evaluate skin for signs of open fracture.

Imaging
- Radiograph: weight-bearing AP and lateral views, as well as oblique view. If there is concern for sesamoid injury, obtain a tangential view of the sesamoid.
- CT/MRI is usually not indicated unless additional injury is noted or there is significant involvement of the first MTP joint.

Initial Treatment
- Open fractures require immediate irrigation and debridement followed by a course of antibiotics.

Treatment Options
Nonoperative Management
- Nearly all phalangeal fractures can be treated nonoperatively.
- Displaced fractures of lesser toes can be treated with closed reduction with traction after digital block. After reduction, splint to adjacent toe (buddy taping) for 2 to 4 weeks. Weight bearing as tolerated in hard-soled shoe for 4 to 6 weeks.
- Nondisplaced fractures of the great toe require immobilization in hard-soled shoe or boot for 2 to 3 weeks, weight bearing as tolerated primarily through heel.
- Sesamoid fractures: cast boot with sesamoid orthotic (dancer's pad) for 6 weeks, then transition to shoe with sesamoid orthotic for an additional 6 weeks.

Operative Management
Codes
ICD-9
  826.0 Fracture of one or more phalanges of the foot
CPT
  28525: Open treatment of fracture of phalanx or phalanges other than the great toe
  28496: Open treatment of fracture of the great toe (proximal or distal phalanx)

Operative Indications
- Rarely indicated. Operative intervention is only recommended for displaced fractures of the great toe.

Surgical Procedure
- Percutaneous pinning with Kirschner wires. Weight bearing as tolerated in hard-soled shoe. K-wires are removed at about 4 weeks post-op.

Suggested Readings
DiGiovanni C, Greisberg J: *Foot and ankle: core knowledge in orthopaedics*, Philadelphia, 2007, Elsevier.

Sander RW, Papp S: Fractures of the midfoot and forefoot. In Coughlin MJ, Mann RA, Saltzman CL: *Coughlin: surgery of the foot and ankle*, ed 8, Philadelphia, 2007, Mosby.

Schenck RC, Heckman JD: Fractures and dislocations of the forefoot: operative and non-operative treatment, *J Am Acad Orthop Surg* 3:70–78, 1995.

TARSAL TUNNEL SYNDROME
History
- Tarsal tunnel syndrome may present with a history of injury or trauma.
- Patients complain of burning, tingling, and numbness over the plantar aspect of the foot, which may radiate distally or proximally. Symptoms increase with protracted walking or standing and resolve with rest, elevation, and loose shoes. Patients may experience severe pain at night.
- Obtain history related to systemic disorders that can affect nerves (i.e., rheumatologic disorders, diabetes, Lyme disease, thyroid disorder).

Physical Examination

- Note valgus or varus heel alignment.
- Palpate course of tibial nerve for thickness, edema, or paresthesias.
- Look for a positive percussion sign (Tinel) or cuff test.
  - **Cuff Test:** This tests for tarsal tunnel syndrome secondary to venous insufficiency. A pneumatic cuff is placed above the ankle and inflated to 60-80mmHg. This occludes venous flow and increases venous pressure around the nerve and is positive if the patient's symptoms are reproduced.

Imaging

- Electromyography (EMG) or nerve conduction study (NCS)
- Radiograph: weight-bearing foot (AP, oblique, lateral) and ankle (AP, mortise, lateral)
- MRI to evaluate for space-occupying lesion

Classification of Origin

- Trauma
- Space-occupying lesion
- Foot deformity

Initial Treatment

Patient Education

- Nonoperative treatment is the first line and mainstay of treatment for tarsal tunnel syndrome, unless acute. Surgical intervention is to be proceeded with much caution and may not alleviate all of the patient's symptoms.

First Treatment Steps

- Primary care providers can initiate ordering diagnostic studies such as MRI or EMG or NCS.
- Refer to orthopaedic surgeon on a nonurgent basis.

Treatment Options

Nonoperative Management

- Most effective when underlying etiology is tenosynovitis or foot deformity
- Includes use of corticosteroid injection, orthotics, NSAIDS, and immobilization (see Tarsal Tunnel Injection, page 311)
- Can consider prescribing medications such as tricyclic antidepressants,

selective serotonin reuptake inhibitors (SSRIs), antiseizure medication, or other antidepressants. Refer patient to pain management or neurologist if not comfortable prescribing these medications.

Operative Management

Codes
ICD-9
355.5 Tarsal tunnel syndrome
CPT
28035 Tarsal tunnel release

Operative Indications
- Recalcitrant symptoms despite appropriate conservative management
- Evidence of space-occupying lesion on MRI

Informed Consent and Counseling
- Risks and complications include continued pain despite release, increased symptoms, numbness dysesthesias, persistent tenderness or paresthesias over the tarsal tunnel, edema, nerve damage, vascular damage, infection, wound complications, difficulty with footwear, and causalgia or complex regional pain syndrome type 2

Anesthesia
- Surgeon and patient discretion, likely general with regional nerve block

Patient Positioning
- Supine or mild Trendelenburg
- Tourniquet optional

Surgical Procedures

Tibial Nerve Release

- Curved medial incision extending above, behind, and below the medial malleolus beginning 10 cm proximal to medial malleolus and 2 cm posterior to tibia
- Incision is deepened to expose flexor retinaculum. Tibial nerve sheath is identified and opened proximally. Flexor retinaculum is then carefully released.
- Terminal branches of tibial nerve should be identified and released
- Wound closed in layers, leaving retinaculum open

- Patient placed in well-molded posterior splint, non–weight bearing

Estimated Postoperative Course
- 10 Days to 2 Weeks Postoperative
  - Splint and sutures removed. May continue to protect incision with CAM boot. Begin gently with range of motion (ROM) exercises to prevent adhesions.
- 3 to 4 Weeks Postoperative
  - Weight bearing as tolerated, increase activities as tolerated. May begin more aggressive therapy as indicated.

Suggested Readings
Antoniadis G, Scheglmann K: Posterior tarsal tunnel syndrome, *Dtsch Arxtebl Int* 105:776–781, 2008.

Coughlin M, Mann R, Saltzman C: *Surgery of the foot and ankle*, ed 8, Philadelphia, 2007, Mosby.

Lau J, Daniels T: Tarsal tunnel syndrome: a review of the literature, *Foot Ankle Inter* 20: 201–209, 1999.

ACHILLES TENDINOPATHY AND RUPTURE
Achilles Tendon Rupture
History
- Sharp unexpected dorsiflexion force to the ankle in conjunction with a strong contraction of the calf (e.g., tripping on a curb, unexpectedly stepping into a hole), pushing off the weight-bearing foot with the knee in extension (e.g., lunging for a tennis shot), and a strong or violent dorsiflexion force on a plantar-flexed ankle (e.g., jumping from a height)
- Sensation of a snap or audible pop in posterior calf followed by acute pain like "got kicked from behind" or sounds "like a gun being shot", difficulty walking, and weakened plantarflexion.

Physical Examination
- Palpable defect approximately 2 to 6 cm from insertion of Achilles tendon
- Increased ankle dorsiflexion ROM and decreased plantarflexion strength compared with uninjured extremity
- **Positive Thompson test:** assesses the continuity of Achilles tendon. Patient is placed in a prone position with both feet extended past end of examination table. The affected calf is squeezed, and reflex plantarflexion is assessed.

A positive test is when there is no reflex plantarflexion with a squeeze of the calf.
- Be sure to palpate for calcaneal tenderness.

Imaging
- Radiographs only if calcaneal bony tenderness
- MRI or ultrasound not necessary to confirm diagnosis with strong history and physical examination findings—may order if considering nonoperative treatment

Initial Treatment
Patient Education
- Acute Achilles ruptures may be treated surgically or nonsurgically with similar outcomes with appropriate patient selection. Nonsurgical treatment has lower complication rates; however, surgical repair has a faster recovery time, quicker return to sport activities, and slightly lower re-rupture rates. Missed or improperly treated ruptures can lead to significant weakness and altered gait mechanics.

 ORTHOPAEDIC WARNING

Quinolone use has been associated with rupture of Achilles tendon most commonly in the elderly and patients using corticosteroids.

First Treatment Steps
- Immobilize affected extremity in plantarflexed position, non–weight bearing
- Refer immediately to orthopaedic surgeon

Treatment Options
Nonoperative Management
- With dynamic ultrasound or MRI imaging, rupture gap must be less than 5 mm with maximum plantarflexion, less than 10-mm gap with foot in neutral dorsiflexion, or greater than 75% apposition of tendon in 20 degrees of plantarflexion
- Good candidates for non-operative management include those with systemic disease, medical comorbidities, smokers, and diabetics, as well as healthy individuals who meet the

Table 8-5. Nonoperative Treatment Protocol for Achilles Tendon Rupture

Initial Evaluation	Ultrasound (U/S) or magnetic resonance imaging (MRI) examination showing < 5 mm gap of tendon ends with maximal plantarflexion, <10 mm gap with neutral, or >75% apposition of tendon ends in 20 degrees PF.
Initial Management	Cast in full PF, non–weight bearing
2-wk evaluation	May transition to pneumatic walking boot or bivalved cast with foot in 20 degrees PF with two 1-cm heel wedges, may be weight bearing. Must wear boot 24 hours/day
4-wk evaluation	On examination, palpable continuity of tendon. If concern tendon not apposed, order repeat U/S or MRI. Patient may remove boot 5 minutes per hour to perform active dorsiflexion to neutral with passive plantarflexion.
6-wk evaluation	On examination, continue to document continuity of tendon. Patient may remove one 1-cm lift. Continue range-of-motion exercises, may initiate more formal physical therapy protocol.
8-wk evaluation	Document continued continuity of tendon. May decrease to zero lifts in boot and discontinue use of boot at night. Continue therapy program.
10-wk evaluation	Discontinue use of boot and transition into a shoe with one 1-cm heel lift to be used for 3 additional months. Continue therapy program, and avoid aggressive sport activity until heel lift is discontinued.

previously mentioned criteria and do not want to have surgery
- Treatment protocol (Table 8-5)

Operative Management
Codes
ICD-9
  727.67 Achilles tendon rupture
CPT
  27650 Acute Achilles rupture repair

Operative Indications
- Greater than 1-cm gap in neutral dorsiflexion
- Patient preference

Informed Consent and Counseling
- Risks include infection and wound complications, which can be catastrophic, re-rupture, keloid formation, sural nerve injury, and adhesions
- Most people are back to sport activity at 6 months postoperatively
- Full recovery in terms of pain, edema, and strength can take a full year to achieve

Anesthesia
- General anesthesia with regional block such as popliteal

Patient Positioning
- Prone or modified lateral
- Nonsterile tourniquet on upper thigh

Surgical Procedure
Primary Repair of Achilles Tendon Rupture
- 10-cm incision made 0.5 cm medial to Achilles tendon and extended proximally to insertion
- Dissection down to peritenon, which is then cut longitudinally to expose ruptured tendon, care is taken not to undermine the skin
- Ankle plantarflexed to approximate tendon ends, hematoma debrided
- Nonabsorbable suture is used to repair the rupture using a modified Kessler, Bunnell, or Krackow stitch
- Peritenon is closed and skin sutured
- Patient placed in non–weight bearing, well-padded, molded posterior splint in plantarflexion

Estimated Postoperative Course
- Early protected weight bearing and use of protective device that allows mobilization is key in successful rehabilitation of Achilles tendon ruptures
- 1 to 2 Weeks Postoperative
  - Postoperative splint removed and wound inspected, well-healed sutures removed. If not, patient placed back into short leg cast for 1 week

- Once sutures removed, patient placed in removable boot with 2 heel wedges and allowed to initiate weight bearing as tolerated
- 4 to 5 Weeks Postoperative
  - Heel wedges are gradually decreased over the course of the next 2 to 3 weeks, until the patient is weight bearing in the boot with no lifts
- 6 to 8 Weeks Postoperative
  - Boot is discontinued after 1 week of weight bearing in boot with no lifts
  - Physical therapy program initiated
  - Patient may increase activities as tolerated after discontinuing use of boot, starting with nonimpact activities. Most people do not return to sport activity until at least 6 months after surgery.

ACHILLES TENDINOPATHY
History
- Due to overuse injuries with primary contributing factors of host susceptibility and mechanical overload
- Associated with advancing age, usually insidious and chronic in nature
- Patient complains of pain in Achilles tendon with activities, thickness or edema of tendon, and impaired performance. May be related to training errors and inappropriate footwear.

Physical Examination
- Tender to palpation, thickened and/or edematous Achilles tendon or bony prominence at posterior calcaneus
- Decreased plantarflexion strength, calf atrophy, palpable gap if chronic or missed rupture
- Antalgic gait
- Assess for heel cord tightness

Imaging
- Radiographs: Weight-bearing foot (AP/oblique/lateral) and ankle (AP/mortise/lateral)
- Ultrasound or MRI to delineate source of pathology or for surgical planning

Classification
- Paratendinopathy—inflammation of the tendon sheath
- Noninsertional—tendinopathy within the substance of the tendon
- Insertional- tendinopathy where the Achilles inserts onto the calcaneus
- Retrocalcaneal bursitis—inflammation of the fluid-filled sac that lies between the Achilles and the calcaneus

Initial Treatment
Patient Education
- This condition is likely chronic and noninflammatory in nature. It responds well to a specific rehabilitation program in which the patient's compliance is crucial in its success. The goal of treatment is symptomatic only. The patient may always have thickened tendon or calcaneal bony prominence unless he or she undergoes surgical intervention. Recovery may follow a prolonged time course, taking 4 to 6 months before noticing improvement and even longer until the patient is back to reasonable activities comfortably.

First Treatment Steps
- Prescribe heel lifts, NSAIDs, rest, ice, and an eccentric physical therapy program (see nonoperative management below).
- Refer to orthopaedic surgeon if you suspect acute rupture or if symptoms are recalcitrant to prescribed treatment program.

Treatment Options
Nonoperative Management
- Mainstay of treatment, especially for patients with no prior formal treatment
- Eccentric loading proven to be beneficial in treatment of symptoms but may take up to 12 weeks to notice improvements in symptoms
- Immobilization in walking cast or boot necessary initially if symptoms severe
- Physical therapy prescription for Alfredson's 12-week Eccentric Loading Protocol
- Follow-up in 4 to 6 months if no significant improvement to discuss possible need for surgical intervention

Operative Management
Codes
ICD-9
726.71 Achilles bursitis or tendonitis

CPT
27654 Achilles debridement mid-substance w or w/o FHL tendon transfer
27680 Achilles debridement, Haglund excision with FHL tendon transfer

Operative Indications
- Symptoms recalcitrant to appropriate conservative treatment
- Missed or chronic Achilles tendon rupture

Informed Consent and Counseling
- Risks include infection and wound complications, which can be catastrophic, painful scar; nerve injury; and continued pain.
- In cases where there is a missed Achilles tendon rupture or more than 50% of the tendon is debrided, a flexor hallucis longus (FHL) tendon transfer is necessary to augment Achilles.

Anesthesia
- General with regional nerve block, likely popliteal

Patient Positioning
- Prone or modified lateral
- Nonsterile tourniquet on upper thigh

Surgical Procedures
Achilles Tendon Reconstruction Using Flexor Hallucis Longus (FHL) Transfer
- Longitudinal incision made medial to Achilles tendon from musculotendinous junction to 2 cm distal to insertion
- Peritenon incised, and Achilles tendon inspected and debrided
- Flexor hallucis longus muscle belly exposed by retracting posterior tibial artery, vein, and nerve and incising deep posterior compartment
- FHL harvested distally through a second longitudinal incision made along the medial border of the foot; pulled through the proximal wound and passed through a calcaneal drill hole made 1 cm distal and 1 cm anterior to Achilles tendon insertion; and FHL secured through the drill hole or

through suture to anterior aspect of Achilles tendon
- Peritenon repaired followed by wound closure
- Patient placed in posterior mold splint in slight plantarflexion

Estimated Postoperative Course
- Postoperative course similar to recovery for acute rupture repair; may be delayed only if tendon transfer used to augment the Achilles tendon
- 1 to 2 Weeks Postoperative
  - Splint and sutures removed; patient placed into cast or boot in 10 to 20 degrees of plantarflexion
- 4 to 6 Weeks Postoperative
  - Place the patient in neutral dorsiflexion boot or cast and initiate weight bearing at 8 weeks postoperatively.
  - Initiate rehabilitation program.
- 12 Weeks Postoperative
  - Transition out of boot into regular shoe with 2.5-cm heel lift for another 3 months.

Suggested Readings
Alfredson H, Pietila T, Jonsson P, et al: Heavy-load eccentric calf muscle training for the treatment of chronic Achilles tendinosis, *Am J Sports Med* 26:360–366, 1998.

Reddy S, Pedowitz D, Parekh S, et al: Surgical treatment for chronic disease and disorders of the Achilles tendon, *J Am Acad Orthop Surg* 17:3–14, 2009.

Saltzman C, Tearse D: Achilles tendon injuries, *J Am Acad Orthop Surg* 6:316–325, 1998.

Tan G, Sabb B, Kadakia A: Non-surgical management of Achilles ruptures, *Foot Ankle Clin N Am* 14:675–684, 2009.

Wilcox D, Bohay D, Anderson J: Treatment of chronic Achilles tendon disorders with flexor hallucis longus tendon transfer/augmentation, *Foot Ankle Intern* 21:1004–1010, 2000.

ANKLE SPRAIN
History
- Inversion injury in plantar-flexed position
- Injury to lateral ligamentous complex including the anterior talofibular ligament (ATFL), calcaneofibular ligament (CFL), and posterior talofibular ligament (PTFL)

- External rotation forces in syndesmotic sprains or high ankle sprain
- Patients complain of pain, swelling, bruising, inability to bear weight, and loss of functional ability

Physical Examination
- Lateral ankle edema and ecchymosis exist.
- Tenderness to palpation occurs over ATFL and CFL.
- **Anterior drawer test** to assess injury to ATFL (Fig. 8-23): The patient is seated with the leg hanging off the side of the bed or table with the knee bent, the tibia is stabilized with one hand, and the foot is translated anteriorly with the other hand at the level of the heel. With sprain or partial rupture of ligaments, pain may be elicited. With a complete tear, the patient may demonstrate a suction sign.
- Conduct an **inversion stress test** to assess injury to the CFL: With the ankle in neutral or slightly dorsiflexed

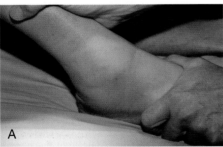
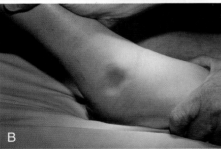

Figure 8-23. Positive anterior drawer test. *(From Clanton TO, McGarvey W: Athletic injuries to the soft tissues of the foot and ankle. In Coughlin MJ, et al (eds): Surgery of the foot and ankle, ed 8, St. Louis 2007, Elsevier.)*

position, invert the ankle by grasping the lateral calcaneus. This may elicit pain with injury to the CFL.
- Use **squeeze test** or **cross-legged test** to assess syndesmotic injury: A positive result occurs when a squeeze of the proximal calf causes pain in the distal syndesmosis. Squeezing the calf will cause separation of the distal fibula and anterior tibiofibular ligament and therefore, if injured, elicits discomfort.

Imaging
- Radiograph: Weight-bearing foot (AP/oblique/lateral) and ankle (AP/mortise/lateral) if indicated per Ottawa Rules for Ankle radiographs (can be any one of the following):
  - Bone tenderness along distal 6 cm of posterior tibia or medial malleolus
  - Bone tenderness along distal 6 cm of the fibula or lateral malleolus
  - Inability to bear weight for four steps
- MRI or CT if ankle sprain symptomatic for more than 6 weeks to assess for osteochondral injury, tendon injury, or missed fracture

Classification System
- Grade 1—ATFL stretched, no frank ligament tear, no laxity on examination
- Grade 2—Moderate injury to ligamentous complex, complete tear of ATFL ± partial tear of CFL; may or may not have increased laxity
- Grade 3—Complete tear of ATFL and CFL ± capsular tear ± PTFL tear

Initial Treatment
Patient Education
- Lateral ligament ankle sprains are the most common musculoskeletal injuries in the United States. Goals of treatment include reduction in pain and edema and prevention of further injury. Inadequate treatment can lead to chronic problems including joint instability, pain, and loss of range of motion.

First Treatment Steps
- Engage in RICE therapy (rest, ice, compression, and elevation)
- Functional immobilization in lace-up or semirigid ankle support devices

such as CAM walking boot for more severe injuries or ASO brace for less severe
- Weight bearing as tolerated unless significant amount of pain
- Referral to orthopaedic surgeon appropriate if concern or evidence of fracture or dislocation, neurovascular compromise, tendon rupture or subluxation, mechanical "locking" of joint, open wound penetrating the joint, and syndesmotic injury

Treatment Options
Nonoperative Management
- Most patients will recover well from an ankle sprain with nonsurgical management with surgical management reserved for high-performance athletes.
- Functional rehabilitation is superior to prolonged immobilization with protection of injured tissue postinjury days 1 to 5 and protected stress in a CAM walker boot days 6 to 32 postinjury
- If patient placed in CAM walker boot, see back in office 2 to 3 weeks postinjury to reassess ability to transition into semirigid device such as ASO
- Initiate physical therapy 2 to 3 weeks postinjury
- If continued or worsening symptoms 6 or more weeks postinjury, consider MRI and/or orthopaedic referral

Rehabilitation
- An effective rehabilitation program involves resumption of preinjury ROM, strength, proprioception, and motor control.
- Physical therapy prescription should include ankle ROM and strengthening, as well as peroneal strengthening and proprioception one to three times a week for 6 weeks.
- The patient may return to normal activity depending on pain and with guidance of a therapist once rehabilitation goals are met.

Prevention
- Use of an ankle brace with activity has been shown to prevent injury with minimal to no performance decrements.

Suggested Readings
Ivins D: Acute ankle sprain: an update, *Am Fam Physician* 74:1714–1720, 2006.

Lin C-W, Hiller C, de Bie R: Evidence-based treatment for ankle injuries: a clinical perspective, *J Man Manip Ther* 18:22–28, 2010.

Maffulli N, Ferran N: Management of acute and chronic ankle instability, *J Am Acad Orthop Surg* 16:608–615, 2008.

Mattacola C, Dwyer M: Rehabilitation of the ankle after acute sprain or chronic instability, *J Athl Train* 37:413–429, 2002.

CAVOVARUS FOOT DEFORMITY
History
- Foot deformity characterized by hindfoot varus and forefoot valgus or pronated position
- Increased pain over lateral border of foot, first metatarsal (MT) head or lateral metatarsal heads
- High arch
- Stress fractures of fifth metatarsal
- Lateral ankle instability
- Family history of similar foot shape
- History of Charcot-Marie-Tooth (CMT)

Physical Examination
- **"Peek-a-boo heel" sign** on standing examination: positive test is when patient's heel pad is visible from the front with feet aligned straight ahead
- May have abnormal callus formation at plantar first MT head and lateral border of foot
- Decreased strength with dorsiflexion and eversion with CMT
- Coleman block testing to assess flexibility of deformity and pronation of forefoot: heel varus is correctable or flexible if hindfoot alignment corrects with use of 2.5- to 4-cm thick Coleman block placed under the lateral border of the foot allowing first, second, and third metatarsal to drop
- May have tenderness over peroneal tendons

Imaging
- Radiographs: weight-bearing ankle (AP/mortise/lateral) and foot (AP/lateral/oblique) (Fig. 8-24)

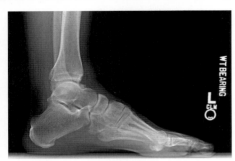

Figure 8-24. Lateral radiograph of cavovarus foot. Note increased calcaneal pitch.

Classification (Table 8-6)

Table 8-6. Classification of Cavovarus Foot Deformity
Neurologic   Hereditary sensory & motor neuropathies   Cerebral palsy   Cerebrovascular accident   Spinal root injury
Traumatic   Compartment syndrome   Peroneal nerve injury   Knee dislocation (neurovascular injury)   Talar neck malunion
Residual Clubfoot
Idiopathic

Initial Treatment
Patient Education
- The goal of treatment is to improve gait and prevent overload that may contribute to ankle instability, peroneal tendinitis, stress fractures, and arthritic joints. Surgery is indicated to rebalance tendons and muscle control to prevent deterioration of the foot.

First Treatment Steps
- Initiate neurologic and genetic testing if indicated
- Initiate orthotic management if flexible deformity
- Refer to orthopaedic surgeon for recurrent symptoms or injury and for surgical evaluation

Treatment Options
Nonoperative Management
- Orthotics—custom versus modifying over-the-counter inserts
- AFO brace—indicated for patients with muscle imbalance

Operative Management
Codes
ICD-9
736.75 Cavovarus deformity of the foot

Operative Indications
- Presence of progressive deformity due to muscular imbalance
- Continued pain or injury despite appropriate conservative management

Informed Consent and Counseling:
- Surgery may involve tendon transfers and corrective osteotomy for fusion, with the goal to improve function and decrease the risk of injury and progressive foot deterioration.
- Risks of surgery include nonunion or malunion of bony procedures and the continued need for brace or orthotic management.
- The patient may require extensive physical therapy after surgery.

Anesthesia
- General with regional nerve block

Patient Positioning
- Supine
- Nonsterile tourniquet on upper thigh

Surgical Procedures
- Combination of soft tissue and bony procedures, which are numerous; indications and surgeon preference dictate type of procedure(s) used
- Soft tissue release and tendon lengthening
- Tendon transfer
- Osteotomies—calcaneal, midfoot, dorsiflexion of 1st ray, talar neck, lateral column shortening
- Fusion
- Claw-toe reconstruction

Suggested Readings
Guyton G: Current concepts review: orthopaedic aspects of Charcot-Marie-Tooth disease, *Foot Ankle Int* 27:1003–1010, 2006.

Manoli A, Graham B: The subtle cavus foot, "The Underpronator," a review, *Foot Ankle Int* 26:256–263, 2005.

Younger A, Hansen S: Adult cavovarus foot, *J Am Acad Orthop Surg* 13:302–315, 2005.

HALLUX RIGIDUS

History
- Osteoarthritis of the first metatarsal-phalangeal joint (MTP joint)
- Insidious onset of pain and stiffness at the great toe MTP joint
- Presence of dorsal bony prominence can cause pain with shoe wear and impingement with activities
- Patient may complain of lateral foot pain due to compensatory overload

Physical Examination
- Decreased motion, especially dorsiflexion
- Pain with motion, initially with terminal dorsiflexion and plantarflexion progressing to pain and crepitus with midrange motion as disease progresses
- Evidence of dorsal bony prominence at MTP joint
- Antalgic gait
- Note evidence of transfer metatarsalgia, lesser toe deformities, or foot malalignment

Imaging
- Radiographs: weight-bearing foot—AP, lateral, and oblique (Fig. 8-25)

Radiographic Classification
- Grade I: mild to moderate osteophyte formation with preservation of joint space

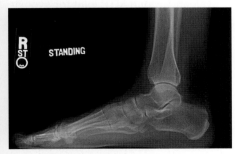

Figure 8-25. Lateral foot x-ray demonstrating dorsal osteophyte formation.

- Grade II: moderate osteophyte with joint space narrowing and subchondral sclerosis
- Grade III: marked osteophyte with severe loss of joint space and subchondral cyst formation

Initial Treatment
Patient Education
- Hallux rigidus is one of the most common disorders of the great toe and the most common form of arthritis in the foot. The exact etiology is unclear because many biomechanical and structural factors may play a role in its development.

First Treatment Steps
- Engage in shoe modifications, activity modifications, ice, and anti-inflammatories.
- Refer to orthopaedic surgeon for surgical consult as needed.

Treatment Options
Nonoperative Management
- Use of shoe with adequate width and height to accommodate dorsal bony prominence
- Carbon fiber plate/Morton's extension or rigid soled shoe
- Intermittent corticosteroid injections

Operative Management
Codes
ICD-9
  735.2 Hallux rigidus
CPT
  28289 Cheilectomy—1st MTP
  28750 Arthrodesis—1st MTP

Operative Indications
- Failed nonoperative treatment

Informed Consent and Counseling
- Risks of surgery include infection, nerve trapped in scar, progression of arthritis, and need for further surgery, such as arthrodesis, if pain continues.
- It is important to discuss the objectives of surgery with the patient. In case of cheilectomy, the arthritic joint still remains; therefore, pain may still be present when stressed.

Anesthesia
■ General with regional or local block

Patient Positioning
■ Supine
■ Nonsterile tourniquet on upper thigh

Surgical Procedures
■ Cheilectomy—bone spur excision, indicated for grade I and grade II arthritis
■ First MTP arthrodesis—indicated for grade III arthritis, arthritis in addition to hallux valgus deformity, failed prior surgical intervention, or underlying rheumatoid arthritis or other neuromuscular conditions

Cheilectomy
■ A dorsal longitudinal incision is made over the first MTP joint. The extensor hood and joint capsule are incised, and deep dissection is done either medial or lateral to the EHL.
■ Thorough synovectomy is performed, and osteophytes are located.
■ The joint is inspected to assess cartilage loss. The metatarsal osteophyte is resected on the dorsal, dorsomedial, and dorsolateral aspects using an osteotome.
■ Articular cartilage irregularities including loose bodies are removed with the goal of achieving 60 degrees of dorsiflexion.
■ Raw bone surfaces are smoothed with a rasp or rongeur and may be coated with a thin film of bone wax.
■ The joint capsule is sutured followed by subcutaneous and skin closure. A dry bulky dressing and a postoperative shoe are applied. The patient may be heel weight bearing or full weight bearing depending on the surgeon's preference.

Estimated Postoperative Course
■ 2 Weeks Postoperative
  • Sutures are removed.
  • The patient may transition back into a regular shoe and start activities as tolerated. Active ROM is encouraged.

■ Maximal medical improvement can take up to 3 to 4 months to achieve.

Suggested Readings
Coughlin M, Mann R, Saltzman C: *Surgery of the foot and ankle*, ed 8, Philadelphia, 2007, Mosby.
Mann R: Disorders of the first metatarsophalangeal joint, *J Am Acad Ortho Surg* 3: 34–43, 1995.
Yee G, Lau J: Current concepts eview: hallux rigidus, *Foot Ankle Int* 29:637–646, 2008.

HALLUX VALGUS
History
■ Lateral deviation of the great toe with medial deviation of the first metatarsal, commonly known as a "bunion"
■ Pain over medial eminence of first metatarsal with shoe wear, especially narrow toe box shoes
■ Other locations of pain include within first MTP joint, plantar aspect of second metatarsal head, and with impingement of the first toe onto the second
■ May be present since childhood and/or worsening deformity over time
■ Cosmetic deformity

Physical Examination
■ Note severity of hallux valgus deformity and presence of pes planus while patient is weight bearing.
■ Note skin changes (erythema, skin breakdown, callus formation).
■ Assess pain over medial eminence, with first MTP joint motion and first TMT joint laxity.
■ Evaluate second MTP joint for synovitis, second toe deformity, and metatarsal head overload.

Imaging
■ Weight-bearing foot radiograph (AP, lateral, oblique) (Fig. 8-26)
■ Measure hallux valgus angle (HVA)—intersection of longitudinal axes of diaphysis of first metatarsal and proximal phalanx
■ Measure intermetatarsal angle (IMA)—angle between diaphysis of first and second metatarsals

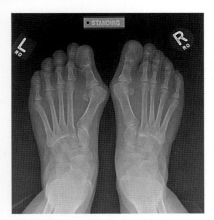

Figure 8-26. Anteroposterior view of bilateral hallux valgus deformities.

Classification
- Mild: HVA less than 30 degrees and IMA less than 10 to 15 degrees
- Moderate: HVA 30 to 40 degrees and IMA 10 to 15 degrees
- Severe: HVA greater than 40 degrees and IMA greater than 15 to 20 degrees

Initial Treatment
Patient Education
- The cause of a bunion is thought to be multifactorial and largely due to shoe/foot size mismatch, some genetic predisposition, and from repetitive forces applied to the first MTP joint. Only surgery can correct the deformity, but patients' symptoms can be significantly relieved with appropriate conservative management.

First Treatment Steps
- Initially advise patient of proper accommodative shoe wear to include wider toe box and use of shoe stretchers.
- Refer to orthopaedic surgeon if patient has failed appropriate conservative treatment.

Treatment Options
Nonoperative Management
- The main goal is symptomatic relief only, but it will not permanently correct the deformity.
- Shoe modifications include shoes with a wider toe box and use of shoe stretcher or ball and ring stretcher.
- Use devices such as toe spacers, bunion sleeve, and padding over medial eminence.

Operative Management
Codes
ICD-9
  735.0 Acquired hallux valgus
CPT
  28296 Hallux valgus—distal/proximal osteotomy
  28297 Hallux valgus—lapidus procedure
  28750 First MTP fusion

Operative Indications
- Pain recalcitrant to appropriate non-operative treatment

Informed Consent and Counseling
- There are more than 100 described bunion surgeries.
- Risks/complications of surgery include reoccurrence of deformity or residual deformity, stiffness at the first MTP joint, and inability to return to level of activity before surgery.
- Surgery should not be done to achieve unlimited shoe wear potential.

Anesthesia
- Surgeon and patient discretion, likely general with regional block

Patient Positioning
- Supine
- Nonsterile tourniquet

Surgical Procedures
- The degree of deformity usually dictates the surgical procedure of choice.
  - Mild to moderate—distal procedure
  - Severe—proximal procedure
  - With concurrent hallux rigidus or underlying rheumatoid arthritis—arthrodesis

Distal Chevron Osteotomy (Fig. 8-27)
- Hardware: Kirschner wire
- Longitudinal incision made over medial eminence with dissection down to joint capsule. Full-thickness

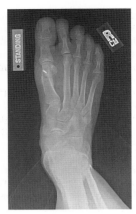

Figure 8-27. Distal chevron osteotomy for hallux valgus correction.

dorsal and plantar skin flaps are created being careful to avoid the dorsomedial and plantar medial cutaneous nerve.
- An L-shaped, distally based capsular flap is made for distal soft tissue release.
- Osteotomy technique: The medial eminence is resected using an oscillating saw parallel to the medial border of the foot. An oscillating saw is used for the horizontal osteotomy in the metaphyseal region with a divergent angle of approximately 60 degrees. Care must be taken to avoid overpenetrating the lateral cortex and entering the soft tissues, which may compromise the metatarsal head blood supply. The osteotomy is displaced approximately 30% of the metatarsal's width.
- The capital fragment is impacted and fixated on proximal fragment, with a Kirschner wire directed from proximal dorsal to distal plantar with care not to penetrate the MTP. Any bony prominence is beveled with a saw.
- The medial capsule is repaired with interrupted absorbable sutures with the toe in neutral position. Skin closure is per surgeon's preference.
- Dry, compressive dressing is applied with a postoperative shoe.

Estimated Postoperative Course
- 1 to 2 Weeks Postoperative
  - Postoperative dressing removed and bunion dressing applied if indicated; change every week for 10 days for 8 weeks
  - Sutures removed 2 to 3 weeks postoperative
  - Immobilization in a postoperative shoe or CAM boot, weight bearing through heel only
- 4 Weeks Postoperative
  - Kirschner wire removed
- 6 to 8 Weeks Postoperative
  - Discontinue bunion dressing, if indicated
  - Transition into full weight bearing in postoperative shoe or CAM boot
  - Initiate ROM at first MTP joint to prevent stiffness and pain
- 10 to 12 Weeks Postoperative
  - Transition into regular shoe as tolerated
  - Increase activities as tolerated

Suggested Readings

Coughlin M, Mann R, Saltzman C: *Surgery of the foot and ankle*, ed 8, Philadelphia, 2007, Mosby.

Easley M, Trnka H-J: Current concepts review: hallux valgus part I: pathomechanics, clinical assessment, and non-operative treatment, *Foot Ankle Int* 28:654–659, 2007.

Easley M, Trnka H-J: Current concepts review: hallux valgus part II: operative treatment, *Foot Ankle Int* 28:748–758, 2007.

POSTERIOR TIBIAL TENDON DYSFUNCTION OR ACQUIRED ADULT FLATFOOT DEFORMITY (AAFD)

History
- Gradual-onset medial hindfoot pain and swelling caused by lateral impingement in the subfibular and sinus tarsi region
- Pain increases with activity
- Gait disturbance to include inability to run, push off, and do heel raise
- Also known as "fallen arches"

Physical Examination
- Flatfoot deformity on affected side to include flattening of medial longitudinal arch, hindfoot valgus, and abduction of midfoot onto hindfoot

- "Too many toes" sign: When examining standing patient from the rear, most of the lesser toes visible because of midfoot abduction
- Edema, thickness, tenderness to palpation over posterior tibial tendon (PTT), subfibular region and sinus tarsi
- Inability to do single heel raise
- Assess ROM of hindfoot for flexible or rigid deformity and dorsiflexion range of motion for equinus contracture

Imaging
- Radiographs: Weight-bearing foot (AP/oblique/lateral) and ankle (AP/mortise/lateral) (Figs. 8-28 and 8-29).
- MRI: not needed to make diagnosis; can be ordered to assess status of soft tissues (i.e., PTT, spring ligament, deltoid ligament)

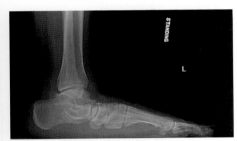

Figure 8-28. Lateral radiograph demonstrating pes planus.

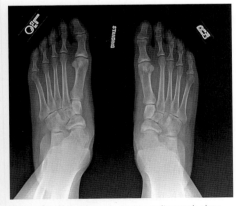

Figure 8-29. Anteroposterior radiograph demonstrating talar uncovering.

Classification System
- Stage I—No deformity
- Stage IIa—Mild/moderate flexible deformity
- Stage IIb—Severe flexible deformity
- Stage III—Fixed deformity
- Stage IV—Includes ankle deformity (lateral talar tilt)
- Stage IVa—Flexible foot deformity
- Stage IVb—Fixed foot deformity

Initial Treatment
Patient Education
- Deformity can be effectively treated nonoperatively, but surgery may be indicated if deformity and pain progress.

First Treatment Steps
- Acute exacerbation treated in CAM boot, NSAIDs, ice
- Refer to orthopaedics for orthotic and surgical management

Treatment Options
Nonoperative Management
- Custom orthotics with flexible deformity with goal to support the longitudinal arch and decrease hindfoot valgus
- Custom ankle bracing to include Arizona or AFO for rigid deformity
- Physical therapy may be beneficial in the early stages

Operative Management
Codes
ICD-9
    734 Flat foot
    905.8 Late effect of tendon injury
CPT
    28300 Medial slide calcaneal osteotomy
    27691 Posterior tibial tendon reconstruction with FDL to navicular
    27687 Gastrocnemius recession

Operative Indications
- Failed appropriate nonoperative management with continued pain and deformity

Informed Consent and Counseling
- Risks to include infection, nerve injury, nonunion or malunion, and persistent pain and deformity

Anesthesia
- General with regional nerve block, likely popliteal

Patient Positioning
- Supine
- Nonsterile tourniquet on upper thigh

Surgical Procedures
- Posterior tibial tenosynovectomy: indicated for stage I
- Flatfoot reconstruction—Medial slide calcaneal osteotomy, FHL augmentation of PTT, gastrocnemius recession, ± lateral column lengthening and medial column fusion: indicated for stage II flexible deformity
- Triple arthrodesis: indicated for rigid deformity

Flatfoot Reconstruction (Fig. 8-30)
- Hardware: Kirschner wires, cannulated screws
- Incision made from posterosuperior to anteroinferior along lateral aspect calcaneus, dissection down to calcaneus with careful consideration of the sural nerve
- Osteotomy performed at 45-degree angle to its longitudinal axis. Posterior segment is translated medially and temporarily fixated with Kirschner wire followed by one to two cannulated screws
- Incision made from tip of medial malleolus extending distally to navicular
- PTT sheath incised and tendon exposed. Tendon examined and debrided as indicated

- Flexor digitorum longus (FDL) located deep to PTT by flexing and extending toes; once located, tendon sheath incised
- FDL traced distally into foot until fibrous connection between the FDL and FHL is reached, where a side-to-side tenodesis is performed
- Krakow suture technique used at distal aspect of FDL
- Dorsomedial aspect of navicular bone exposed in anticipation of tendon transfer. FDL passed inferior to superior through the navicular and appropriately tensioned using nonabsorbable suture
- Gastrocnemius recession then performed as indicated
- All incisions sutured; posterior mold/sugar tong splint applied

Estimated Postoperative Course
- 2 Weeks Postoperative
  - Postoperative dressing removed, sutures removed
  - Patient placed in non–weight-bearing short leg cast or removable CAM boot
- 6 Weeks Postoperative
  - Initiate weight bearing in CAM boot
  - Rehabilitation exercises to include ankle dorsiflexion and plantarflexion
- 12 Weeks Postoperative
  - Transition from CAM to tennis shoe with ASO ankle brace as indicated
  - Allowed to initiate non–weight-bearing exercise
  - Evaluate need for custom orthotics

Suggested Readings
Coughlin M, Mann R, Saltzman C: *Surgery of the foot and ankle*, ed 8, Philadelphia, 2007, Mosby.
Deland J: Adult-acquired flatfoot deformity, *J Am Acad Orthop Surg* 16:399–406, 2008.
Haddad S, Myerson M, Younger A, et al: Adult acquired flatfoot deformity, *Foot Ankle Int* 32: 95–111, 2011.
Pinney S, Lin S: Current concept review: acquired adult flatfoot deformity, *Foot Ankle Int* 27:66–75, 2006.

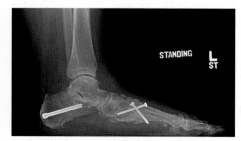

Figure 8-30. Lateral weight-bearing radiograph demonstrating calcaneal osteotomy.

SUBTALAR JOINT DISLOCATION
History
- Results from high-energy trauma (e.g., motor vehicle crash, fall from height, sport activity)

- Pain and deformity to affected extremity
- Relatively uncommon injury, less than 1% of all dislocations

Physical Examination
- Inspect for open wounds.
- Determine type of deformity present: medial, lateral, anterior, or posterior.
- Assess neurovascular status to include a dorsalis pedis pulse and sensation to superficial peroneal nerve, deep peroneal nerve, sural, saphenous, and tibial nerves.
- Assess for associated injuries.

Imaging
- Radiographs: initial and postreduction—ankle (AP/mortise/lateral) and foot (AP/lateral/oblique) (Fig. 8-31AB)
- CT scan: evaluation for osteochondral injuries and occult trauma

Classification
- Dislocation at the talonavicular joint with intact calcaneocuboid and tibiotalar joints
- Medial: inversion force, most common
- Lateral: eversion force, usually associated with concomitant fractures
- Anterior
- Posterior

Initial Treatment
Patient Education
- Injury is associated with post-traumatic restricted subtalar joint ROM and

arthritis. Symptomatology seems to be directly correlated with severity of initial injury.

First Treatment Steps
- Immediate referral to emergency department for prompt evaluation and reduction.
- Postreduction follow-up with orthopaedic surgeon.

Treatment Options
Nonoperative Management
- Closed reduction under sedation: Traction is placed on the foot and heel in line with the deformity. Countertraction is applied with the knee in flexion to relax the gastrocnemius. For medial dislocations, the foot is abducted and ankle is dorsiflexed. For lateral dislocations, the foot is adducted and the ankle is dorsiflexed.
- Immobilize patient in non–weight-bearing short leg cast 4 to 6 weeks, followed by protected mobilization and weight bearing.

Operative Management
Codes
ICD-9
    838.01 Closed dislocation of tarsal joint
CPT
    27846 Open treatment of ankle dislocation, w or w/o percutaneous skeletal fixation, w/o repair or internal fixation

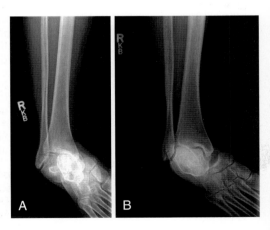

Figure 8-31. Subtalar dislocation anteroposterior view (**A**) and oblique view. Note dislocation at talonavicular joint (**B**).

27848 Open treatment of ankle dislocation, w or w/o percutaneous skeletal fixation; with repair or internal or external fixation

Operative Indications
- If unsuccessful closed reduction and/or open dislocation

Informed Consent and Counseling
- Associated foot and ankle injuries are common and can lead to future pain and morbidity.
- Restriction of subtalar joint motion and progression of post-traumatic arthritis are common.

Anesthesia
- General anesthesia

Patient Positioning
- Supine

Surgical Procedures
- Irrigation and debridement with rigid fixation such as ORIF and/or external fixator, if needed

Estimated Postoperative Course
- Immobilization in non–weight-bearing short leg cast for 4 to 6 weeks followed by protected immobilization and weight bearing
- Physical therapy as needed after cast removal to improve range of motion of subtalar joint

Suggested Readings
Bibbo C, Anderson B, Davis WH: Injury characteristics and clinical outcomes of subtalar dislocations: a clinical and radiographic analysis of 25 cases, *Foot Ankle Int* 24:158–163, 2003.
DeLee J, Curtis R: Subtalar dislocation of the foot, *J Bone and Joint Surg* 64-A:433–437, 1982.
Heppenstall R, Farahvar H, Balderston R, et al: Evaluation and management of subtalar dislocations, *J Trauma* 20:494–497, 1980.

TARSAL FRACTURES
Calcaneus Fracture
History
- High-energy, axial load such as fall from height or motor vehicle crash
- Pain in heel, inability to bear weight
- Most common tarsal bone fracture, approximately 2% of all fractures

Physical Examination
- Edema and hematoma of hindfoot and ankle, possible deformity
- Tenderness to palpation in heel
- Associated injuries possible (e.g., low back pain/injury)

Imaging
- Radiographs: ankle (AP/mortise/lateral) and foot (AP/oblique/lateral) and Harris view (Fig. 8-32)
- CT: used to evaluate fracture for preoperative planning

Classification
Sanders Classification
- Type I: extra-articular, nondisplaced
- Type II: one displaced fracture line
- Type III: two displaced fracture lines
- Type IV: three or more displaced fracture lines

Initial Treatment
Patient Education
- Calcaneus fractures are notoriously bad injuries with a high probability of developing post-traumatic arthritis. The goal of operative intervention is to restore anatomy and prevent severity of arthritis in the future.

First Treatment Steps
- Immobilize affected extremity in non–weight-bearing posterior and stir-up splint.
- Refer to orthopaedic surgeon for management.

Treatment Options
Nonoperative Management
- Indications: nondisplaced or minimally displaced fractures; local or systemic contraindications to surgery
- Non–weight-bearing splint, cast, or CAM boot for 6 weeks, followed by weight bearing in boot for additional 4 to 6 weeks
- Subtalar joint range of motion initiated after 2 to 6 weeks of treatment

Operative Management
Codes
ICD-9
  825.0 Closed fracture of calcaneus

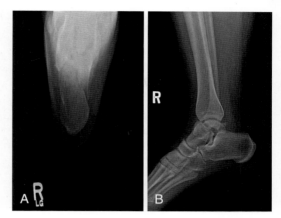

Figure 8-32. Harris view (**A**) and Lateral radiograph of calcaneus fracture (**B**).

CPT
  28415 ORIF calcaneus fracture

Operative Indications
- Displaced intra-articular fracture with joint displacement greater than 1 mm
- Extra-articular fractures with significant hindfoot valgus/varus or considerable flattening, broadening, or shortening of the heel
- Primary subtalar fusion in case of highly comminuted fractures where restoration of joint is impossible

Informed Consent and Counseling
- Risks of surgery include but are not limited to surgical wound infection, malunion/nonunion, and nerve injury.
- The patient may need subtalar fusion in the future if he or she has persistent pain and evidence of post-traumatic osteoarthritis of subtalar joint.
- Maximal medical improvement can take up to 1 year to achieve.

Anesthesia
- General with ankle or popliteal block

Patient Positioning
- Lateral decubitus on noninjured side
- Nonsterile tourniquet on upper thigh

Surgical Procedure
- ORIF calcaneus—minimally invasive approach

- ORIF calcaneus—extended lateral approach
- Primary subtalar arthrodesis

ORIF Calcaneus—Minimally Invasive Approach
- Hardware: 6.5-mm Schanz screw with handle, Kirschner wires, cortical screws
- Percutaneous leverage is used to reduce the main tuberosity fracture fragment.
- A 6.5-mm Schanz screw with a handle is placed into the main portion of tuberosity fragment parallel to its upper aspect. The handle is used to manipulate the fracture fragments to achieve fluoroscopic-guided anatomic reduction.
- Fracture fragments are fixed with three to six cortical screws introduced via stab incisions. One or two screws are placed into the thalamic portion toward sustenaculum tali to achieve maximum stability.
- Wound closure and splinting in a well-molded posterior non–weight-bearing splint.

Estimated Postoperative Course
- 1 to 2 Weeks Postoperative
  - First office visit and wound check. Sutures removed 10 to 14 days postoperatively

- Placed into immoveable device such as CAM walker boot or bivalve cast
- Strictly non–weight bearing, may initiate gentle ROM of ankle.
- 6 Weeks Postoperative
  - Initiate weight bearing in a CAM boot.
  - Initiate non–weight bearing ROM subtalar joint out of boot
- 12 Weeks Postoperative
  - Transition from boot to tennis shoe.
  - Increase therapy to include weight-bearing ROM and strengthening and gait training.
  - The patient may initiate non–weight-bearing exercise; no impact for additional 4 to 6 weeks

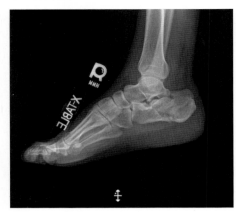

Figure 8-33. Lateral view, talar body fracture.

TALUS FRACTURE
History
- Axial load on plantarflexed foot—talar head fracture
- High-velocity trauma—talar neck fracture
- Ankle inversion, dorsiflexion—lateral process fracture, "snowboarder's fracture"
- Ankle pain, swelling, inability to bear weight

Physical Examination
- Note edema or tenderness over affected area (e.g., talonavicular joint, proximal dorsal foot).
- Assess for deformity or change in normal ankle contours.
- Assess for associated injuries.

Imaging (Fig. 8-33)
- Radiographs: Foot (AP/lateral/oblique) and ankle (AP/lateral/mortise). May consider Canale's view (foot in maximum equinus, pronated 15 degrees, beam directed at 75-degree angle from horizontal plane) and Broden's view (foot in neutral flexion with leg internally rotated 30 to 40 degrees. The beam is centered over the lateral malleolus; radiographs are taken at 40, 30, 20, and 10 degrees toward patient's head) for further evaluation.
- CT: A scan provides better fracture detail, which is useful in assessing

comminution, success of reduction, and congruency of subtalar joint.

Classification
- Talar head
- Talar neck: Hawkins classification (Table 8-7)
- Talar body

Table 8-7. Hawkins Classification of Talar Neck Fractures
Type I: Nondisplaced
Type II: Displaced with subtalar joint subluxation
Type III: Displaced with dislocation of ankle and subtalar joint
Type IV: Displaced with dislocation at talonavicular joint

Initial Treatment
Patient Education
- Treatment of talus fractures provides a difficult challenge because of the large amount of articular surface present, vulnerable blood supply, and crucial biomechanical role in function of the foot and ankle. Injury to the talus puts patients at high risk for osteoarthrosis and osteonecrosis.

First Treatment Steps
- Immobilization in non–weight-bearing posterior/stirrup lower leg splint

- Referral to orthopaedic surgery for further management

Treatment Options
Nonoperative Management
- Indications: talar neck fracture Hawkins type I; stable talar head fracture; talar osteochondral fractures less than 10 mm; nondisplaced talar body fractures less than 2 mm fracture gaping; types I and III lateral process fracture
- Immobilization in non–weight bearing short leg cast for 6 to 8 weeks

Operative Management
Codes
ICD-9
825.21 Closed fracture of talus
CPT
28445 ORIF talus

Operative Indications
- Unstable talar fracture or risk of significant morbidity with nonoperative treatment

Informed Consent and Counseling
- Talar fractures can be difficult to treat and can lead to disability despite the appropriate treatment.
- Recovery may require prolonged course of immobilization and non–weight bearing.

Anesthesia
- General with regional nerve block

Patient Positioning
- Supine
- Nonsterile tourniquet on upper thigh

Surgical Procedures
- ORIF talar neck fracture
- ORIF talar head fracture
- ORIF talar body fracture
- ORIF versus excision of lateral process fracture

Estimated Postoperative Course
- 1 to 2 Weeks Postoperative
  - Wound check and suture removal
  - Placed into non–weight-bearing CAM boot or cast

- 6 to 8 Weeks Postoperative
  - Transition into weight bearing in CAM boot
- 12 Weeks Postoperative
  - Transition from CAM boot to tennis shoe, likely with ASO ankle brace for additional 4 to 6 weeks
  - Patient can gradually increase activities
  - Therapy if indicated for ankle and subtalar joint range of motion and strengthening

Suggested Readings
Ahmad J, Raikin S: Current concepts review: talar fractures, *Foot Ankle Int* 27:475–482, 2006.
Higgins T, Baumgaertner M: Diagnosis and treatment of fractures of the talus: a comprehensive review of the literature, *Foot Ankle Int* 20:595–605, 1999.
Rammelt S, Zwipp H: Calcaneus fractures, *Trauma* 8:197–212, 2006.

ORTHOPAEDIC PROCEDURES
Ankle Injection/Aspiration
CPT Code
20605

Indications
- Arthritis, synovitis, crystal arthropathies

Contraindications
- Infection
- Local skin rash

Equipment Needed
- Sterile gloves
- Topical bactericidal solution
- 18-gauge needle for aspiration, 25-gauge needle for injection
- 5 to 10 mL syringe
- Injectate: 1% lidocaine without epinephrine (4 to 8 mL) and corticosteroid (Celestone or Solumedrol) (1 mL)
- Sterile bandage

Procedure (Fig. 8-34)
1) Place patient in supine position with the ankle relaxed
2) Palpate the anterior joint line between anterior tibial tendon and anterior border of medial malleolous.
3) Prepare the skin with a bactericidal agent at the injection site.

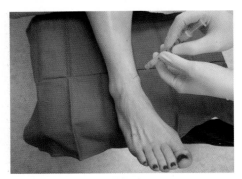

Figure 8-34. See text for the ankle injection/ aspiration procedure.

4) Using sterile technique, insert needle into identified joint space, aiming posterolateral. Once the needle is in the joint space, there will be reduced resistance, allowing aspiration and/or easy injection of medication.
5) Apply sterile dressing.

Aftercare Instructions
1) Monitor for local erythema, edema, increased pain, or systemic symptoms. Notify clinician.
2) Local anesthetic effect will wear off within a few hours, and corticosteroid will take effect within 3 to 5 days. Patients may experience steroid flare where symptoms may be worse for the first 24 to 48 hours. This can be treated with NSAIDs and ice.
3) The patient should remain in the office for 30 minutes after injection to monitor for adverse effects.
4) He or she should avoid strenuous activity for 48 hours after injection.

Plantar Fasciitis Injection
CPT Code
  20550

Indications
■ Plantar fasciitis not resolved with stretching and inserts

Contraindications
■ Foot infection
■ Local skin rash

■ Allergy to any injection material
■ Multiple previous injections to the same area

Equipment Needed
■ Sterile gloves
■ Bactericidal solution
■ 25-gauge needle
■ 5 to 10 mL syringe
■ Injectate: 1% lidocaine without epinephrine (2 to 3 mL), corticosteroid (1 mL of Celestone or Solumedrol)
■ Sterile bandage

Procedure (Fig. 8-35)
1) Place the patient in supine or lateral recumbent position on the examination table.
2) Palpate insertion of plantar fascia on the medial, plantar calcaneus.
3) Prepare the medial aspect of the plantar heel with bactericidal solution.
4) Using sterile technique, insert a 25-gauge needle perpendicular to the skin from the medial aspect directly down to midline of the foot. Aspirate to ensure needle is not in a vessel and then slowly inject medication evenly as the needle is slowly withdrawn. Use caution to avoid injecting the calcaneal fat pad.
5) Apply sterile dressing.

Aftercare Instructions
1) Monitor for local erythema, edema, increased pain, or systemic symptoms and notify clinician of any symptoms.

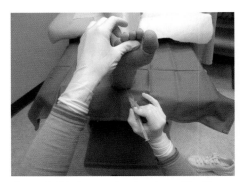

Figure 8-35. See text for the plantar/fasciitis injection procedure.

2) Local anesthesia will wear off within a few hours, and the corticosteroid will take effect within 3 to 5 days. Patients may experience steroid flare where symptoms may be worse for the first 24 to 48 hours. This can be treated with NSAIDs and ice.
3) The patient should remain in the office for 30 minutes after injection to monitor for adverse effects.
4) Avoid strenuous activity for at least 48 hours after injection.

Morton's Neuroma Injection
CPT code:
   64455, 64632

Indications
- Pain, paresthesias, and/or burning sensation into toes of affected interdigital nerve
- Positive Mulder click or pain with squeeze of the metatarsal heads
- Continued pain despite other appropriate treatment to include NSAIDs, ice, and orthotics

Contraindications
- Local skin irritation or infection
- Allergy to anesthetic or steroid

Equipment Needed
- Topical cleansing agent (e.g., Betadine)
- Sterile gloves
- Syringe, 3 to 5 mL
- 25-gauge needle, 1.5 inch
- Injectate:1 mL Lidocaine (1%) or Bupivacaine (0.25% or 0.5%) and 1 mL steroid (e.g., Celestone, Solumedrol)
- Clean dressing (gauze and tape)

Procedure (Fig. 8-36)
1) Place patient in supine position with foot in relaxed neutral position.
2) Palpate area of tenderness and mark location.
3) Apply Betadine.
4) Insert needle on dorsal surface, pointed distal to proximal, at 45-degree angle to skin at marked site until reaching area of fullness. Be careful not to puncture through plantar skin.
5) Aspirate and then inject steroid/anesthetic medication.

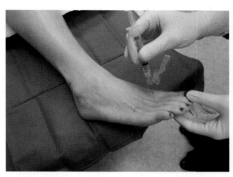

Figure 8-36. See text for the Morton neuroma injection procedure.

6) Withdraw needle, and apply clean dressing.

Aftercare Instructions
1) Patients should remain in the office for 30 minutes after injection to monitor for adverse effects.
2) Patients should avoid any strenuous activity for at least 48 hours after injection.
3) Caution patients on possible steroid flare where symptoms may be worse for the first 24 to 48 hours. This can be treated with NSAIDs and ice.
4) Call the office with any complaints of local erythema or systemic reaction.

Tarsal Tunnel Injection
CPT code
   64450

Indications
- Pain, paresthesias, and/or burning sensation over the tibial nerve distribution
- Positive Tinel sign over tibial nerve
- Continued pain despite other appropriate treatment to include NSAIDs, ice, and orthotics

Contraindications
- Local skin irritation or infection
- Allergy to anesthetic or steroid

Equipment Needed
- Topical cleansing agent (e.g., Betadine)
- Sterile gloves
- Syringe, 3 to 5 mL

- 25-gauge needle, 1 to 1.5 inch
- Injectate: 1 to 2 mL Lidocaine (1%) or Bupivacaine (0.25% or 0.5%) and 1 mL steroid (e.g., Celestone or Solumedrol)
- Clean dressing (gauze and tape)

Procedure (Fig. 8-37)
1) Place patient in lateral recombinant position.

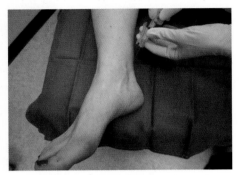

Figure 8-37. See text for the tarsal tunnel injection procedure.

2) Percuss posterior to medial malleolus to locate area of pain, mark. Also identify PTT.
3) Apply Betadine.
4) Insert needle, pointed distally, approximately 2 cm proximal to marked location with needle at 30-degree angle to the skin.
5) Aspirate and then inject steroid/anesthetic medication.
6) Withdraw needle, and apply clean dressing.

Aftercare Instructions
1) Patients should remain in the office for 30 minutes after injection to monitor for adverse effects.
2) Patients should avoid any strenuous activity for at least 48 hours after injection.
3) Caution patients on possible steroid flare where symptoms may be worse for the first 24 to 48 hours. This can be treated with NSAIDs and ice.
4) Call the office with any complaints of local erythema or systemic reaction.

Pediatrics 9
Scott Yang

INTRODUCTION
Development and Growth
- Developmental milestones (Table 9-1)

Structure and Function of Bone
- Basic bone anatomy
  - Epiphysis—This region of bone is closest to a joint and lined with articular cartilage.
    - Ossification of the child's epiphysis depends on age and location: Distal femoral, proximal tibial, and proximal humeral epiphysis are ossified at birth.
    - Ossification of the elbow epiphysis follows a sequence in pneumonic. Remember CRITOE and 1,3,5,7,9,11 for a rough age guideline for evaluating elbow radiographs:
    - C—capitellum: ossifies around 1 year
    - R—radial head: ossifies around 3 years
    - I—internal (medial) epicondyle: ossifies around 5 years
    - T—trochlea: ossifies around 7 years
    - O—olecranon: ossifies around 9 years
    - E—external (lateral) epicondyle: ossifies around 11 years
      - Fractures through the epiphysis cannot be seen by plain radiograph until they are ossified.

- Metaphysis—the region of spongy bone that is the transition zone to the shaft of the long bone.
- Diaphysis—the shaft of a long bone.

Skeletal Growth
- Skeletal growth over the lifetime is not constant—the rate of growth is highest in the first 4 years and levels off until adolescence.
- Growth proportion varies by anatomic region (i.e., proximal tibial physis contributes more to tibial length than distal tibial physis).
- Longitudinal growth of limbs occurs via endochondral ossification.
  - Endochondral ossification occurs when cartilage cells mature → hypertrophy → calcify → and are replaced by mature bone.
  - Endochondral ossification occurs at the physis, or growth plate, of each bone.
- Physeal anatomy
  - In long bones, the physis is located near a joint, lying in between the epiphysis and metaphysis.
  - Physis contains four continuous zones starting adjacent to the epiphysis to the metaphysis: resting zone (near epiphysis), proliferating zone, hypertrophic

Table 9-1. Developmental Milestones

MILESTONE	AGE (MO)	CONSIDER FURTHER EVALUATION IF:
Rolls from back to stomach	3.6 ± 1.4	Not rolling by 6 mo
Sits unsupported	6.3 ± 1.2	Not sitting by 8 mo
Pull to stand	8.1 ± 1.5	
Walk	11.7 ± 2	Not walking by 18 mo
Run	15 ± 3	

(Modified from Palmer F: Keys to developmental assessment. In McMillan J, editor: *Oski's pediatrics,* ed 3, Philadelphia, 2006, Lippincott Williams & Wilkins, p 789.)

zone and provisional calcification zone (near metaphysis) (Table 9-2).

■ Fractures in children take special consideration due to growth considerations because fractures in the growth plate may cause growth disturbances and potential for limb length inequality and deformity from asymmetric growth.

■ The Salter-Harris classification is for growth plate injuries (Table 9-3).

Table 9-2. Physeal Zones

ZONE	RESTING ZONE	PROLIFERATING ZONE	HYPERTROPHIC ZONE	PROVISIONAL CALCIFICATION ZONE
Actions in the zone	Resting immature chondrocytes supply necessary cells for growth	Chondrocytes grow and divide, and arrange into columns, develop extracellular matrix	Chondrocytes hypertrophy, produce type X collagen, which is important for extracellular matrix calcification	Chondrocytes die, cartilage matrix becomes calcified, which leads to vascular invasion and invasion of osteoblasts & osteoclasts for bone formation
Clinical Pearls	Injury to this zone causes growth arrest	Achondroplastic dwarves have a genetic mutation that prevents cartilage growth in this zone	-Weakest part of physis, fractures tend to propagate through this region. -Slipped capital femoral epiphysis occurs in this weak zone -Rickets (vitamin D deficiency) prevents calcification of cells past this zone	Scurvy (severe vitamin C deficiency) causes failure of collagen cross-linking in the transition between this zone and the metaphysis leading to brittleness of this region

Table 9-3. Salter Harris Classification for Growth Plate Injuries

TYPE	FIGURE	DESCRIPTION	SIGNIFICANCE
I		Fracture line through the physis only (zone of hypertrophy)	-Low chance of growth disturbance -Occurs most commonly in hypertrophic zone of physis
II		Fracture line through the physis and extending to include a portion of the metaphysis	-Most common -Variable growth disturbance— depends on location (i.e., rare in wrist but high in distal femur)
III		Fracture line through the physis and exiting through the epiphysis into a joint	-Variable growth disturbance -Anatomic reduction important as fracture involves joint
IV		Vertical fracture line through the epiphysis, physis, and metaphysis	-Physeal bar formation possible as fracture line traverses cartilage reserve zone of physis -Anatomic reduction important as fracture involves joint
V		Crush injury to the physis	-Rare, hard to distinguish from nondisplaced Salter Harris type I -High chance of growth disturbance

COMMON PEDIATRIC INJURIES
Pediatric Wrist Fractures
History
- Background: Pediatric distal radius and ulna fractures are common injuries. Younger children generally sustain metaphyseal buckle fractures, whereas older children can sustain distal radius and ulna physeal fractures.
- A fall onto an outstretched hand is the most common mechanism. Most fractures occur with a hyperextended wrist leading to dorsal displacement of the distal fracture fragment.
- The patient may report pain and may have a wrist deformity or swelling.

Physical Examination
- Inspect for significant edema and deformity of the wrist.
- Palpate for significant tenderness at fracture site.
- Perform a careful neurovascular examination.
  - High-energy injuries can be associated with carpal tunnel syndrome.
- Assess the extremity proximal and distal to the injury site to rule out other associated injuries.

Imaging: Figure 9-1
- Take posteroanterior (PA) and lateral radiographs of the wrist.
- Consider radiographs of the hand, forearm, and elbow to rule out adjacent injuries.

Classification System
- Salter Harris classification for physeal injuries
- Nondisplaced versus displaced metaphyseal fractures
  - Nondisplaced fractures can be treated in a splint or cast without reduction.
  - Displaced fractures require closed reduction.

Initial Treatment
- Low-energy trauma and nondisplaced: splint or casting in the outpatient setting

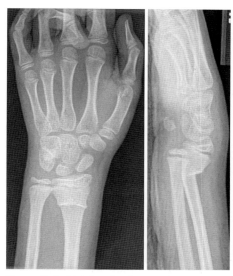

Figure 9-1. Distal radius fracture in an 8-year-old boy.

- Higher-energy trauma + displaced injury: closed reduction and splinting under conscious sedation in the emergency department

Patient Education
- Distal radius and ulna fractures are common injuries in children. The patient can expect to be immobilized in a splint or cast for approximately 3 to 4 weeks. General results of treatment are good if acceptable alignment of fracture is obtained.
- Physeal arrest is rare, although it can occur in up to 10% of physeal distal radius and ulna fractures.

First Treatment Steps
- For nondisplaced fractures, apply a sugar tong splint without manipulation of the fracture. Provide the patient with an appropriately fitting sling.
- Displaced fractures: Apply a temporary volar splint in a position of comfort. Arrange for the patient to be seen in an acute care setting that will allow for reduction and sedation.

Treatment Options
Codes
ICD-9 813.4 Closed fracture of the distal radius
CPT: 25606 Closed reduction of distal radius fracture

Nonoperative Management
- Closed manipulation and reduction of dorsally displaced distal radius and ulna fracture
  - After adequate anesthesia is established, the displaced fracture is reduced with slight traction (excessive traction may be counterproductive due to tightening of thick periosteum in children), re-creation of the injury force by wrist dorsiflexion, and then volar pressure of the distal fragment. The reduction is held in place manually and confirmed with fluoroscopy. A sugar tong splint or long arm cast with a three-point mold is then applied to hold the reduction in place.
  - Displacement of the fracture in the splint/cast can occur, and hence serial radiographs are recommended within the first week after injury and subsequent weeks per discretion of the clinician.
  - Mild residual dorsal angulation (<30 degrees) in children after reduction can remodel with time.
  - The splint or cast should be held in place for at least 3 weeks. Radiographs should be obtained within 1 week after reduction to confirm that displacement has not occurred. Cast can be discontinued around 1 month when the fracture has healed and the patient is nontender at the injury site.

Operative Management
Operative Indications
- Rare for this injury. Reserved for open fractures, fractures with significant neurovascular compromise, or irreducible fractures

Suggested Readings
Bae DS: Pediatric distal radius and forearm fractures, *J Hand Surg Am* 33(10):1911–1923, 2008.
Beatty E, Light TR, Belsole RJ, Ogden JA, et al: Wrist and hand skeletal injuries in children, *Hand Clin* 6(4):723–738, 1990.
Campbell RM Jr: Operative treatment of fractures and dislocations of the hand and wrist region in children, *Orthop Clin North Am* 21(2):217–243, 1990.
de Putter CE, van Beeck EF, Looman CW, et al: Trends in wrist fractures in children and adolescents, *J Hand Surg Am* 36(11):1810–1815, 2011.
Dolan M, Waters PM: Fractures and dislocations of the forearm, wrist, and hand. In Green NE, Swiontkowski MF, editors: *Skeletal trauma in children,* Philadelphia, 2009, Saunders, pp 159–205.

PEDIATRIC FOREARM FRACTURES
History
- Background: Pediatric forearm fractures include fractures of the diaphysis of the radius and/or ulna. Forearm bony anatomy is unforgiving of significant displacement or malrotation with regard to subsequent range of motion and function.
- Common mechanisms include a fall onto an outstretched hand or direct blow to the forearm.
- Severe pain or neurovascular problems should prompt suspicion for compartment syndrome of the forearm.
- The patient may report forearm pain, swelling, or deformity.

Physical Examination
- Inspect for edema and rotational deformity (a key component to the injury).
  - Inspect for the apex of the deformity, which serves as a clue for malrotation: An apex dorsal deformity suggests a pronation deformity of the distal fragment, whereas an apex volar deformity suggests a supination deformity of the distal fragment.
- Palpate for significant tenderness at the fracture site.
- Perform a careful neurovascular examination.

Imaging: Figure 9-2
- Anteroposterior (AP) and lateral radiographs of forearm (full length)
- Wrist and elbow radiographs to rule out associated injuries (injuries to the wrist, distal radioulnar joint, radial head dislocation)

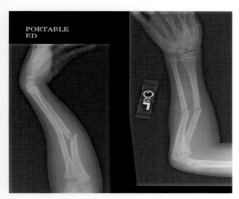

Figure 9-2. Both bone forearm fracture in a 9-year-old boy.

- Evaluate images for the apex of the deformity and clues to malrotation including the relationship between the bicipital tuberosity and radial styloid (which should be facing opposite to each other in the normal forearm)

Initial Treatment
Patient Education
- Forearm fractures are common injuries in children. These injuries must be reduced in near anatomic alignment, or limited range of motion and deformity may develop. Most preadolescents can be treated with casting. Children approaching maturity may be considered for operative open reduction and internal fixation.

First Treatment Steps
- The patient's forearm should be immobilized with a temporary splint until transport to a facility that can offer adequate anesthesia (conscious sedation or general anesthesia) can be arranged.
- All patients with displaced radius and ulna fractures should undergo manipulative reduction or fixation.

Treatment Options
Nonoperative Management
- Nonoperative management with closed manipulation under sedation/anesthesia is the mainstay of treatment.
- The deformity should be reduced, paying particular attention to the fact that forearm injuries often require reduction of a rotational deformity.
- A long arm cast or sugar tong splint with the elbow at 90 degrees with a flat ulna and interosseous mold can be used to hold the reduction.
- The patient should be followed up weekly for repeat radiographs, and cast immobilization should be continued for 6 weeks.

Operative Management
Codes
ICD-9: 813.2 Closed fracture of radius and ulna
CPT: 25575 ORIF both bone forearm fracture, flexible IM nailing of both bone forearm fracture

Operative Indications
- Adolescents approaching skeletal maturity should be treated with rigid internal fixation.
- Younger children with displaced fractures for which closed treatment fails to hold acceptable alignment can be treated with flexible intramedullar nailing.

Informed Consent and Counseling
- Decreased forearm rotation can occur with nonanatomic reductions.
- Risk of infection and nerve damage can occur with surgical approaches for open reduction and internal fixation.

Anesthesia
- General

Patient Positioning
- Supine with operative extremity placed on a hand table. A tourniquet is applied to the operative extremity.

Surgical Procedures
- ***Intramedullary nailing of forearm fracture***
  - Using C-arm guidance, an appropriate start point is determined for insertion of elastic nail. A nail of 2 to 2.5 mm in diameter is usually used. In the radius, the entry point is 2 cm proximal to the distal physis along the radial border. A small incision is made and bluntly spread down to

bone to prevent injury to the radial sensory nerve. The nail is inserted and passed down the shaft of the radius with the bone held reduced. In the ulna the entry point is 2 cm distal to the apophyseal plate (proximal, along the dorsoradial side). The nails are cut within 6 mm from the bone. A bivalved long arm cast is placed.
- Open reduction and internal fixation of forearm fracture
  - See p. 99, the section on Forearm (Radius and Ulna) Fractures and Dislocations

Estimated Postoperative Course
- Postoperative days 10 to 14—Repeat radiographs
- Postoperative 6 weeks—Repeat radiographs, discontinue cast; if healing, gradual progression to activities

Suggested Readings
Dolan M, Waters PM: Fractures and dislocations of the forearm, wrist, and hand. In Green NE, Swiontkowski MF, editors: *Skeletal trauma in children,* Philadelphia, 2009, Saunders, pp 159–205.

Flynn JM, Jones KJ, Garner MR, Goebel J: Eleven years experience in the operative management of pediatric forearm fractures, *J Pediatr Orthop* 30(4):313–319, 2010.

Garg NK, Ballal MS, Malek IA, et al: Use of elastic stable intramedullary nailing for treating unstable forearm fractures in children, *J Trauma* 65(1):109–115, 2008.

Herman MJ, Marshall ST: Forearm fractures in children and adolescents: a practical approach, *Hand Clin* 22(1):55–67, 2006.

Rodriguez-Merchan EC: Pediatric fractures of the forearm, *Clin Orthop Relat Res* Mar (342): 65–72, 2005.

RADIAL HEAD SUBLUXATION (NURSEMAID'S ELBOW)
History
- Background: Nursemaid's elbow is radial head subluxation with an annular ligament tear and interposition of annular ligament between the radial head and capitellum.
- This is a common injury in young children, where a longitudinal traction force is placed on the child's extended and pronated forearm (i.e., child being helped up onto a sidewalk).
- Children affected are usually younger than 5 years old.

- Initially the condition is painful, but it eventually subsides, although the child will guard the extremity with activities.
- The patient or parents may report that the arm is not being used.

Physical Examination
- Inspect for how the child holds the arm, which is usually flexed and pronated.
- Inspect for use of the arm. Pseudoparalysis is possible in very young children due to pain.
- Palpate for tenderness along the radial head. Also palpate throughout the upper extremity to rule out other injuries.
- Perform neurovascular examination and document.

Imaging
- AP and lateral radiographs of elbow to rule out other injuries

Initial Treatment
Patient Education
- Nursemaid's elbow is a common elbow injury in young children. The vast majority of patients improve with closed reduction without future problems.

First Treatment Step
- If the patient is uncomfortable, immobilize him or her in a posterior splint with the arm in a position of comfort until reduction can be performed.

Treatment Options
Nonoperative Management
Codes
ICD-9: 832.2 Nursemaid's elbow
CPT: 24605 Closed reduction of elbow dislocation

Closed Reduction of Radial Head Subluxation (Figure 9-3)
- Under adequate anesthesia, child's forearm is supinated and maximally flexed with the clinician's thumb placed over the radial head.
- A palpable click is often felt on reduction.
- There is no need to immobilize after reduction if this is a first-time reduction. If this is a repeat injury, consider cast immobilization.

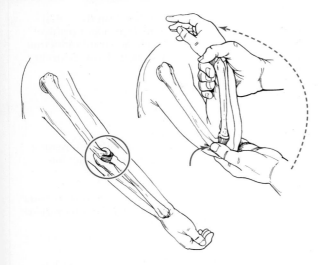

Figure 9-3. Closed reduction of nursemaid's elbow. *(From Flynn JM, Kolze EA: Upper extremity injuries. In Dormans JP, editor: Core knowledge in orthopaedics: pediatric orthopaedics, Philadelphia, 2005, Mosby, p 76.)*

Suggested Readings
Chuong W, Heinrich SD: Acute annular ligament interposition into the radiocapitellar joint in children (nursemaid's elbow), *J Pediatr Orthop* 15(4):454–456, 1995.

Dolan M, Waters PM: Fractures and dislocations of the forearm, wrist, and hand. In Green NE, Swiontkowski MF, editors: *Skeletal trauma in children*, Philadelphia, 2009, Saunders, pp 159–205.

Lewis D, Argall J: Reduction of pulled elbows, *Emerg Med J* 20(1):61-62, 2003.

PEDIATRIC SUPRACONDYLAR HUMERUS FRACTURES

History
- Background: Common elbow injury in children, with location of fracture site above the condyles of the elbow
- Common mechanism of injury is fall onto an outstretched hand or direct blow to the elbow
- Patient may report elbow pain, deformity, or swelling

Physical Examination
- Inspect for deformity and edema, refusal to use the injured arm
- Palpate forearm and evaluate for compartment syndrome
- Perform and document a neurovascular examination (critical as major vessels and nerves cross the elbow)

Imaging: Figure 9-4
- AP, lateral, and oblique radiographs of elbow
  - For nondisplaced or occult fractures, evaluate for the presence of elevated anterior and posterior fat pads on the lateral radiograph.
  - The anterior humeral line should intersect the capitellum on the lateral radiograph in a normal elbow.

Classification System
- Flexion- and extension-type injuries depending on whether the arm was flexed or extended at the time of injury; majority of injuries are of the extension type

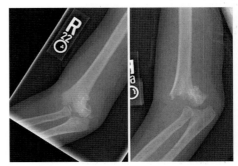

Figure 9-4. Type III supracondylar humerus fracture in a 5-year-old girl.

- Gartland classification (extension-type injuries)—type I: nondisplaced, type II: angulated with an intact posterior cortex, type III: displaced with no intact cortex

Initial Treatment
Patient Education
- Supracondylar humerus fractures are the most common elbow injuries in young children, with a 10% to 15% neurovascular injury rate in displaced fractures. These injuries should be evaluated and treated urgently in an emergency department where a pediatric orthopaedist is available. The standard of care is to pin displaced fractures.

First Treatment Step
- Place in a temporary posterior long arm splint in a position of comfort and send to the emergency department for evaluation.

Treatment Options
Nonoperative Management
- Type I injuries: Immobilize initially in a posterior long arm splint and then transition to a long arm cast with the elbow at 90 degrees. Avoid hyperflexion.
- Type II injuries without significant angulation, intact medial cortex, and in which the anterior humeral line intersects the capitellum: Immobilize initially in a splint and then transition to a cast as indicated earlier.

Operative Management
Codes
ICD-9: 812.41 Closed fracture of supracondylar humerus
CPT: 24538 Closed reduction and percutaneous pinning of supracondylar humerus fracture

Operative Indications
- Any fracture with significant displacement should be treated with closed reduction and percutaneous pinning.

Informed Consent and Counseling
- Risks of neurovascular injury from pinning can occur, especially to the ulnar nerve with medial-based pins.

Most nerve injuries from the initial trauma are neuropraxia and resolve with time. Despite accurate reduction, risk of malunion and elbow deformity can occur.

Anesthesia
- General anesthesia

Patient Positioning
- Supine with the patient's arm resting on a draped fluoroscopy machine

Surgical Procedures
- ***Closed reduction and percutaneous pinning of displaced supracondylar humerus fracture***
  - The patient's arm is prepped and draped as proximally as possible. The fluoroscopy machine is then draped, and the patient's arm is placed on the base of the fluoroscopy machine.
  - Gentle traction is applied to the arm, and varus/valgus angulation is corrected with fluoroscopic guidance. The elbow is then flexed to reduce the extended fracture. The reduction is held in place until pinned.
  - Two to three lateral 0.062-inch pins are placed from the lateral condyle engaging the medial diaphyseal cortex to hold the fracture in place.
  - The arm is splinted in a long arm posterior splint in approximately 70 degrees of elbow flexion.

Estimated Postoperative Course
- Postoperative days 7 to 10—Repeat radiographs of elbow in splint.
- Postoperative week 3—Repeat radiographs of elbow, splint, and pin removal if radiographs demonstrate acceptable alignment. Start range of motion at 3 weeks with activity restriction, with gradual progression based on healing.
- Postoperative month 3—Repeat radiographs and clinical evaluation of range of motion.

Suggested Readings
Abzug JM, Herman MJ: Management of supracondylar humerus fractures in children: current concepts, *J Am Acad Orthop Surg* 20(2): 69–77, 2012.

Brauer CA, Lee BM, Bae DS, et al: A systematic review of medial and lateral entry pinning versus lateral entry pinning for supracondylar fractures of the humerus, *J Pediatr Orthop* 27(2):181–186, 2007.

Green NE, Van Zeeland NL et al. Fractures and dislocations about the elbow. In Green NE, Swiontkowski MF, editors: *Skeletal trauma in children,* Philadelphia, 2009, Saunders, pp 207–282.

Omid R et al: Supracondylar humeral fractures in children, *J Bone Joint Surg Am* 90(5): 1121–1132, 2008.

Woratanarat P, Angsanuntsukh C, Rattanasirri S, et al: Meta-analysis of pinning in supracondylar fracture of the humerus in children, *J Orthop Trauma* 26(1):48–53, 2012.

PEDIATRIC FEMUR FRACTURES

Age Range
- Age 0 to 6 months
- Age 6 months to 5 years
- Age 5 years to 11 years
- Age older than 11 years

History
- Background: Femur fractures in children can be related to both low-energy and high-energy mechanisms, including torsional-type injuries and motor vehicle accidents. Child abuse is not an uncommon mechanism of fracture in younger children (30% in children younger than 4 years old).
- Patient characteristics (age and patient size); fracture characteristics (spiral, transverse, comminuted); and mechanism of injury are all important in determining appropriate treatment.
- Patients present with pain and deformity and an impaired ability to bear weight on the affected lower extremity.

Physical Examination
- If a high-energy mechanism occurred, a thorough trauma evaluation is necessary.
- Inspect for evidence of open injury and identify abrasions, edema, and deformity.
- Palpate throughout the lower extremity to evaluate for other injuries.
- Perform and document a neurovascular examination.

Imaging: Figure 9-5 AB. Note differences in age and severity of mechanism.
- AP and lateral radiographs of the femur

Initial Treatment

Patient Education
- The appropriate treatment of pediatric femur fractures includes many variables. Most low-energy mechanism injuries can be treated in a closed fashion in young children. Internal fixation options in older children include intramedullary stabilization options. Common complications can include leg length inequality, malrotation, and angular malunion.

First Treatment Steps
- Initiate a pediatric trauma evaluation for high-energy injuries.
- Immobilize the extremity in a temporary posterior long leg splint.

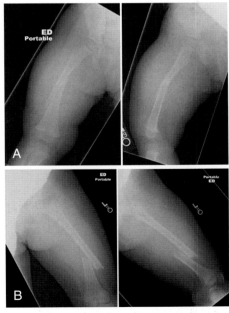

Figure 9-5. A, Spiral femur fracture in a toddler from a fall. **B,** Transverse femur fracture in a 10-year-old from a motor vehicle accident.

Treatment Options

Nonoperative Management

- **0 to 6 months:** Apply a Pavlik harness and immobilize the patient for 2 to 3 weeks. Rapid healing with exuberant callous formation is expected.
- **6 months to 5 years:** Apply a spica cast under anesthesia **(CPT Code 29325).** Reduce the fracture with fluoroscopic guidance and then apply a spica cast positioning the injured extremity in approximately 45 degrees hip flexion and 45- to 60-degree knee flexion. Repeat radiographs within 2 weeks, and continue spica cast for approximately 6 weeks until healing.

Operative Management

Codes

ICD-9: 821.01 Closed fracture of shaft of femur

CPT: 27506 Intramedullary stabilization of femoral shaft fracture

Operative Indications

- Surgical treatment should be considered in all displaced femoral shaft fractures in the appropriate age group (older than 5 years).

Informed Consent and Counseling

- The risk of malunion, leg length discrepancy, and malrotation exists for any treatment type.

Anesthesia

- General anesthesia

Patient Positioning

- Supine positioning on a fracture table

Surgical Procedures

- *5 to 11 years*
  - *Flexible intramedullary nailing (for patients < 108 lb)*
    - The appropriate-sized nail is planned on the basis of radiographs and should be selected to be less than 40% of the narrowest portion of the femoral canal. The patient is placed supine on the fracture table, and closed reduction is obtained with gentle traction under C-arm guidance. The nails are manually contoured

such that the apex of the bow is at the fracture site. A fluoroscope is used to identify the nail entry point on the lateral femur approximately 3 cm above the physis. A small stab incision is made along the lateral aspect of the distal femur, and a drill is used to open the femoral cortex. The nail is inserted to the level of the fracture. The opposite medial cortex is drilled at the same level and opened analogous to the lateral side, and a second nail is passed up to the level of the fracture. Each nail is then inserted in diverging directions past the fracture site sequentially while the fracture is held reduced. The nails are advanced until they just pass the proximal femoral physis. The nails are then cut (within 1 cm off the cortex of insertion site) and bent. Wounds are then closed.

- *> 11 years*
  - *Trochanteric entry with intramedullary nailing.*
    - The patient is placed supine on a fracture table. C-arm images are obtained of the proximal femur before prepping to ensure adequate images are obtained. The fracture is reduced using traction on the fracture table. A small incision is made proximal to the greater trochanter, and a guidewire is used to determine the appropriate start point just lateral to the tip of the greater trochanter. The guidewire is drilled into the greater trochanter under C-arm guidance in the AP and lateral planes to verify accurate placement. An entry reamer is used to open the proximal femoral canal over the guidewire. A reaming guidewire is then placed down the intramedullary canal past the fracture site ending proximal to the physis. The appropriate length nail is then measured with the measuring guide. The femur is then reamed to the appropriate width. An intramedullary nail is then placed down the reaming

guidewire with the fracture held reduced in place. The reaming guidewire is removed. Using C-arm guidance, proximal and distal nail interlocking screws are placed through stab incisions. Wounds are then irrigated and closed.

Estimated Postoperative Course
- Postoperative day 0: Ensure hemodynamic stability and monitor in the hospital. Patients generally may start partial weight bearing unless there is concern for fracture stability postoperatively.
- Postoperative days 10 to 14: Check the wound and take radiographs.
- Postoperative weeks 6 to 8: Repeat radiographs and clinical evaluation, and progress activities gradually if healing.
- Postoperative months 3 to 6: Gradual progression to normal activities follows.

Suggested Readings
Anglen JO, Choi L: Treatment options in pediatric femoral shaft fractures, *J Orthop Trauma* 19(10):724–733, 2005.

Bopst L, Reinberg O, Lutz N, et al: Femur fracture in preschool children: experience with flexible intramedullary nailing in 72 children, *J Orthop* 27(3):299–303, 2007.

Hosalkar HS, Pandya NK, Cho RH, et al: Intramedullary nailing of pediatric femoral shaft fracture, *J Am Acad Orthop Surg* 19(8):472–481, 2011.

Kocher MS, Sink EL, Blasier RD, et al: Treatment of pediatric diaphyseal femur fractures, *J Am Acad Orthop Surg* 17(11):718–725, 2009.

Shilt J: Fractures of the femoral shaft. In Green NE, Swiontkowski MF, editors: *Skeletal trauma in children,* Philadelphia, 2009, Saunders, pp 397–423.

PEDIATRIC TIBIA/FIBULA FRACTURES

Types of Fractures
- Fractures of the proximal tibial metaphysis
- Fractures of the tibial and fibular shafts
- Isolated fractures of the tibial shaft
- Fractures of the distal tibial metaphysis

History
- The mechanism of injury commonly includes motor vehicle accidents, falls, and sports.
- Pain is the most reliable clinical history.
- In young children, inability to walk may be the clue, especially in nondisplaced toddler spiral fractures of the tibia.
- Incidence peaks at 3 to 4 years (mostly spiral fractures) and 15 to 16 years (mostly transverse fractures).
- Direct and indirect forces can contribute to tibia fractures in which direct injuries cause transverse or segmental fractures while indirect forces can cause oblique fractures.

Physical Examination
- Inspect for deformity and open fracture.
- Palpate throughout the tibia if the deformity is not obvious (nondisplaced fractures are common in young children with a low-energy mechanism).
- Palpate compartments because of risk of compartment syndrome, especially in a high-energy mechanism.
- Perform and document a neurovascular examination.

Imaging
- Obtain AP and lateral radiographs of the tibia/fibula (Fig. 9-6).
- Image surrounding joints (ankle, knee).

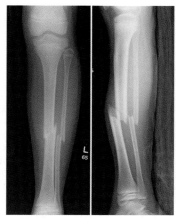

Figure 9-6. Tibial and fibular shaft fracture in a 12-year-old boy.

Classification System

- Fractures of the proximal tibial metaphysis (common in children 3 to 6 years; most fractures are nondisplaced or greenstick with tendency to develop posttraumatic valgus)
- Fractures of the tibial and fibular shafts (complete both bone fractures are associated with higher energy mechanisms and direct blows)
- Isolated fractures of the tibial shaft or fibular shaft (tibial shaft—torsional injuries without significant displacement or shortening due to intact fibula; fibular shaft—direct-impact injuries)
- Fractures of the distal tibial metaphysis (rare injuries that generally heal without significant malalignment)

Initial Treatment

Patient Education

- Tibia/fibula fractures represent a wide spectrum of injury severity and are common fractures in children. In general most low-energy mechanism injuries are expected to heal well with closed treatment. Higher-energy mechanism injuries can be associated with open fractures and a higher rate of subsequent disability.

First Treatment Steps

- Pediatric trauma evaluation is necessary for high-energy injuries.
- Apply a long leg posterior splint to prevent further damage to soft tissues.
- Open fractures need to be débrided in the operating room.

Treatment Options

Nonoperative Management

Fractures of the Proximal Tibial Metaphysis

- Closed manipulation to correct valgus angulation under anesthesia and application of a long leg cast with knee extended is the treatment of choice.
- Immobilize for 4 to 6 weeks in a cast.
- Monitor weekly radiographs for first 3 weeks and then spread out future radiographs.
- Remove cast when fracture is healed. Progress knee range of motion and activities as tolerated.

- Valgus deformity of less than 15 degrees generally remodels and improves with time.

Fractures of the Tibial and Fibular Shafts, Isolated Fractures of the Tibial Shaft, Fractures of the Distal Tibial Metaphysis

- Closed fractures should be treated with immobilization in a cast.
- Obtain closed reduction and long leg casting with approximately 30 degrees of knee flexion.
- Acceptable alignment is 5 degrees varus/valgus, 5 degrees flexion/extension, less than 1 cm shortening, and less than 50% translation.
- Immobilize for 4 to 6 weeks in long leg cast, and instruct patient not to bear weight.
- Monitor weekly radiographs for first 3 weeks, and then spread out future radiographs.
- Transition to short leg cast or patellar tendon-bearing cast with healing fracture for 2 more weeks.

Operative Management

Codes

ICD-9:

  823.01 Proximal tibial metaphysis fracture
  823.20 Fracture of tibial shaft
  832.21 Fracture of fibular shaft
  832.22 Fracture of fibula with tibia

CPT:

  27752 Closed reduction of tibia/fibula fracture
  27759 Intramedullary fixation of tibia fracture

Operative Indications

- Any open fracture or compartment syndrome should undergo débridement and fasciotomy, respectively.
- Failure to adequately maintain closed reduction in pediatric tibia fracture should be considered for operative stabilization (rare).

Informed Consent and Counseling

- Tibia fractures can develop rotational or angular malunion, as well as length discrepancy to the contralateral leg. Proximal metaphyseal fractures tend to angulate toward valgus, whereas isolated tibial fractures tend to angulate in varus after initial casting. Repeat manipulations may be necessary to maintain some reductions, and if these fail operative management is indicated.

Anesthesia
- General anesthesia

Patient Positioning
- Supine on a regular table, tourniquet applied to proximal thigh

Surgical Procedures
Closed reduction and flexible intramedullary nailing of tibia fracture (Fig. 9-7).
- The appropriate-sized nail is planned on the basis of radiographs, and should be selected to be less than 40% of the narrowest portion of the tibial canal. The patient is placed supine on a regular table and closed reduction is obtained under C-arm guidance. The nails are manually contoured such that the apex of the bow is at the fracture site. A fluoroscope is used to identify the nail entry point on the anteromedial proximal tibia approximately 2 cm distal to the proximal physis. A small stab incision is made along the anteromedial proximal tibia, and a drill used to open the tibial cortex. The nail is inserted to the level of the fracture. The opposite anterolateral cortex is drilled at the

same level and opened analogous to the medial side, and a second nail is inserted up to the level of the fracture. Each nail is then inserted in diverging directions past the fracture site sequentially while the fracture is held reduced. The nails are advanced until they are several centimeters proximal to the distal tibial physis. The nails are then cut (within 1 cm off the cortex of insertion site) and bent. Wounds are then closed. A long leg cast is placed to protect the fixation, and the patient remains non–weight bearing.

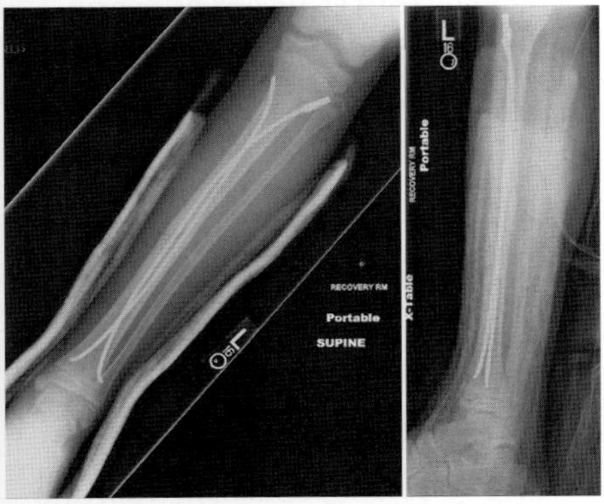

Estimated Postoperative Course
- Postoperative days 10 to 14—return for clinical evaluation and radiographs in the cast
- Postoperative weeks 6 to 8—cast removed; radiographs should show signs of healing
- Postoperative months 3 to 6—gradual progression to normal activities

Suggested Readings
Mashru RP, Herman MJ, Pizzutillo PD: Tibial shaft fractures in children and adolescents, *J Am Acad Orthop Surg* 13(5):345–352, 2005.
Sankar WN, Jones KJ, David Horn B, Wells L: Titanium elastic nails for pediatric tibial shaft fractures, *J Child Orthop* Nov;1(5):281–286, 2007.
Shannak AO: Tibial fractures in children: follow-up study, *J Pediatr Orthop* 8(3):306-310.
Thompson GH, Son-Hing J: Fractures and dislocations of the tibia and fibula. In Green NE, Swiontkowski MF, editors: *Skeletal trauma in children*, Philadelphia, 2009, Saunders, pp 471–506.

Figure 9-7. Tibial and fibular shaft fracture in a 12-year-old boy treated with flexible intramedullary nails.

COMMON PEDIATRIC DISORDERS
Adolescent Idiopathic Scoliosis
History
- Adolescent idiopathic scoliosis is abnormal curvature of the adolescent spine, with greater than 10 degrees coronal plane deformity and rotational deformity not associated with other conditions.
- Back pain may or may not be present.
- Patients may complain of rib hump and shoulder asymmetry.
- Menarche status (for growth spurt) and family history (positive in 30%) should be assessed.

Physical Examination

- Inspect the body for cutaneous lesions or congenital malformations to rule out nonidiopathic scoliosis.
- Inspect for shoulder symmetry, forward-bending rib hump, direction and level of curve, pelvic obliquity, and kyphosis/lordosis (Fig. 9-8).
- Perform thorough neurologic examination including abdominal reflexes.
- Assess body for general assessment of maturity (breast appearance, axillary hair, facial hair).

Imaging: Figure 9-9

- Full-length standing PA and lateral scoliosis radiographs
  - Assess location and degree of curvature.
  - Assess Risser grade on iliac apophysis (grade 1: 25% ossified, 2: 50%

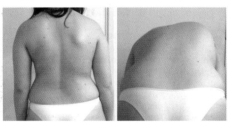

Figure 9-8. Common deformity in adolescent idiopathic scoliosis. Note shoulder asymmetry and rib hump.

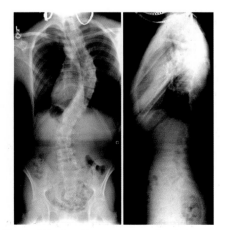

Figure 9-9. Standing scoliosis radiographs.

ossified, 3: 75% ossified, 4: 100% ossified, 5: 100% ossified and fused). Ossification progresses from lateral to medial, with higher grades indicating progression to skeletal maturity.

Classification System

- Lenke classification (Fig. 9-10)

Initial Treatment

Patient Education

- Adolescent idiopathic scoliosis is an abnormal curvature in the spine with the age of onset after 10 years. There is a higher female to male prevalence in the general population. Risk of progression is associated with curve magnitude, younger age, and time remaining until skeletal maturity.

First Treatment Step

- Patient education of the condition is the first step. All curves will benefit from more than one evaluation to document progression or nonprogression of the curve. Most curves can be observed or braced, with the exception of large curves in the skeletally immature patient.

Treatment Options

Nonoperative Management

- Observation is indicated for skeletally immature patients with curves less than 25 degrees or patients with nonprogressive curves near maturity.
  - Patients should be observed serially with radiographs every 6 months to 1 year.
- Bracing is indicated for skeletally immature patients with curves greater than 25 degrees that are progressing, or with curves 30 to 40 degrees.
  - Full-time bracing with a thoracolumbar orthosis is recommended until the patient reaches Risser grade 4.

Operative Management

Codes
ICD-9: 737.30 Idiopathic scoliosis
CPT:
  22842—Posterior spinal instrumentation 3 to 6 vertebral segments
  22843—Posterior spinal instrumentation 7 to 12 vertebral segments

Type	Proximal Thoracic	Main Thoracic	Thoracolumbar / Lumbar	Curve Type
			Curve Type	
1	Non-Structural	Structural (Major*)	Non-Structural	Main Thoracic (MT)
2	Structural	Structural (Major*)	Non-Structural	Double Thoracic (DT)
3	Non-Structural	Structural (Major*)	Structural	Double Major (DM)
4	Structural	Structural (Major*)	Structural	Triple Major (TM)
5	Non-Structural	Non-Structural	Structural (Major*)	Thoracolumbar / Lumbar (TL/L)
6	Non-Structural	Structural	Structural (Major*)	Thoracolumbar / Lumbar - Main Thoracic (TL/L - MT)

STRUCTURAL CRITERIA
(Minor Curves)

Proximal Thoracic: - Side Bending Cobb ≥ 25°
- T2 - T5 Kyphosis ≥ +20°

Main Thoracic: - Side Bending Cobb ≥ 25°
- T10 - L2 Kyphosis ≥ +20°

Thoracolumbar / Lumbar: - Side Bending Cobb ≥ 25°
- T10 - L2 Kyphosis ≥ +20°

*Major = Largest Cobb Measurement, always structural
Minor = all other curves with structural criteria applied

LOCATION OF APEX
(SRS definition)

CURVE	APEX
THORACIC	T2 - T11-12 DISC
THORACOLUMBAR	T12 - L1
LUMBAR	L1-2 DISC - L4

Modifiers

Lumbar Spine Modifier	CSVL to Lumbar Apex		Thoracic Sagittal Profile T5 - T12	
A	CSVL Between Pedicles		— (Hypo)	< 10°
B	CSVL Touches Apical Body(ies)		N (Normal)	10°- 40°
C	CSVL Completely Medial		+ (Hyper)	> 40°

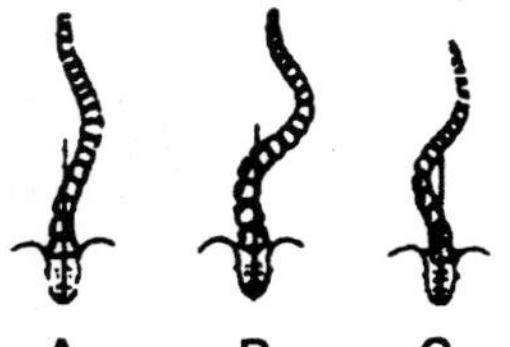

Curve Type (1-6) **+** Lumbar Spine Modifier (A, B, or C) **+** Thoracic Sagittal Modifier (−,N, or +)

Classification (e.g.1B+):_____

Figure 9-10. Lenke classification of adolescent idiopathic scoliosis. *(From Pierz, K, Dormans JP: Spinal disorders. In Dormans JP, editor:* Core knowledge in orthopaedics: pediatric orthopaedics, *Philadelphia,2005, Mosby, p 277.)*

22844—Posterior spinal instrumentation 13 or more vertebral segments

26610—Arthrodesis, posterior or posterolateral technique, single level (thoracic)

26612—Arthrodesis, posterior or posterolateral technique, single level (lumbar)

26614—Arthrodesis, posterior or posterolateral technique, each additional level

Informed Consent and Counseling
- Surgery for adolescent idiopathic scoliosis is major surgery, with high blood loss and possible observational monitoring in the intensive care unit postoperatively.

Complications of spine surgery include infection, nerve damage/cord injury (rare), pseudoarthrosis, and hardware-related complications.

Anesthesia
- General anesthesia

Patient Positioning
- Prone positioning on a Jackson table with neuro-monitoring setup

Surgical Procedures
Posterior Spinal Instrumentation and Fusion
- This is the most common procedure for adolescent idiopathic scoliosis

The patient is positioned prone, and posterior exposure of the spine is carried out with a midline incision, carefully exposing the spinous processes and lamina of the instrumented levels by subperiosteal dissection and cautery of paraspinal musculature. For pedicle screw instrumentation, the vertebrae are exposed to show the transverse process and superior articular facet. Pedicle screws are inserted on the basis of a thorough understanding of vertebral anatomy because screw trajectories differ on the basis of both location in the spine and intrinsic patient anatomy. Osteotomies and facetectomies are performed to allow for correction of deformity. Segmental instrumentation is performed, and rods are contoured and affixed to reduce the spinal deformity. The wound is irrigated thoroughly and closed.

Estimated Postoperative Course
- Postoperative days 0 to 1—Close hemodynamic monitoring in the intensive care unit (ICU) due to possibility of large-volume blood loss
- Postoperative days 2 to 5—Normalization in the hospital, work on improving mobility until safe discharge from the hospital
- Postoperative days 14 to 21—Wound evaluation, remove stitches, standing scoliosis radiographs
- Postoperative week 6—Routine follow-up, standing scoliosis radiographs. Progress activities as tolerated; follow-up visits spaced out

Suggested Readings
Cuartas E, Rasouli A, O'Brien M, Shufflebarger HL: Use of all-pedicle screw constructs in the treatment of adolescent idiopathic scoliosis, *J Am Acad Orthop Surg* 17(9): 550–561, 2009.

Kim HJ, Blanco JS, Ridman RF: Update on the management of idiopathic scoliosis, *Curr Opin Pediatr* 21(1):55–64, 2009.

Lenke LG, Betz RR, Harms J, et al: Adolescent idiopathic scoliosis: a new classification to determine extent of spinal arthrodesis, *J Bone Joint Surg Am* 83:1169–1181, 2001.

Sponseller PD: Bracing for adolescent idiopathic scoliosis in practice today, *J Pediatr Orthop* 31(1 Suppl):S53–60, 2011.

DEVELOPMENTAL DYSPLASIA OF THE HIP
History
- Definition: Developmental dysplasia of the hip (DDH) is a dislocation of the hip joint that is present at birth.
- Dysplasia is generally caused by abnormal forces acting on the hip in utero leading to abnormal development of the acetabulum, and in severe cases it leads to eventual hip dislocation because of insufficient bony coverage for the femoral head.
- Risk factors include family history of DDH, breech positioning before birth, female, and large gestational weight.

Physical Examination
Newborn
- Barlow test is performed by flexing (90 degrees) and adducting the thigh, then applying posteriorly directed force. Test is positive if the hip dislocates.
- Ortolani test is performed by flexing (90 degrees) and adducting the thigh, then applying an anteriorly directed pressure along the greater trochanter while simultaneously abducting the hip. Test is positive if a clunk is felt to indicate relocation of the hip.

Infant/Toddler
- Asymmetric or limitation of abduction could indicate hip dysplasia.
- Evaluate for asymmetric thigh folds and the Galeazzi sign.
  - Galeazzi sign: The child's hips and knees are flexed to 90 degrees and adducted to midline. The height of the knees is compared with one another. The test is positive if one knee appears shorter than the other knee, indicating DDH on the shorter side.
- Walking children can have leg length discrepancy, Trendelenburg gait, and excessive lumbar lordosis.

Imaging: Figure 9-11
Newborn to 6 months: The acetabulum and femoral head do not readily appear on radiographs until 6 months. Hence, ultrasound is the preferred modality for evaluation at this age.

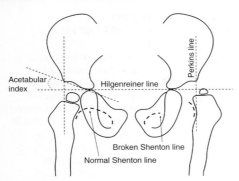

Acetabular index
Hilgenreiner line
Perkins line
Broken Shenton line
Normal Shenton line

Figure 9-11. Radiographic assessment of hip dysplasia. *(From Erol B, Dormans JP: Hip disorders. In Dormans JP, editor: Core knowledge in orthopaedics: pediatric orthopaedics, Philadelphia, 2005, Mosby, p 232.)*

- Ultrasound is indicated when screening for patients with risk factors for DDH when the diagnosis is in question or to evaluate the efficacy of Pavlik harness treatment in children younger than 6 months old.
- *6 months and older:* Radiographic evaluation is appropriate in this age group. An AP view of the pelvis is reviewed for several criteria illustrated in Table 9-4 and Figure 9-11.

Treatment Options
Patient Education
- Hip dysplasia is a condition in which the hip is not concentrically reduced at the time of birth. If left untreated, abnormal forces and contact from developmental dysplasia can lead to a

progressive problem that impairs normal development of the acetabulum. It is important to develop a treatment plan once a diagnosis has been established.

Initial Treatment
The goal of treatment is to achieve a concentric reduction of the femoral head on the acetabulum.

Newborn to 6 Months
- A Pavlik harness is the initial treatment. Reassess ultrasound in 2 weeks for reduction. If the hip is not reduced on ultrasound, the patient may need a closed reduction under anesthesia. If reduced, continue using the Pavlik harness and wean by 6 to 12 weeks.
  - Risks of femoral nerve palsy exist from excessive hip flexion, avascular necrosis with excessive hip abduction, and brachial plexus palsy from shoulder straps.

6 Months to 2 Years
- Closed reduction and casting under anesthesia
  - Risks of avascular necrosis exist with excessive hip abduction and cast-related complications including skin breakdown and irritation.
  - Technique for closed reduction of the hip.
    - Gentle traction is applied manually to the leg, and the hip is brought into approximately 120 degrees flexion and then abduction. After a reduction is felt, the hip is considered stable if it remains reduced with adduction greater than 30 degrees past maximal abduction and less than 90 degrees of flexion. An arthrogram of the hip is performed to confirm adequate reduction. Percutaneous adductor tenotomy is considered to relieve pressure on the reduction if the adductors are tight in the reduced position. A hip spica cast is then applied.
      - Skin traction may be considered before closed reduction to relieve muscular contraction.

Table 9-4. Radiographic Assessment of Hip Dysplasia

RADIOGRAPHIC LANDMARK	ABNORMAL IF:
Intersection of Hilgenreiner line and Perkin line	Femoral head not located in the medial lower quadrant
Shenton line	Break in the continuity of the line
Acetabular index	>25 degrees (age dependent—can be higher in newborn)

- Confirm reduction with radiograph or single-cut CT.
- If hip does not remain reduced in a cast, open reduction should be performed.

2 Years and Older
- Open reduction is the initial treatment. By this point, chronic dislocation is difficult to reduce due to significant acetabular dysplasia.
- Consideration of femoral shortening osteotomy should be made to avoid excessive pressure on the proximal femur after reduction.
- Acetabular coverage is often deficient, and remodeling potential is lower at this age; hence pelvic osteotomy should be considered to provide adequate femoral head coverage.

Operative Management
Codes
ICD-9: 754.3 Congenital dislocation of hip
CPT: 27257 Closed reduction of congenital hip dislocation
27258 Open reduction of congenital hip dislocation
29325 Application of hip spica cast

Operative Indications
- Open reduction under anesthesia for dysplasia diagnosed in children older than 2 years old or those who failed attempts at closed reduction

Informed Consent and Counseling
- Open reduction and spica cast are associated with risks depending on the approach. If using a medial approach to the hip, there is a risk of medial femoral circumflex artery disruption. If using an anterior approach to the hip, there is a risk of damage to iliac crest apophysis and lateral femoral cutaneous nerve. There is always a risk of avascular necrosis with reduction and application of a spica cast.

Anesthesia
- General anesthesia

Patient Positioning
- Supine positioning on standard operating room table

Surgical Procedures
Open Reduction of the Hip via a Medial Approach
- Prepare the skin for the entire operative leg and hemipelvis. Create an oblique skin incision approximately 5 cm long, 1 cm distal and parallel to the inguinal crease, and centered over the adductor longus. The deep fascia is incised, and the saphenous vein is avoided if possible or ligated. The pectineus muscle is identified and retracted inferomedially. The femoral neurovascular structures are retracted laterally. The femoral circumflex vessels are also then retracted laterally. The psoas tendon is divided and allowed to retract proximally. The capsule is opened in line to the acetabular margin. The transverse acetabular ligament is identified and released. Next, the ligamentum teres is removed allowing for reduction of the femoral head. The hip is held reduced, and the wound is closed. A hip spica is then applied with the hip in 90 to 100 degrees of flexion, 30 to 40 degrees of abduction, and neutral rotation.

Open Reduction of the Hip via an Anterior Approach
- Prepare the skin for the entire operative leg and hemipelvis. Place a bump under the operative hip. An incision is made in a curvilinear fashion starting at a point two thirds above the greater trochanter and the iliac crest and immediately crossing the anterior inferior iliac spine. The apophysis of the iliac crest is exposed. The interval between the tensor fascia lata and sartorius is bluntly developed, being careful to avoid the lateral femoral cutaneous nerve. The iliac apophysis is split sharply down to bone and exposed subperiosteally, allowing for retraction of the sartorius medially and the tensor fascia lata laterally. The rectus femoris is identified deep to this interval, reflected from its origin, and tagged. The hip capsule is then dissected with a periosteal elevator and then opened sharply with a knife (T-shaped incision). The ligamentum teres is then cut with scissors. The hip is then reduced under direct

visualization. Additional procedures such as pelvic osteotomies can be added at this point if the femoral head coverage is inadequate. The wound is closed, and a hip spica cast is applied.

Estimated Postoperative Course
- Postoperative days 10 to 14—First clinical visit, evaluate cast hygiene, patient and parent education
- Postoperative week 6—Radiographs to evaluate hip reduction, removal of spica cast
- Postoperative months 2 to 3— Radiographs to evaluate hip reduction, mobilize gradually

Suggested Readings

Bohm P, Brzuske A: Salter innominate osteotomy for the treatment of development dysplasia of the hip in children: results of seventy-three consecutive osteotomies after twenty-six to thirty-five years of follow-up, *J Bone Joint Surg Am* 84(A)-2:178–186, 2002.

Erol B, Dormans J: Hip disorders. In Dormans JP, editor: *Core knowledge in orthopaedics: pediatric orthopaedics,* Mosby, 2005, Philadelphia.

Herring JA, Sucato DJ: Developmental dysplasia of the hip. In Herring JA, editor: *Tachdjian's pediatric orthopaedics,* ed 4, Philadelphia, 2008, Saunders.

Ramsey P et al: Congenital dislocation of the hip, *J Bone Joint Surg Am* 58(7):1000–1004, 1976.

LEGG-CALVE-PERTHES DISEASE
History
- Background: Legg-Calve-Perthes disease (LCPD) is avascular necrosis of the femoral head without a known etiology, possibly from a temporary interruption to the blood supply to the capital femoral epiphysis. Initially, the capital femoral epiphysis undergoes necrosis leading to relative decreased size compared with the unaffected side and radiographic physeal irregularity. Then the epiphysis appears fragmented and begins to resorb and collapse. With collapse, the femoral head can migrate proximally and laterally to uncover the lateral portion of the head. The femoral head then remodels until maturity.
- The age of a child affected is usually between 4 and 10.
- The limping child has mild or no pain. Pain is usually activity related and can be located from hip/groin all the way to the knee.

Physical Examination
- Inspect child's gait—is he or she limping?
- Inspect for leg length discrepancy (from contractures or femoral head collapse).
- Assess hip range of motion: loss of internal rotation and abduction.

Imaging
- Obtain AP and frog leg lateral views of the hip (Fig. 9-12AB).
- Depending on the course of the disease, findings on radiographs vary (Table 9-5).

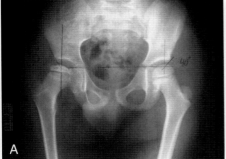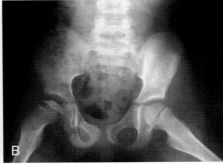

Figure 9-12. Anteroposterior and frog-leg lateral radiographs of Legg-Calve-Perthes disease of the right hip (initial stage). *(From Erol B, Dormans JP: Hip disorders. In Dormans JP, editors:* Core knowledge in orthopaedics: pediatric orthopaedics, *Philadelphia, 2005, Mosby, p 239.)*

Table 9-5. Radiographic Findings in Legg-Calve-Perthes Disease

STAGE	FINDINGS
Initial (avascular necrosis)	-Smaller ossific nucleus of femoral head, lateralization of the femoral head relative to the acetabulum -Later, subchondral fractures and increased density of the femoral head
Fragmentation	Areas of radiolucencies in the femoral head (resorbed areas)
Reossification	Radiolucent areas replaced by new bone
Remodeling	Gradual remodeling of the reossified femoral head and acetabulum

Classification System

- Herring lateral pillar classification is the most commonly used and most prognostic radiographic classification. Radiographs are taken in the early fragmentation stage and evaluated for lucencies in the lateral pillar of the femoral head (Table 9-6).
  - The lateral pillar is the lateral 15% to 30% of the femoral head width.

Initial Treatment
Patient Education

- LCPD is caused by a disruption to blood flow to the femoral head. The mechanism is still not completely understood. The femoral head undergoes a process of remodeling over time. The younger the child is when the disease first presents, the better the remodeling prognosis. Prognosis also depends on the severity of the femoral head involvement.
- The patient may experience loss of range of motion and early hip degenerative changes with an aspherical femoral head at maturity.

First Treatment Steps

- Identify the stage of the disease and classify the severity of femoral head involvement.
- Rule out other hip pathologies including infection.

Treatment Options

- Goal of treatment: maintain range of motion and containment of femoral head in the acetabulum.

Nonoperative Management

- Children younger than age 8 at the onset of disease with all Herring lateral pillar grades can be treated with nonoperative management.
  - Pain control with nonsteroidal anti-inflammatory drugs (NSAIDs) and observation is the mainstay of treatment.
  - Use of an abduction orthosis (Atlanta Scottish Rite brace) is controversial. An orthosis can be used in mild disease part time during the day until reossification is verified on radiographs (>9 months).

Table 9-6. Lateral Pillar Classification

LATERAL PILLAR GROUP	CHARACTERISTICS	PROGNOSIS
A	Lateral pillar not involved	Good; spherical femoral head at maturity
B	>50% of the lateral pillar height maintained	Mixed; improved outcomes when children affected with disease at earlier age
C	<50% of the lateral pillar height maintained	Poor; aspherical femoral head at maturity

- Physical therapy is necessary to maintain hip range of motion.

Operative Management

Codes

ICD-9: 732.1 Juvenile osteochondrosis of the pelvis and hip

CPT: 27145 Osteotomy, iliac, acetabular or innominate bone

    27151 Osteotomy, iliac, or innominate bone; with femoral osteotomy

    27165 Osteotomy, intertrochanteric or subtrochanteric including Internet fixation and/or cast

Operative Indications

- Age older than 8 years at onset of disease with Herring lateral pillar grade B or B/C border, without severe motion loss
- Femoral varus osteotomy and salter innominate acetabular osteotomy can be considered for realignment and containment.
  - The concept is that the femoral head spherical congruity can be restored if the femoral head can be contained in the acetabulum to allow for subsequent remodeling.

Informed Consent and Counseling

- Complications with femoral osteotomy: abductor limp, failure of remodeling leading to persistent varus angulation, leg length discrepancy
- Complications with salter innominate osteotomy: hip stiffness

Anesthesia

- General anesthesia

Patient Positioning

- Supine positioning on a radiolucent table with a bump under the hip

Surgical Procedures

Proximal Femoral Varus Osteotomy

- An incision is made longitudinally centered just distal to the greater trochanter, and the fascia lata is split. The vastus lateralis fascia is incised using an L-shaped incision along the vastus ridge. The vastus lateralis is retracted anteriorly, and the proximal femur is exposed subperiosteally under this. A degree of desired varus correction is planned, and a transverse osteotomy cut is made just proximal to the lesser trochanter. Then the chisel for the blade plate is introduced into the proximal fragment, and the proximal fragment is tipped into varus into the desired amount of varus correction. A wedge of medial bone is then removed to allow for the desired amount of varus. The blade plate is then inserted into the chiseled portion and affixed to the distal fragment.

Salter Innominate Pelvic Osteotomy

- Several pelvic osteotomies exist and are beyond the scope of this text. The salter osteotomy is a rotational osteotomy of the acetabulum aimed to gain anterior and lateral coverage for the femoral head by rotating through the pubic symphysis. The entire extremity to inferior rib cage is prepped. An anterior approach to the hip as previously described in developmental dysplasia of the hip section is used. The inner and outer tables are subperiosteally dissected using periosteal elevators to the sciatic notch, and retractors are placed into the sciatic notch from the inner and outer tables overlapping each other. Subperiosteal dissection into the notch is crucial to avoid neurovascular injury to the gluteal vessels/nerves and the sciatic nerve. A gigli saw is passed on top of the retractors using a right-angle clamp and pulled to create a cut from the sciatic notch to the anterior inferior iliac spine (AIIS). This cut creates a proximal and distal pelvic fragment. A bone graft from the iliac wing is removed with a saw laterally, along a path just above the AIIS to the iliac tubercle. The graft is shaped to a 30-degree triangular wedge. The distal pelvic fragment is then hinged anterolaterally with towel clamps. The graft wedge is then placed in the osteotomy gap and affixed with two threaded pins from proximal to distal stopping short of the triradiate cartilage. The iliac apophysis is then closed, and threaded pins are cut above the apophysis. The exposure is then closed in the usual fashion. A hip spica cast is applied.

Estimated Postoperative Course
- Postoperative days 10 to 14—Evaluate cast hygiene, and educate the patient and parent.
- Postoperative week 6—Obtain radiographs to evaluate healing osteotomy, and remove spica cast. If the osteotomy has healed, remove the pins (for pelvic osteotomy). A physical therapist should gradually mobilize the hips.
- Postoperative months 2 to 3: Obtain radiographs to evaluate healing osteotomy, and mobilize as tolerated.

Suggested Readings
Herring JA, Neustadt JB, Williams JA, et al: The lateral pillar classification of Legg-Calvé-Perthes disease, *J Pediatr Orthop* 12(2): 143-150.

Herring JA: Legg-Calvé-Perthes disease. In Herring JA, editor: *Tachdjian's pediatric orthopaedics,* ed 4, Philadelphia, 2008, Saunders.

Stulberg SD, Cooperman DR, Wallenstein R, et al: The natural history of Legg-Calvé-Perthes disease, *J Bone Joint Surg Am* 63(7):1095–1108, 1981.

Thompson GH, Price CT, Roy D, et al: Legg-Calvé-Perthes disease, *Instr Course Lect* 51: 367–384, 2002.

Thompson GH: Salter osteotomy in Legg-Calve-Perthes disease, *J Pediatr Orthop* 31 (2 Suppl):S192–197, 2011.

SLIPPED CAPITAL FEMORAL EPIPHYSIS (SCFE)
History
- Definition: SCFE is the displacement of the femoral neck and shaft from the femoral epiphysis, in which the femoral neck moves anterior-superior relative to the epiphysis.
- It usually occurs during a period of rapid growth in adolescence (ages 12 to 15).
- Obesity, mechanical (i.e., femoral neck retroversion), and endocrine factors (i.e., hypothyroidism, hypogonadism) are all proposed risk factors.
- Patients present with either acute onset of severe pain to the hip region (acute SCFE) or more commonly several months' duration of insidious vague groin and thigh pain (chronic SCFE).
- Minimal to no trauma before significant pain distinguishes acute SCFE from Salter-Harris type I injury to the proximal femoral epiphysis.

Physical Examination
- Generally obese child
- Chronic SCFE:
  - Inspect for antalgic gait with limp, limb externally rotated at rest
  - Assess obligatory external rotation with hip flexion due to anatomic distortion of proximal femur
- Acute SCFE:
  - Inspect for refusal to bear weight, limb shortened and externally rotated

Imaging: Figure 9-13
- Obtain AP pelvis and lateral hip radiograph.
- Irregularity of the proximal femoral physis can be seen.
- Klein's line—A line drawn along the superior femoral neck on the AP radiograph intersects the lateral epiphysis normally and does not intersect in SCFE.
- CT scans can help evaluate for displacement if radiographic findings are subtle, or to characterize proximal femoral deformity as a result of SCFE.

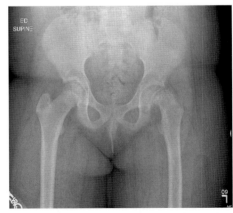

Figure 9-13. Acute on chronic slipped capital femoral epiphysis in a 12-year-old girl.

Classification System
- Onset of symptoms:
  - Acute—prodromal symptoms less than 3 weeks before sudden acute severe pain without significant trauma. No remodeling of the proximal femur on radiographs
    - Up to 47% risk of avascular necrosis of the femoral head
  - Chronic—prodromal symptoms more than several months of vague groin and thigh pain. Remodeling of the femoral neck on radiographs
  - Acute on chronic—prodromal symptoms more than 3 weeks, although sudden acute severe pain and radiographic evidence of minor prior femoral neck remodeling
- Clinical function:
  - Stable—pain tolerable enough for patient to bear weight
  - Unstable—pain intolerable, patient unable to bear weight; higher incidence of avascular necrosis in unstable group

Initial Treatment
Patient Education
- SCFE is a separation of the proximal femur from the proximal femoral growth plate. It can occur on both hips. The cause is unknown, although obesity is a risk factor. The most devastating result is the risk of avascular necrosis, especially in acute, unstable, or significantly displaced slips, as well as risk of early osteoarthritis from proximal femoral deformity in significantly displaced slip.

First Treatment Steps
- Evaluate other hip because up to 25% of slips are bilateral.
- Rule out fracture/dislocation of affected hip.
- Once a diagnosis of SCFE has been confirmed by radiographs, a pediatric orthopaedist should be involved in formulating a definitive management plan. The patient should be admitted to the hospital for bed rest and pain control until fixation.

Treatment Options
Nonoperative Management
- Spica casting for patients with chronic SCFE has fallen out of favor due to associated risks including recurrent slip and chondrolysis.

Operative Management
Codes
ICD-9: 820.01 Closed fracture/separation of epiphysis from femoral neck
CPT: 27176 In-situ pinning of SCFE

Informed Consent and Counseling
- Technical risk of screw penetration into the hip joint

Anesthesia
- General anesthesia

Patient Positioning
- Patient is positioned supine on a fracture table, with the operative leg in neutral position. The other leg can be positioned flexed and abducted in a leg holder to clear it from fluoroscopic view. For acute and unstable slips, *gentle* reduction of the hip on the traction table is sufficient.

Surgical Procedures
In Situ Screw Fixation of the Hip:
Figure 9-14
- Before prepping the operative leg, it is important to be able to obtain adequate fluoroscopic AP and lateral views of the hip.
- Ideal screw placement is perpendicular to the physis and in the center of the epiphysis.
- A guidewire is placed on the skin to estimate the trajectory of the screw in the AP and lateral planes. The trajectories are marked on the skin with a marking pen.
- The guidewire is inserted through a small stab incision and placed through the femoral neck, physis, and epiphysis using fluoroscopic guidance, being careful not to penetrate the hip joint. The guidewire length is measured using a depth gauge to estimate the screw length.
- A drill and tap are used over the guidewire to prepare for screw insertion.

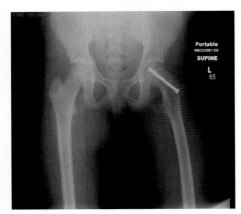

Figure 9-14. In situ screw fixation of slipped capital femoral epiphysis.

- A cannulated partially threaded screw is then inserted over the guidewire, with at least three screw threads passing the epiphysis.
- The skin is closed in the usual fashion. The patient may be discharged on toe-touch weight bearing on crutches.

Estimated Postoperative Course
- For stable slips, patients can bear weight as tolerated.
- For unstable slips, patients remain partial weight bearing for up to 6 weeks.
- Postoperative days 10-14—Perform clinical evaluation, check wounds, and obtain radiographs.
- Postoperative week 6—Perform clinical evaluation, obtain radiographs, and progress with weight bearing as tolerated.

Suggested Readings
Goodman WW, Johnson JT, Robertson WW Jr, et al: Single screw fixation for acute and acute-on-chronic slipped capital femoral epiphysis, *Clin Orthop Related Res* Jan;(322): 86–90, 1996.

Larson AN, Sierra RJ, Yu EM, et al: Outcomes of slipped capital femoral epiphysis treated with in situ pinning, *J Pediatr Orthop* 32(2):125-130, 2012.

Loder RT, Richards BS, Shapiro BS, et al: Acute slipped capital femoral epiphysis: the importance of physeal stability, *J Bone Joint Surg Am* 75(8):1134–1140, 1993.

Loder RT, Aronsson DD, Dobbs MB, Weinstein SL: Slipped capital femoral epiphysis, *Instr Course Lect* 50:1141–1147, 2001.

PES PLANOVALGUS (FLAT FEET)
History
- Definition: loss of medial foot arch
- Commonly presents as painless flexible deformity in early childhood
- Flexible flat foot is common in toddlers, and prevalence decreases by preschool years
- Foot arch develops around 5 to 6 years of age
- Parents often concerned about appearance of deformity, asymmetric shoe wear, and potential future disability
- Important to rule out other conditions including tarsal coalition, equinus, and congenital vertical talus before diagnosis of flat feet
- Higher prevalence in children with ligamentous laxity and obesity

Physical Examination
- Assess if flat foot is rigid or mobile (Fig. 9-15).
  - If arch is restored by the patient standing on tiptoe, deformity is flexible.
  - Rigid flat foot is always pathologic and can indicate other conditions such as tarsal coalition.
- Assess the flexibility of the subtalar joint by inverting and everting the heel with a hand cupped on the calcaneus.
- Assess for contracture of the heel cord, which can also predispose to flat feet. This is often associated with callous formation along the head of the talus.
- Perform a **Silfverskiold test** for tight heel cord: Check ankle dorsiflexion with knee in flexion and extension. If improved ankle dorsiflexion with knee flexion exists, then gastrocnemius is tight. If equivalent ankle dorsiflexion with knee flexion and extension exists, then the Achilles tendon is tight.

Imaging
- Radiographs are not routinely necessary for the evaluation of flat feet unless they are associated with pain or rigid deformity exists.

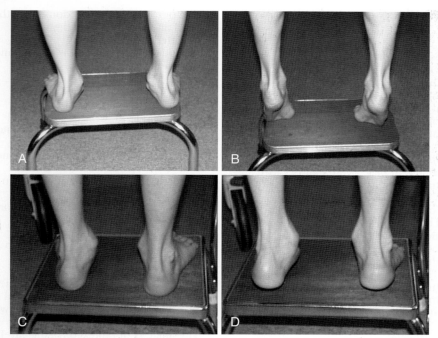

Figure 9-15. Flexible flat foot and rigid flat foot. **A** and **B,** Flexible flat foot. Note inversion of hindfoot with plantarflexion. **C** and **D,** Rigid flat foot. Note hindfoot does not invert with plantarflexion. *(From Wallach D, Davidson RS: Pediatric lower limb disorders. In Dormans JP, editor:* Core knowledge in orthopaedics: pediatric orthopaedics, *Philadelphia, 2005, Mosby, pp 212.)*

- In rigid deformity consider a CT scan to evaluate for tarsal coalition.

Classification System
- Mild flat foot: arch depressed on standing but visible
- Moderate flat foot: arch obliterated on standing though present when non–weight bearing
- Severe flat foot: arch not present when non–weight bearing, with convex medial border of the foot

Initial Treatment
Patient Education
- Flat foot has two characteristic components to the deformity in which the hindfoot is in valgus and the forefoot is in supination, leading to loss of the medial foot arch.
- Most cases of mobile flat feet do not require specific treatment, and no future adverse sequelae is the norm in asymptomatic flexible flat foot.

First Treatment Steps
- First, rule out rigid and significantly painful flat foot. Reassure patient and parents that no significant future disability is substantiated by the presence of the asymptomatic flat foot.
- If mild or moderate flat foot and mostly asymptomatic or with mild symptoms of foot strain, consider arch support or heel cups.

Treatment Options
Nonoperative Management
- Nonoperative management with reassurance and consideration of arch supports is the mainstay of treatment of mild to moderate flat foot.

Operative Management
Codes
ICD-9: 734 Flat foot
CPT: 28300 Lateral column lengthening via calcaneal osteotomy

27685 Lengthening or shortening of tendon, leg or ankle

Operative Indications
- Operative management is indicated for older children with severe or painful flat feet.
- If the patient has severe flat feet without significant pain and appearance is bothersome for child and parents, consider medial calcaneal displacement osteotomy or lateral column lengthening.
- If patient has severe flat feet with significant pain, consider subtalar fusion.

Informed Consent and Counseling
- Long-term results of arch reconstruction are lacking, and treatment should be aimed toward joint-sparing procedures if possible.
- There is a risk of graft failure or nonunion (for lateral column lengthening), and infection and continued pain should be discussed.

Anesthesia
- General anesthesia

Patient Positioning
- The patient is positioned supine on a regular table, with a bump under the ipsilateral hip. A tourniquet is applied to the operative extremity.

Surgical Procedures
Lateral Column Lengthening
- An oblique incision is made along the lateral ankle anterior and parallel to the peroneus brevis. The peroneal tendons are released from their sheaths to allow for retraction.
- The sinus tarsi is exposed, and the calcaneocuboid joint is visualized.
- An oblique osteotomy of the calcaneus is made using an oscillating saw starting at the inferior aspect of the calcaneus 2 cm proximal to the calcaneocuboid joint and exiting the junction between the anterior and middle facets.
- An osteotome is used to open the osteotomy, and a tricortical iliac crest graft is impacted in the osteotomy. A Steinman pin can be used to affix the graft for additional fixation.

- The peroneal brevis tendon is lengthened and repaired, and the wound irrigated and closed.
- A padded short leg cast is placed and bivalved.

Achilles Tendon Lengthening
- If the Silfverskiold test shows tight Achilles tendon, lengthening is indicated as an adjunct to lateral column lengthening procedure.
- A longitudinal skin incision anteromedial to the Achilles tendon is made along the tendon to just proximal to the tendon insertion.
- The paratenon sheath is incised along the tendon.
- Two incisions are made along the tendon: (1) distally just proximal to the tendon insertion, an incision directed from anterior to posterior (two thirds the width of the tendon); and (2) proximally along the medial two thirds from medial to lateral (two thirds the width of the tendon).
- The ankle is dorsiflexed (being careful not to be too aggressive) to the desired position.
- A short leg cast is applied.

Estimated Postoperative Course
- Non–weight bearing for 6 to 8 weeks
- Postoperative days 10 to 14—Routine follow-up, patient and parent education
- Postoperative 6 to 8 weeks—Cast and pin removal, with standing radiographs at that time. Use arch supports to supplement walking out of cast.

Suggested Readings
Bordelon RL: Hypermobile flatfoot in children. Comprehension, evaluation, and treatment, *Clin Orthop Relat Res* 181:7–14, 1983.

Koutsogiannis E: Treatment of mobile flat foot by displacement osteotomy of the calcaneus, *J Bone Joint Surg Br* 53:96–100, 1971.

Mosca VS: Calcaneal lengthening for valgus deformity of the hindfoot. Results in children who had severe, symptomatic flatfoot and skewfoot, *J Bone Joint Surg Am* 77:500–512, 1995.

Staheli LT, Chew DE, Corbett M, et al. The longitudinal arch: a survey of eight hundred and eighty-two feet in normal children and adults, *J Bone Joint Surg Am* 69(3):426–428, 1987.

CLUBFOOT (EQUINOVARUS DEFORMITY)

History
- Background: Congenital deformity of the foot, in which foot is shaped like a "club"
- Deformity present at birth and hypothesized to be caused by several factors including intrauterine restriction, genetics, and neuromuscular conditions
- Can be unilateral or bilateral

Physical Examination
- Assess position and flexibility of foot:
  - The hindfoot is in equinus and the subtalar joint is in varus (inversion and adduction). The posterior tibial tendon and Achilles tendon are tight.
  - The midfoot is adducted and plantarflexed.
- Evaluate hips for dysplasia because intrauterine "packing" problems are commonly associated.

Imaging
- Imaging is not required in the diagnosis or management of clubfoot.

Initial Treatment
Patient Education
- Clubfoot occurs in approximately 1 in 1000 births, and although many theories on etiology exist there is no definitive answer regarding etiology. Nonoperative treatment is the initial treatment of choice, although Achilles tendon releases are often necessary to help with contracture. Parental patience is key because patients postcasting will require long-term foot bracing to prevent recurrence of deformity.

First Treatment Step
- Patients can start their first Ponseti cast in the first week of life

Treatment Options
Nonoperative Management
Serial Ponseti Casting
- In children younger than 2 years old, the majority of the deformity can be corrected with four to six long leg casts in a sequence described by Ponseti.
- Sequence: C.A.V.E
  - C—Cavus: The first cast is used to elevate the first ray into alignment with other rays.
  - A—Adductus: A second to third cast is used to decrease the adduction deformity of the forefoot. Counter-pressure should be applied to the head of the talus to ensure abduction around the talus.
  - V—Varus: A second to third cast is also used to gradually decrease varus of the hindfoot.
  - E—Equinus: A fourth cast is used to correct any equinus of the calcaneus.
  - Each cast should be left on for 5 to 7 days before the next cast change. Once appropriate cavus, adductus, and varus are achieved, it is often necessary to perform percutaneous Achilles tenotomy to correct hindfoot equinus, after which point the final cast can be applied for 3 weeks.
  - Check perfusion of toes after each cast change to ensure that the cast has not been applied too tightly.

Operative Management
Codes
ICD-9: 754.51 Congenital talipes equinovarus
CPT: 27605 Tenotomy, percutaneous, Achilles tendon
28262 Capsulotomy, midfoot; extensive

Operative Indications
- Hindfoot equinus after Ponseti casting → percutaneous Achilles tenotomy
- Recalcitrant clubfoot or long-standing clubfoot not amenable to Ponseti technique → surgical release of clubfoot

Informed Consent and Counseling
- Surgical release of clubfoot can be associated with wound problems, damage to nerves and vessels, overcorrection or undercorrection of deformity, recurrence of deformity, stiffness, and weakness.

Anesthesia
- Local anesthesia for percutaneous Achilles tenotomy
- General anesthesia for open release of resistant clubfoot

Patient Positioning
- Supine position with knee flexed and ankle maximally dorsiflexed for percutaneous Achilles tenotomy
- Prone position with knee extended for surgical release of clubfoot, with tourniquet applied to the upper thigh

Surgical Procedures
Percutaneous Achilles Tenotomy
- The patient is placed supine, and 1% lidocaine is injected into a region approximately 2 cm proximal to the calcaneal insertion of the Achilles tendon.
- An assistant holds the foot in dorsiflexion, which accentuates the Achilles tendon.
- A #11 blade is inserted from the medial side, anterior to the Achilles tendon. The blade is oriented such that on insertion the sharp portion of the blade does not touch the Achilles tendon (parallel to the tendon).
- Once the blade is passed gently past the entire width of the tendon, the blade is gently twisted 90 degrees such that it is perpendicular to and facing the tendon.
- Gentle pressure is placed with a thumb over the tendon until release is complete, which should allow for approximately 15 degrees more dorsiflexion.
- Pressure over the small stab wound is applied until bleeding is stopped, and a long leg cast is applied with increased dorsiflexion. This cast is the final cast in the Ponseti method that addresses equinus.

Surgical Release of Clubfoot
- Soft tissue release of multiple contracted structures may be necessary in older children where Ponseti method will not work due to secondary adaptive changes from long-term clubfoot.

- Intraoperative assessment of tight structures determines which soft tissues need to be released.
- A Cincinnati incision is made. This large incision starts medially along the talonavicular joint, courses posteriorly above the calcaneal tuberosity, and progresses laterally at the level of the talonavicular joint. Parts of the incision can be used if selective releases are being carried out.
- Posterior structures are assessed first, and the Achilles tendon is lengthened with a Z-plasty. If the ankle is still tight in equinus, release the posterior ankle joint capsule by simple incision being careful to protect peroneal tendons and posteromedial neurovascular structures.
- Medial structures are assessed next if further correction is necessary. The posterior tibial neurovascular bundle lies between the flexor digitorum longus and flexor hallucis longus and should be protected throughout the case. Identifying tight structures, the posterior tibial tendon, abductor hallucis muscle, flexor digitorum, and flexor hallucis longus can be lengthened. If this does not provide adequate correction of hindfoot varus and forefoot adduction, then release the talonavicular joint capsule and subtalar joint capsule.
- Lateral structures are assessed next and, rarely, if anatomic alignment cannot be achieved a completion of the talonavicular and subtalar joint capsule release can be performed on the lateral side.
- The subtalar joint is reduced to create a straight lateral border of the foot and held in place with a 0.062 k-wire passing from the posteromedial talus, navicular, medial cuneiform, and the first web space.
- Wound closure is performed, and a bulky soft dressing is applied.

Estimated Postoperative Course
- Percutaneous Achilles tenotomy
  - The final Ponseti cast after tenotomy should be left on for 3 weeks, after which it can be removed.

- A Denis-Browne boot with derotation bar is used continuously for 3 months and then gradually changed to nighttime only wear up to 3 years old.
- Surgical release of clubfoot
  - Postoperative week 1: dressing removed, wound evaluated, long leg cast applied
  - Postoperative week 4: pins removed, cast changed
  - Postoperative week 12: cast removed

Suggested Readings

Cooper DM, Dietz FR: Treatment of idiopathic clubfoot: a thirty-year follow-up noted, *J Bone Joint Surg Am* 77A:1477–1489, 1995.
Davidson R: Posteromedial and posterolateral release for the treatment of resistant clubfoot. In Wiese/SW, editor: *Operative techniques in orthopaedic surgery,* Philadelphia, 2010, Lippincott Williams & Wilkins.
Ponseti IV, Zhivkov M, Davis N, et al: Treatment of the complex idiopathic clubfoot, *Clin Orthop Relat Res* 251:171–176, 2006.
Roye DP Jr, Roye BD: Idiopathic congenital talipes equinovarus, *J Am Acad Orthop Surg* 10(4):239–248, 2002.

PEDIATRIC SPORTS MEDICINE

Little Leaguer's Elbow

History
- History of repetitive throwing/pitching, which places valgus stress along the flexor-pronator origin (medial epicondyle) and the medial epicondylar apophysis
- Medial elbow pain and swelling, decreased throwing distance and effectiveness

Physical Examination
- Inspect for medial elbow swelling.
- Palpate for medial elbow tenderness and overgrowth.

Imaging
- Elbow AP, lateral, oblique radiographs
  - A spectrum of findings of the medial epicondyle apophysis: irregular ossification, enlargement, or partial avulsion
- Magnetic resonance imaging (MRI) helpful in detecting area of injury

Initial Treatment
Patient Education
- Little Leaguer's elbow is a result of repetitive microtrauma to the flexor-pronator mass, leading to inflammation along the medial epicondyle and at the medial epicondylar apophysis. Most patients improve with rest and activity modification, and a throwing rehabilitation and evaluation of pitching mechanics may be helpful. To prevent injury, the recommended per-game pitch counts are 8 to 10 years, 50 pitches; 11 to 14 years, 75 pitches; 15 to 16 years, 90 pitches; and 17 to 18 years, 105 pitches.

First Treatment Step
- 4 to 6 weeks of rest from throwing

Treatment Options
Nonoperative Management
- Anti-inflammatories for pain control
- 4 to 6 weeks of complete rest from throwing
- Structured throwing program starting at 6 to 8 weeks with gradual progression if pain free
- Return to throwing at around 12 weeks
- Recalcitrant symptoms indicative of inadequate rest

Codes
ICD-9: 719.42 Pain of joint upper arm

Suggested Readings
Chen FS, Diaz VA, Loebenberg M, et al: Shoulder and elbow injuries in the skeletally immature athlete, *J Am Acad Orthop Surg* 13:172–185, 2005.
Klingele KE, Kocher MS: Little League elbow: valgus overload injury in the paediatric athlete, *Sports Med* 32(15):1005–1015, 2002.
Kocher MS, Waters PM, Micheli LJ: Upper extremity injuries in the paediatric athlete, *Sports Med* 30(2):117–135, 2000.
Wei AS, Khana S, Limpisvasti O, et al: Clinical and magnetic resonance imaging findings associated with Little League elbow, *J Pediatr Orthop* 30(7):715–719, 2010.

LITTLE LEAGUER'S SHOULDER

History
- Definition: Chondral injury to the proximal humerus physis

- Repetitive microtrauma to the proximal humeral physis to blame for injury
- Recent increase in throwing regimen precedes pain
- Shoulder pain that is activity related, worse with throwing activities
- Decreased ball control and velocity

Physical Examination
- Pain and tenderness along the shoulder near the physis
- Weakness with resisted abduction and internal rotation
- Decreased range of internal rotation

Imaging: Figure 9-16
- AP and axillary radiographic views of the shoulder
  - Radiographs may show physeal widening of the proximal humeral epiphysis, metaphyseal demineralization, and fragmentation
- MRI of shoulder may be helpful to rule out other pathology if diagnosis unclear; may show edema around physis

Initial Treatment
Patient Education
- Little Leaguer's shoulder is an overuse type injury to the pediatric shoulder. Most patients get better with rest and activity modification for several months with gradual progression to a throwing program. Physeal injury, which is rare, can lead to growth arrest. Abnormal pitching mechanics may contribute, and supervised throwing mechanics evaluation may be helpful. To prevent injury, the recommended per-game pitch counts are 8 to 10 years, 50 pitches; 11 to 14 years, 75 pitches; 15 to 16 years, 90 pitches; and 17 to 18 years, 105 pitches.

First Treatment Step
- Initially, rest from throwing for 2 to 3 months is the mainstay of treatment.

Treatment Options
Nonoperative Management
- Rest and activity modification for 2 to 3 months
- Anti-inflammatory medications for pain control
- Gradual return to activity after rest, with evaluation of pitching mechanics and preventing excessive pitch count

Codes
ICD-9: 732.3 Juvenile osteochondrosis of the upper extremity

Suggested Readings
Chen FS, Diaz VA, Loebenberg M, Rosen JE, et al: Shoulder and elbow injuries in the skeletally immature athlete, *J Am Acad Orthop Surg* 13:172–185, 2005.

Keeley DW, Hackett T, Keirns M, et al: A biomechanical analysis of youth pitching mechanics, *J Pediatr Orthop* 28(4):452–459, 2008.

Kocher MS, Waters PM, Micheli LJ: Upper extremity injuries in the paediatric athlete, *Sports Med* 30(2):117–135, 2000.

McFarland EG, Ireland ML: Rehabilitation programs and prevention strategies in adolescent throwing athletes, *Instr Course Lect* 52:37–42, 2003.

DISCOID MENISCUS
History
- Definition: abnormal development of meniscus leading to enlarged and discoid-shaped meniscus
- Majority of cases involve lateral meniscus

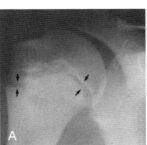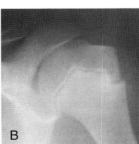

Figure 9-16. Little Leaguer's shoulder. **A,** Widening of the proximal humeral physis compared with **(B)** unaffected side. (*From Wilkins K: Shoulder, section J: injuries of the proximal humerus in the skeletally immature athlete. In DeLee JC, Drez D, Miller MD, et al, editors: DeLee and Drez's orthopaedic sports medicine, Philadelphia, 2010, Saunders, p 1093.*)

- Frequently an incidental finding because most cases are asymptomatic
- Young child can present with lateral knee catching or popping, with or without pain

Physical Examination
- Inspect for any blocks to knee range of motion.
- Palpate the lateral joint line for tenderness.
- Perform the *McMurray test* to evaluate for painful pop/click along the joint line.
  - One hand stabilizes the medial knee at the joint line while the other hand holds the sole of the foot. The knee is in full flexion, then simultaneously extended and internally rotated. If click or pain occurs, the test suggests a lateral meniscus tear.
- Perform a varus stress test to evaluate for LCL laxity because the lateral knee joint line may be widened to accommodate a larger lateral meniscus.

Imaging
- AP, Lateral radiographs of the knee
  - May show widening of lateral compartment compared with medial
- MRI of the knee
  - Best study to evaluate discoid meniscus
  - A discoid meniscus appears as three consecutive sagittal 3-mm cuts without a bow-tie appearance of the anterior and posterior horns

Classification System
- Stable—posterior meniscofemoral ligament is intact securing the discoid meniscus
- Unstable (Wrisberg type)—posterior meniscofemoral ligament is lacking, leading to hypermobile discoid meniscus

Initial Treatment
Patient Education
- Discoid meniscus is present in 3% to 5% of the population, and in most cases is asymptomatic and does not require treatment. However, discoid menisci may have a propensity to develop tears or, if unstable, cause pain

and mechanical symptoms such as knee locking and popping.

First Treatment Steps
- Establish diagnosis on the basis of an examination and MRI of stable or unstable type.
- An initial trial of nonoperative management is appropriate for all cases with anti-inflammatories.
- Surgical treatment is reserved for persistent range of motion loss/locking and pain.

Treatment Options
Nonoperative Management
- Rest and anti-inflammatory medications with observation is the mainstay of nonoperative treatment.

Operative Management
Codes
ICD-9: 717.5 Derangement of meniscus, not elsewhere classified
CPT: 29881 Knee arthroscopy and partial meniscectomy (medial or lateral)
29882 Knee arthroscopy with meniscus repair (medial or lateral)

Operative Indications
- Persistent loss of range of motion/ locking or pain

Informed Consent and Counseling
- Knee stiffness, failure of meniscal stabilization after surgery can occur postoperatively

Anesthesia
- General anesthesia

Patient Positioning
- Supine position with a lateral thigh post and tourniquet to the thigh

Surgical Procedures
Arthroscopic Partial Lateral Meniscectomy and Saucerization:
Figure 9-17
- The patient is positioned supine on a regular table with a lateral post along the thigh. A tourniquet is placed along the proximal thigh. The leg is exsanguinated by elevation only, and the tourniquet pressure is elevated. A

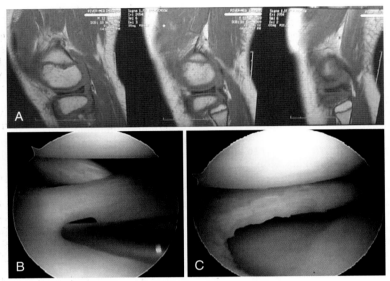

Figure 9-17. Discoid lateral meniscus. **A,** Magnetic resonance imaging showing lack of bow-tie appearance of lateral meniscus. **B,** Arthroscopy: complete discoid lateral meniscus. **C,** Arthroscopy: saucerization of discoid lateral meniscus. *(From Brockmeier S, Rodeo S. Knee, Section B: Meniscal injuries. In DeLee JC, Drez D, Miller MD et al, editors: DeLee and Drez's orthopaedic sports medicine, Philadelphia, 2010, Saunders, pp 1615.)*

small stab incision directed toward the notch is made along the lateral joint line just lateral to the inferior aspect of the patellar tendon and used as a viewing portal. The arthroscope is inserted into this portal, and inflow is established. An inferomedial portal is established for the working portal.

- A diagnostic arthroscopy is performed, and if the discoid meniscus is unstable, a posterolateral approach to the knee is made in preparation for an inside-out suture repair of the meniscus.
  - A 3-cm lateral joint line incision is made in line with the posterior aspect of the fibular head.
  - The interval between the biceps femoris and IT band is found, and a retractor is placed into this interval. The peroneal nerve lies posterior to the biceps femoris.
- Using a combination of biters and shavers, the lateral meniscus is saucerized to leave an approximately 15-mm rim of meniscus. The discoid meniscus is stabilized as needed with an inside-out suture fixation.

Estimated Postoperative Course
- Toe touch weight bearing for 4 weeks if meniscal stabilization was performed
- Postoperative day 0—Start knee range of motion
- Postoperative days 10 to 14—Wound check
- Postoperative weeks 4 to 6—Clinical examination for range of motion; progress activities as tolerated

Suggested Readings

Atay OA, Doral MN, Leblebicioglu G, et al: Management of discoid lateral meniscus tears: observations in 34 knees, *Arthroscopy* 19(4):346–352, 2003.

Carter CW, Hoellwarth J, Weiss JM: Clinical outcomes as a function of meniscal stability in the discoid meniscus: a preliminary report, *J Pediatr Orthop* 32(1):9–14, 2012.

Good CR, Green DW, Griffith MH, et al: Arthroscopic treatment of symptomatic discoid meniscus in children: classification, technique, and results, *Arthroscopy* 23(2):157–163, 2007.

Kramer DE, Micheli LJ: Meniscal tears and discoid meniscus in children: diagnosis and treatment, *J Am Acad Orthop Surg* 17: 698–707, 2009.

PEDIATRIC MUSCULOSKELETAL INFECTION
Introduction
- Musculoskeletal infection in the child has a wide spectrum of severity, and each patient's approach is different.
- Osteomyelitis (infection of the bone) and septic arthritis (infection of the joint) are the focus of this topic discussion.
- Infants younger than 18 months have contiguous metaphyseal and epiphyseal circulation, making simultaneous osteomyelitis and septic arthritis common in this group.
- The metaphyseal outflow circulation is turbulent in children, predisposing this region to osteomyelitis.
  - The hip, ankle, and shoulder are common sites where septic arthritis can occur adjacent to bone infection due to the intracapsular location of the metaphysis.

OSTEOMYELITIS
History
- Definition: Osteomyelitis is infection of the bone.
- Timing and severity of symptoms include the following:
  - Acute hematogenous osteomyelitis (AHO)—Child often presents with sudden illness and localized symptoms within a matter of a few days
  - Subacute osteomyelitis (SO)—Child presents with more than 2 weeks of vague or moderate symptoms
  - Chronic osteomyelitis (CO)—Child presents with months to years of mild symptoms, likely as a result of inadequately treated acute infection
- Evaluate for constitutional symptoms such as fevers, chills, and malaise. Children often appear obviously sick in acute severe cases.
- The patient is unable to bear weight and has worsening pain in the affected extremity.
- Patients and family should be queried about recent systemic and respiratory infections and recent travel history.

Physical Examination
- Fever is higher than 38.5° C.
- Inspect for inability to bear weight or use the affected extremity or pseudoparalysis of the affected extremity.
- Palpate for swelling, warmth, and significant tenderness in affected extremity.
- It may be difficult to localize, so always consider referred pain from a more distant site in children.

Imaging
- Obtain AP and lateral radiographs of the affected extremity.
  - Soft tissue swelling is seen early, and cortical erosion and destruction is seen late.
- Ultrasound is useful to determine deep soft tissue swelling and subperiosteal fluid collections.
- Bone scan is useful when osteomyelitis is suspected, although location is in question.
- MRI allows clear visualization of osteomyelitis and associated abscesses (Fig. 9-18).

Laboratory Evaluation
- Peripheral complete blood cell count (CBC) with differential, erythrocyte sedimentation rate (ESR), C-reactive protein (CRP), and blood cultures

Classification System
- Timing and severity classify osteomyelitis into three major categories: AHO, SO, and CO.
- Age is important in addition to the classification as common causative organisms differ per age group: neonatal (0 to 8 weeks), infant and early child (younger than 3 years), child (greater than 3 years), adolescent (greater than 12 years) (Table 9-7).

Initial Treatment
Patient Education
- Osteomyelitis is an infection to the bone. Adequate treatment of osteomyelitis may take considerable time and effort, including long-term antibiotics, surgical débridement, and reconstructive procedures.

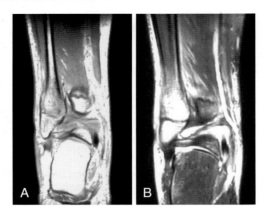

Figure 9-18. Magnetic resonance imaging of osteomyelitis of the fibula. *(From Copley LA, Dormans JP: Musculoskeletal infections. In Dormans JP, editor: Core knowledge in orthopaedics: pediatric orthopaedics, Philadelphia, 2005, Mosby, p 337.)*

Table 9-7. Common Pathogens by Age

AGE	ORGANISM (TOP 3)
Neonatal (0-8 wk)	*Staphylococcus aureus*, Group B *Streptococcus, Staphylococcus epidermidis*
Infant & Early Child (<3 yr)	*Staphylococcus aureus, Kingella kingae, Streptococcus pneumonia*
Child (>3 yr)	*Staphylococcus aureus*, Group A *streptococcus*
Adolescent (>12 yr)	*Staphylococcus aureus, Neisseria gonorrhoeae*

First Treatment Steps

- In all cases of AHO, the patient should be admitted to the hospital for a thorough workup, empiric antibiotics, medical management, and possible surgical débridement.
- For cases of SO, completion of a thorough workup to confirm the diagnosis should be made. Consideration of a bone biopsy should also be made to confirm the diagnosis, and then the patient should be treated with appropriate antibiotics.
- For cases of CO, a thorough workup including possible MRI and bone biopsy should be obtained. A plan for surgical débridement and reconstruction should be made after confirmation of diagnosis.

Treatment Options

Nonoperative Management

- All types of osteomyelitis have a component of antibiotic therapy with or without adjunctive surgical débridement.

- Some cases of AHO (if identified early without abscess formation) and most cases of SO can possibly be treated with antibiotics alone.

Operative Management

Codes
ICD-9: 730.0 Acute osteomyelitis
730.1 Chronic osteomyelitis
CPT: 11044 Débridement of skin, subcutaneous tissue, muscle, and bone

Operative Indications
- Limited response to antibiotics alone, presence of subperiosteal or intraosseous abscess

Informed Consent and Counseling
- Risk of chronic osteomyelitis, growth disturbance, and avascular necrosis
- The need for more than a single procedure for adequate débridement of the infection
- Multisystem involvement of infection and side effects of long-term antibiotics

Anesthesia
- General anesthesia

Patient Positioning
- Supine positioning is the norm in most extremity cases.

Surgical Procedures
Surgical Débridement of Osteomyelitis
- Operative débridement is the goal in complex cases of AHO and almost all cases of CO, and approaches vary by anatomic location of the infection.
- Serial débridement may be necessary, as well as the placement of local antibiotic cement beads.
- Common themes regardless of location and approach are drainage of pus and abscess and débridement of necrotic tissue.
- It is important to perform a careful biopsy if diagnosis is unclear before aggressive débridement to rule out aggressive malignancies.

Estimated Postoperative Course
- At least 6 weeks of antibiotics is the norm, at the discretion of the pediatric infectious disease specialist.
- Postoperative days 0 to 7—Continued clinical and laboratory evaluation
- Postoperative days 10 to 14—Wound evaluation
- Postoperative week 6 onwards— Gradual increase in time between follow-up visits as improvement is seen

Suggested Readings
Copley LA, Dormans JP: Musculoskeletal infections. In Dormans JP, editor: *Core knowledge in orthopaedics: pediatric orthopaedics,* Philadelphia, 2005, Mosby.
Song KM, Sloboda JF: Acute hematogenous osteomyelitis in children, *J Am Acad Orthop Surg* 9:166–175, 2001.
Stanitski CL: Changes in pediatric acute hematogenous osteomyelitis management, *J Pediatr Orthop* 24(4):444-445, 2004.

SEPTIC ARTHRITIS
History
- Definition: Septic arthritis is infection of a joint space.
- Most cases of septic arthritis occur in children younger than 5 years.
- Most cases are monoarticular with the hip, knee, ankle, elbow, wrist, and shoulder the most commonly affected sites in decreasing frequency.
- Hematogenous seeding of the joint is the most common mechanism.
- As in osteomyelitis, historical features include sudden inability to use or bear weight on the affected extremity. Recent sick contacts and illnesses should be assessed.

Physical Examination
- Fever is higher than 38.5° centigrade.
- Inspect for inability to bear weight or use the affected extremity.
- Palpate for edema, warmth, and significant tenderness in the joint.
- Assess passive range of motion of the joint, which is painful in septic arthritis.

Imaging
- AP and lateral radiographs for the affected joint
  - Effusion will be present in acute cases.
  - Rule out trauma.
- Ultrasound—helpful to identify effusion, especially in the hip

Laboratory Evaluation
- As in osteomyelitis, all patients should have CBC with differential, ESR, CRP, and blood cultures drawn.
- Fevers, inability to bear weight on the affected limb, ESR greater than 40 mm/hour, WBC greater than 12,000/mL. If three of these criteria are met, there is a 93.1% probability of septic arthritis. If four of these criteria are met, there is a 99.6% probability of septic arthritis.

Initial Treatment
Patient Education
- Septic arthritis is an infection of the joint space that can lead to damage from severe inflammation. Cartilage and joint destruction can occur if treatment is not initiated expeditiously. Parents should expect at least 4 weeks of antibiotic therapy.

First Treatment Steps
- The patient should be evaluated in the emergency department and receive no food or drink (kept non per os [NPO]) in case urgent joint decompression is necessary.
- An aspiration of the joint should be performed and sent for synovial profile (cell count), and a Gram stain with culture should be obtained.
- Empiric intravenous antibiotics should be started to include gram-positive coverage for the most common pathologies *(Staphylococcus aureus)*. Joint decompression should start as soon as possible to prevent joint damage.

Treatment Options
Nonoperative Management
- There is little role for nonoperative management of septic arthritis once a diagnosis has been made.

Operative Management
Codes
- ICD-9: 711.0 Pyogenic arthritis
- CPT: 29871 Arthroscopic lavage of knee for infection

Operative Indications
- Consideration of formal irrigation and débridement should be given for all septic joints.

Informed Consent and Counseling
- Risk of joint damage without decompression of the affected joint
- Possible need for serial procedures to adequately eradicate infection

Anesthesia
- General anesthesia

Patient Positioning
- Supine positioning is the norm in most extremity cases.

Surgical Procedures
Arthroscopic Joint Lavage and Débridement of the Knee
- The patient is positioned supine on a regular table with a lateral post along the thigh. A tourniquet is placed along the proximal thigh. The leg is exsanguinated by elevation only, and the tourniquet pressure is elevated. A small stab incision directed toward the notch is made along the lateral joint line just lateral to the patellar tendon inferolateral and used as a viewing portal. The arthroscope is inserted into this portal, and inflow is established. An outflow portal is made along the medial joint line just medial to the patellar tendon using a small stab incision directed toward the notch. This portal can also be used to débride inflamed synovium using an arthroscopic shaver as well. Copious irrigation is allowed through the knee to lavage the infection.

Open Joint Arthrotomy and Lavage
- The approach to the particular site of infection varies by the type of joint infected and is beyond the scope of this text. In general, the joint is opened and copious saline is used to lavage the joint to decrease the bacterial burden and reduce the effects of proteolytic enzymes from inflammation.

Estimated Postoperative Course
- At least 4 weeks of antibiotics is the norm, at the discretion of the pediatric infectious disease specialist.
- Postoperative days 0 to 7: Immediately postsurgically, a temporary splint may be applied to immobilize the joint and allow for rest. After the patient's comfort improves, therapy should be started to initiate motion of the joint to prevent stiffness.
- Postoperative days 10 to 14: Check the wound, remove sutures, perform clinical assessment of joint, and continue to work on range of motion.
- Postoperative weeks 2 to 6: There should be a gradual increase in time between follow-up visits as improvement is seen.

Suggested Readings

Copley LA, Dormans JP: Musculoskeletal infections. In Dormans JP, editor: *Core knowledge in orthopaedics: Pediatric orthopaedics,* Philadelphia, 2005, Mosby.

Copley LA: Infections of the musculoskeletal system. In Herring JA, editor: *Tachdjian's pediatric orthopaedics,* ed 4, Philadelphia, 2008, Saunders.

Kocher MS, Zurakowski D, Kasser JR, et al: Differentiating between septic arthritis and transient synovitis of the hip in children: an evidence-based clinical prediction algorithm, *J Bone Joint Surg Am* 81:1662-1670, 1999.

Perlman MH, Patzakis MJ, Kumar PJ, Holtom P: The incidence of joint involvement with adjacent osteomyelitis in pediatric patients, *J Pediatr Orthop* 20:40–43, 2000.

10 Orthopaedic Tumors and Masses

Gregory Domson

INTRODUCTION

- Orthopaedic oncology is a field of orthopaedic surgery that specializes in the diagnosis and treatment of both benign and malignant tumors of the bones and soft tissues of the extremities, pelvis, and spine. Although definitions vary, a tumor can be thought of simply as any mass in the soft tissues or bone that otherwise should not be there. For example, a tumor may be a neoplasm, which is an abnormal proliferation of abnormal cells; a hamartoma, which is an abnormal proliferation of normal cells; or simply an infection causing a masslike effect. The focus of this chapter will be the common neoplasms encountered by the musculoskeletal oncologist.
- Musculoskeletal neoplasms can first be divided into benign and malignant entities. Benign neoplasms are proliferations of abnormal cells that have no potential to metastasize to other areas of the body. Locally, some benign neoplasms can be aggressive and cause significant problems. However, despite its local activity, if a neoplasm has the ability to travel to a distant organ (such as the lungs or lymph nodes) it is considered malignant.

MALIGNANT BONE DISEASE

- There are many categories of malignant neoplasms. Some of these include carcinomas (from epithelial origin), adenocarcinomas (from epithelial cells with secretory properties), lymphomas (arising from lymphocytes), leukemia (from bone marrow cells), and melanomas (from transformed melanocytes). A sarcoma is a malignant neoplasm that arises from cells of mesenchymal origin.

Mesenchymal tissues include those found in the limbs and pelvis: bone, cartilage, muscle, fat, vessels, and nerves. Sarcomas are exceedingly rare. Every year in the United States there are fewer than 10,000 new cases of bone sarcoma and fewer than 15,000 new soft tissue sarcomas.

- Malignant bone disease often causes bone destruction or lysis. A permeative or moth-eaten pattern of lysis (Fig. 10-1), in which the bone is aggressively destroyed with indistinct margins, is usually displayed. A more geographic pattern, in which there is a clear margin between normal and abnormal bone, is seen with benign tumors (Fig. 10-2).

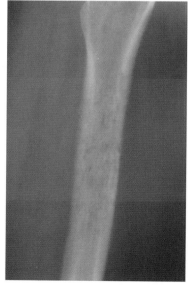

Figure 10-1. A permeative pattern of destruction from a metastatic lesion in the diaphysis of a femur.

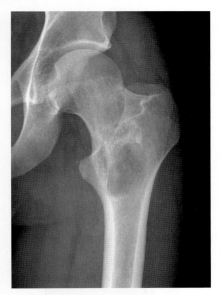

Figure 10-2. A geographic pattern of bone lysis seen in a simple bone cyst of the femur.

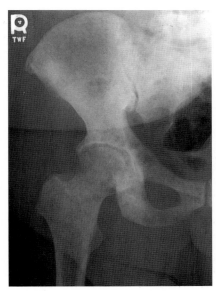

Figure 10-3. A mixed lytic and blastic pattern of metastasis seen with widespread breast cancer.

Metastatic Disease

- Metastatic carcinoma to bone is 25 times more likely to occur than primary bone sarcoma. The five primary carcinomas that most commonly metastasize to bone are breast, prostate, lung, kidney, and thyroid. In contrast to the small numbers of primary bone sarcoma, there are more than a million new cases of these five carcinomas in the United States every year. Metastatic carcinoma most commonly occurs in the thoracic and lumbar spine (theoretically because of the valveless Batson's venous system there) but can occur in virtually any bone. It commonly presents as pain and can lead to weakened bone and pathologic fractures (fractures that occur at normal physiologic loads).

- Metastatic breast cancer is common in women with advanced disease. Radiographically, it is classically a mixed lytic and blastic lesion; that is, it causes lysis of bone and formation of bone (Fig. 10-3). It typically responds to radiation therapy but commonly requires surgical stabilization. Metastatic prostate cancer is also radiosensitive

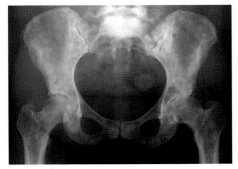

Figure 10-4. Widespread blastic metastases throughout the pelvis, lumbar spine, and femurs.

but typically is a purely blastic process (Fig. 10-4). Lung, kidney, and thyroid disease usually cause purely lytic and destructive lesions (Fig. 10-5). Renal cell carcinoma and thyroid disease are extremely vascular lesions that often require embolization before open surgical treatment.

- Because of the overwhelming preponderance of potentially metastatic carcinoma, any lytic bone lesion in a patient older than 40 years of age should be

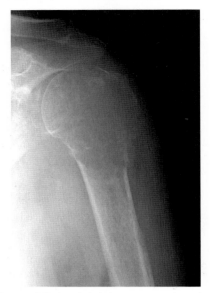

Figure 10-5. Purely lytic lung metastasis to the proximal humerus.

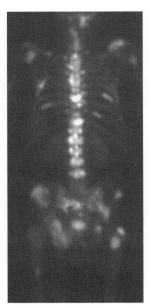

Figure 10-6. A bone scan demonstrating widespread adenocarcinoma metastases.

considered metastatic disease until proven otherwise. Workup for these patients should include radiographs of the entire affected bone, magnetic resonance imaging (MRI) of the area to assess soft tissue extent, a bone scan to assess other skeletal disease, and a computed tomography (CT) scan of the chest, abdomen, and pelvis in an attempt to identify the primary site (Fig. 10-6). Often a biopsy will still be necessary to secure a definitive tissue diagnosis.

- Surgical treatment of metastatic disease can be challenging. Painful lesions in weight-bearing bones should be aggressively stabilized, but many lesions may not have definite surgical indications, especially in patients with limited life spans. A team approach with medical oncology, radiation oncology, orthopaedic oncology, and the patient should be used to optimize treatment and outcomes. Unfortunately, bone metastasis is an ominous finding with little chance of cure.
- Although much rarer, other malignancies such as melanoma, colon, bladder, and cervical cancer can all metastasize to bone and should be suspected in patients with a positive medical history. Metastatic bone disease in children is not common but can be seen with neuroblastoma and Wilms tumor.

Multiple Myeloma

- Multiple myeloma, a malignant disease of monoclonal plasma cells, is the second most common cause of lytic lesions in adults. It is more common in men in their 60s and in African Americans. The bone lesions are well-defined, punched-out lytic areas that can be seen in any bone (Fig. 10-7) and are often seen in the skull. Patients will often have anemia (from bone marrow replacement by tumor), hypercalcemia (from the bone lysis), and a monoclonal protein spike on urine and serum protein electrophoresis. Treatment is multimodal, requiring medical oncology, radiation oncology, and orthopaedics.

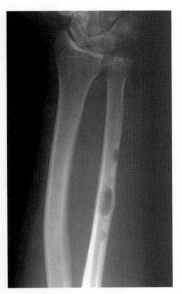

Figure 10-7. Multiple, well-defined, "punched out" lesions seen in multiple myeloma.

LYMPHOMA

- Metastatic disease and multiple myeloma account for the vast majority of malignant lesions of bone in adults and should be the first and second entities on any differential diagnosis. Lymphoma that arises primarily in bone, although rare, can also be seen. It is often in younger and middle-age adults and classically has a large soft tissue mass with little bony change or destruction. Surgery for lymphoma of bone is for biopsy and bone stabilization only; definitive treatment with high cure rates is a combination of chemotherapy and radiation.

Primary Sarcoma of Bone

- Except for chondrosarcoma (which is seen almost exclusively in adults) the primary sarcomas of bone occur more commonly in the pediatric population. Therefore, entities like osteosarcoma and chondrosarcoma should be considered at the bottom of the differential diagnosis of malignant bone lesions in adults (behind metastatic disease, multiple myeloma, and lymphoma). Primary sarcoma should be at the top

of the differential diagnosis of aggressive lesions in children. The primary sarcomas below account for the most common entities.

- Secondary sarcomas of bone are rarely seen but should be considered when there is a lytic lesion or a mass in a bone with preexisting Paget's disease or previous radiation therapy (osteosarcoma is the most common variant). Enchondromas and osteochondromas can transform into chondrosarcomas less than 1% of the time. Rarely, secondary sarcomas can arise from bone infarcts or fibrous dysplasia.

Osteosarcoma

- Osteosarcoma is the most common primary sarcoma of bone. It is a high-grade disease that has a bimodal age distribution; it arises mostly in children but also in the elderly (often secondary to a preexisting condition like Paget's disease). It can occur in any bone but is most common around the knee. Radiographically, it is classically a mixed lytic and blastic lesion with a soft tissue mass characterized by a "sunburst," radial pattern of osteoid formation (Fig. 10-8). Pathologically, the

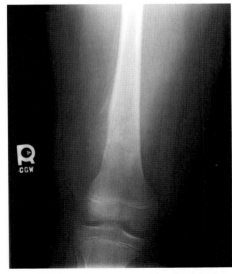

Figure 10-8. Osteosarcoma of the distal femur. Note the blastic soft tissue mass.

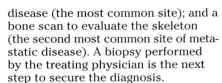

tumor is required to have malignant cells producing osteoid (Fig. 10-9).

- The workup for osteosarcoma should include an MRI of the entire bone to assess tumor extent (Fig. 10-10), assist with preoperative planning, and rule out any skip metastases (anatomically separate areas of tumor in the same bone); a CT scan of the chest to evaluate the lungs for metastatic

disease (the most common site); and a bone scan to evaluate the skeleton (the second most common site of metastatic disease). A biopsy performed by the treating physician is the next step to secure the diagnosis.

- Treatment for osteosarcoma is typically multidrug chemotherapy, followed by wide excision of the lesion (80% to 90% of cases are limb salvage; see Fig. 10-11), followed by more chemotherapy. Five-year survival rates are currently approaching 80%. Chemotherapy can have ototoxic and cardiotoxic side effects.

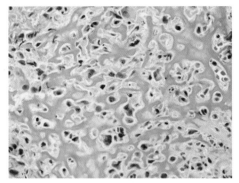

Figure 10-9. High-power view of osteosarcoma. Malignant cells are evident among the pink bands of osteoid.

Ewing's Sarcoma

- Ewing's sarcoma is the second most common primary sarcoma in children. Pathologically, it is a high-grade tumor composed of monotonous, small round blue cells (Fig. 10-12). The majority of Ewing's sarcomas have a characteristic t(11,22) translocation that results in the formation of the EWS-FLI1 oncogene.
- Ewing's sarcoma is often seen in flat bones and the metaphyseal-diaphyseal

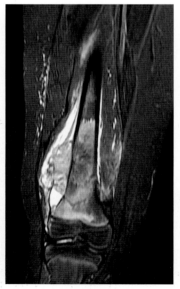

Figure 10-10. Coronal magnetic resonance imaging of the osteosarcoma seen in Figure 10-8.

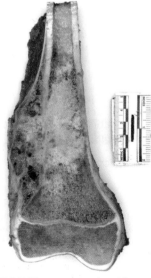

Figure 10-11. The gross specimen from Figure 10-8 after chemotherapy and limb salvage surgery.

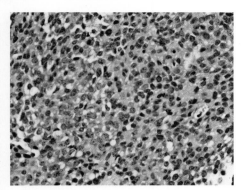

Figure 10-12. High-powered view of Ewing sarcoma showing the uniform, small, round, blue cells.

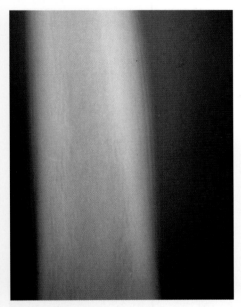

Figure 10-13. Plain radiograph showing the layered, periosteal reaction known as "onion skinning."

regions of long bones. Classically, it has an "onion skin" appearance (multiple thin layers of periosteal reaction at the site of the tumor; see Fig. 10-13). The workup for Ewing sarcoma is the same as for osteosarcoma, but the prognosis is slightly worse. Treatment involves chemotherapy and local treatment. Most tumors are surgically

excised, but because Ewing sarcoma is sensitive to radiation, it can be used to treat tumors that are otherwise unresectable.

Chondrosarcoma

- Chondrosarcoma is a primary bone tumor of chondroid origin. Except for clear cell chondrosarcoma (a rare variant seen in the epiphysis of younger patients), chondrosarcomas are seen almost exclusively in adults. They can range from low-grade (grades 1 and 2) to aggressive, high-grade (3) tumors. On radiographs (especially with lower-grade lesions) they often display the punctate calcifications and rings and whorls classic for cartilaginous tissue. They sometimes arise from preexisting benign cartilaginous tumors like enchondromas (Figs. 10-14 and 10-15) and osteochondromas.
- Chondrosarcomas can arise in any bone and are often seen in the pelvis, where they carry a worse prognosis. The workup for a chondrosarcoma

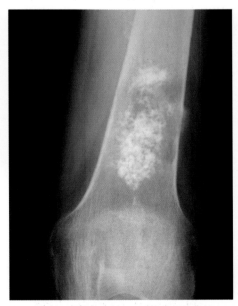

Figure 10-14. Plain radiograph of a chondrosarcoma arising from an enchondroma. Note the lucency and periosteal reaction around the stippled calcification of the enchondroma.

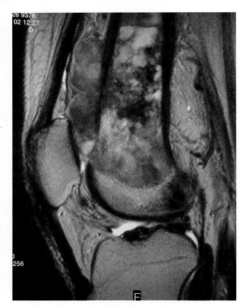

Figure 10-15. Sagittal magnetic resonance image showing the anterior soft tissue mass of the chondrosarcoma from Figure 10-14.

includes an MRI of the affected area, a bone scan, and a chest CT. Chondrosarcomas are not responsive to chemotherapy or radiation, so wide surgical excision is the treatment of choice.

BENIGN BONE TUMORS
- Benign tumors are much more common than malignant bony disease. Benign tumors are characterized by a geographic pattern of bone destruction and often have a well-defined rim of reactive bone around the lesion, "walling it off." According to the Enneking/ Musculoskeletal Tumor Society staging system, they can be stage 1 or latent lesions, which are asymptomatic and often found incidentally; they can be stage 2 or active lesions, which are symptomatic and usually require treatment; or they can be stage 3 or aggressive lesions, which can mimic a malignant tumor with local destruction and activity.
- Benign tumors can be classified into bone forming, cartilage forming, and others. Careful examination of plain

radiography can reveal clues to the lesion's histology and help in subclassifying and diagnosing the tumor. An MRI is then used to define the anatomic extent of disease and aid in preoperative planning.

Benign Bone-Forming Tumors
Bone Island
- A bone island, or enostosis, is a benign formation of histologically normal cortical bone that is usually seen as an incidental finding on radiography done for other reasons. Enostoses are commonly seen in the pelvis bones on CT scans (Fig. 10-16). Typically, they are small punctate areas of dense bone. They may have mild activity on bone scan. Rarely, they can become large or symptomatic. Treatment is benign neglect. An autosomal dominant disorder in which multiple bone islands can be seen is called osteopoikolosis or spotted bone disease.

Osteiod Osteoma
- Osteoid osteoma is a benign bone tumor seen in young people (usually teenagers) presenting as pain, worse at night, that responds to nonsteroidal antiinflammatory drugs. The actual tumor is a small nidus composed of osteoblasts and osteoid that creates a reactive area of dense cortical bone easily identified on plain films and CT scan (Figs. 10-17 and 10-18). They often occur around the proximal femur and acetabulum but can occur in any bone.

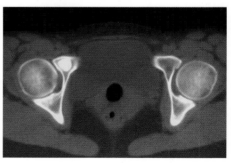

Figure 10-16. Computed tomography scan of the pelvis showing the dense cortical bone of a bone island.

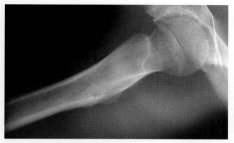

Figure 10-17. Plain radiograph of an osteoid osteoma of the femur. Note the lucent nidus.

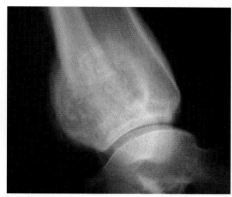

Figure 10-19. A benign, bone-forming osteoblastoma of the distal tibia.

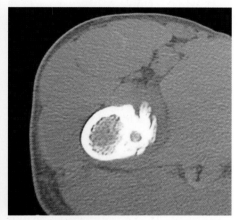

Figure 10-18. A computed tomography scan of the osteoid osteoma in Figure 10-17 shows the reactive bone formation around the nidus.

They often arise in the posterior elements of the spine, where they are the most common cause of painful scoliosis (found on the concave side at the apex of the curve). The natural history is to gradually burn out, so long-term treatment with NSAIDs is an option, but most patients choose a radiofrequency ablation of the nidus with good results.

Osteoblastoma

- Osteoblastomas (Fig. 10-19) are also known as giant osteoid osteomas. Pathologically, they are virtually identical. Osteoblastomas are more aggressive than osteoid osteomas and cause a geographic pattern of destruction with expansile remodeling. Stage 3 lesions can mimic malignant disease. They can be found in any bone (like osteoid osteomas, they too are seen in the posterior elements of the spine). The workup should include plain films, an MRI of the area, and possibly a biopsy in the aggressive lesions to rule out malignancy. Treatment is curettage of the lesion and reconstruction of the defect, often with bone graft.

Benign Cartilage-Forming Tumors

Enchondroma

- Enchondromas are extremely common benign areas of mature hyaline cartilage that occur in the metaphyseal and diaphyseal areas of virtually any bone (Fig. 10-20). It is theorized that they arise from persistent rests of cartilage from the physis. They are usually incidental and can be treated with serial radiographs to follow for the rare instance of malignant degeneration. Sometimes, they can occupy large portions of the intramedullary canal and raise the possibility of a low-grade chondrosarcoma. The most reliable indicator of malignancy is pain at the site of the lesion, but this can be clinically difficult to distinguish from other musculoskeletal conditions. In cases of possibly painful enchondromas, it is advisable to refer the patient to a

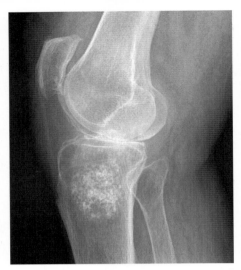

Figure 10-20. The enchondroma in the proximal tibia shows the classic, stippled, or "rings and arcs" calcification.

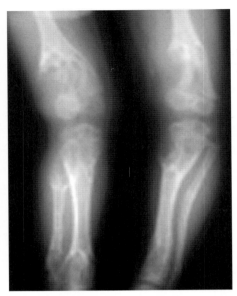

Figure 10-21. A severe case of Ollier's disease, or enchondromatosis, of bilateral lower extremities.

musculoskeletal oncologist for treatment. Enchondromas in the hand are often more aggressive clinically (although it is extremely uncommon for malignant degeneration) and can be treated with curettage and bone graft.

- Ollier disease, also known as *enchondromatosis,* is an autosomal dominant condition characterized by multiple enchondromas throughout the skeleton (Fig. 10-21). The patients often have growth disturbances and are of short stature. Because of the sheer number of lesions, there is a significant chance one of them will become malignant over the course of the patient's lifetime.

Osteochondroma

- Osteochondromas, otherwise known as *exostoses,* are common benign bone tumors that present as exophytic boney masses (Fig. 10-22). They are thought to be aberrations of the growth plate and can be pedunculated (with a well-defined stalk) or sessile (having a more broad-based attachment to the underlying bone). All osteochondromas have corticomedullary continuity; that

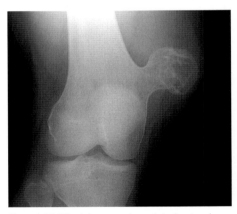

Figure 10-22. A large pedunculated osteochondroma of the distal femur.

is, the medullary canal of the bone flows into the osteochondroma without interruption. The surface of osteochondromas is made up of a cartilage cap that is subject to the same growth regulation as any physis. Therefore, osteochondromas will grow until skeletal maturity, and then the cap tends to become thin and growth ceases. There is a small chance that the cartilage cap can degenerate into a (usually low-grade) chondrosarcoma. Treatment is excision for symptomatic lesions.

- Multiple hereditary exostosis (MHE), also known as osteochondromatosis, is an autosomal dominant disorder with many exostoses. Patients have growth disturbances (especially around the elbows, forearms, and ankles) and are of short stature. Like with Ollier disease, the chance of malignant transformation is much higher due to the numerous lesions.

Periosteal Chondroma
- A periosteal chondroma is a benign cartilaginous tumor on the surface of a bone that is often painful. On plain radiography it appears as a "scalloped-out" lesion on the surface of cortical bone with a thin rim of reactive bone around the actual cartilaginous tissue (Fig. 10-23). Microscopically it is benign lobules of cartilage. Treatment is curettage of the lesion and bone grafting of the defect if necessary.

Chondroblastoma
- Chondroblastoma is a rare, benign proliferation of chondroblasts seen almost exclusively as a well-defined lytic lesion (occasionally with stippled calcifications) in the epiphyseal region of bone (Fig. 10-24). Benign fetal chondroblasts with characteristic "chicken

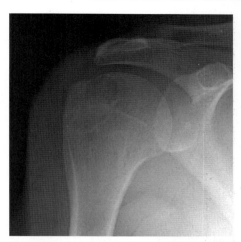

Figure 10-24. A chondroblastoma of the proximal humerus. Note the well-defined lucency in the epiphysis and the reactive bone laterally.

wire" calcification are seen under the microscope. It is most commonly seen in patients between the ages of 15 and 25. In patients with open physes the other entity to consider is a Brodie's abscess. Treatment is curettage and bone grafting. Occasionally chondroblastoma can metastasize to the lungs in a "benign fashion." These lesions are usually treated successfully with wedge resection.

Chondromyxoid Fibroma
Chondromyxoid fibroma is a rare, benign cartilaginous tumor characteristically seen in the metaphysis of the proximal tibia (although it can be seen in any bone) as a multiloculated lesion with a sclerotic rim that resembles a "soap bubble" (Fig. 10-25). These fibromas have a trimodal appearance under the microscope (hence the name) with characteristic spindle cells that have cytoplasmic projections resembling boat propellers. They can be locally aggressive and should be treated with curettage and bone grafting.

Giant Cell Tumor of Bone
- Giant cell tumor of bone is a benign bone tumor that arises in the metaphyseal-epiphyseal region of bone (and almost always extends to

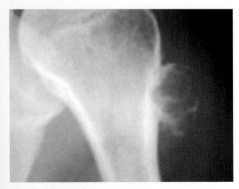

Figure 10-23. A periosteal chondroma of the proximal humerus. Note the surface lesion and the thin periosteal rim of bone.

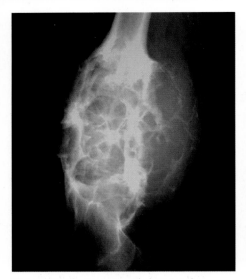

Figure 10-25. An extremely large and aggressive chondromyxoid fibroma of the femur displaying the classic "soap bubble" appearance.

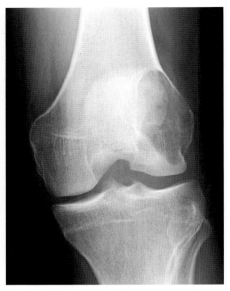

Figure 10-26. A giant cell tumor of the distal femur. Note the involvement of the epiphysis and metaphysis.

the subchondral region) in patients in their third through fifth decades of life. It is a lytic lesion usually without any sclerotic rim that can be aggressive and is often associated with a soft tissue mass (Figs. 10-26 and 10-27). Microscopically, there are large osteoclast-like giants cells with many nuclei in a stroma of mononuclear cells (Fig. 10-28). Like with chondroblastoma, "benign metastases" to the lung can occur and a chest radiograph to evaluate these patients is advisable (especially with lesions of the distal radius, which tend to be more aggressive).

- Because of their epiphyseal location, giant cell tumors can be challenging to treat. Curettage, high-speed burring, and some adjuvants (e.g., argon beam, cryotherapy, phenol) can reduce the rate of local recurrence and the defect can be filled with cement and/or bone graft. However, some aggressive disease requires wide excision and more complex reconstructions like joint replacement or fusion depending on the location and extent of disease.

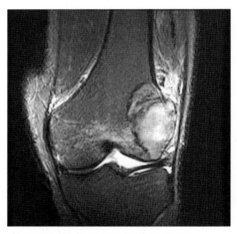

Figure 10-27. A T2-weighted magnetic resonance image of the giant cell tumor from Figure 10-26.

Fibrous Lesions
Nonossifying Fibroma

- Nonossifing fibroma, or NOF, is a benign, eccentric, metaphyseal lesion often seen as an incidental finding on radiographs done for another reason.

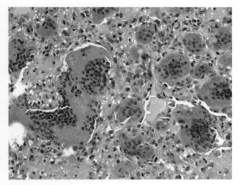

Figure 10-28. A high-power micrograph of a giant cell tumor demonstrating the large, multinucleated giant cells.

The lesion presents as a well-defined area of radiolucency with a sclerotic border found on the endosteal surface of bone in children and teenagers (Fig. 10-29). The natural history is to fill in with bone over time, and NOFs can usually be treated expectantly. However, some lesions are large and can cause pain and even pathologic fracture. In these instances, curettage, bone grafting, and fixation is often necessary.

Fibrous Dysplasia
- Fibrous dysplasia is a benign fibro-osseous proliferation during skeletal maturation that can occur in any bone but is most commonly seen in the femur and tibia. 80% of cases are isolated to a single bone (monostotic). Severe polyostotic cases are often associated with pigmented skin lesion and endocrine abnormalities (often precocious puberty), a syndrome called *McCune Albright disease.*
- Radiographically, fibrous dysplasia displays symmetric cortical thinning and expansile remodeling down the long axis of the bone leading to the "long lesion in a long bone" description of the disease (Fig. 10-30). The matrix of the tumor on radiographs is classically described as "ground glass" and represents the microscopic areas of dysplastic bone (in an "alphabet soup" or "Chinese letters" configuration) in a benign fibrous stroma.
- Fibrous dysplasia can weaken the bone, cause pain, and lead to fractures. Multiple fractures of the proximal femur over time lead to deformity and the classic "shepherd's crook" appearance. Asymptomatic lesions can be observed. Symptomatic lesions can be curetted and bone grafted.

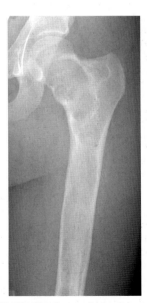

Figure 10-30. The "ground glass" appearance of fibrous dysplasia. Note the involvement of the entire bone.

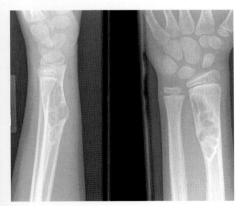

Figure 10-29. Anteroposterior and lateral views of a large nonossifying fibroma of the radius.

Unfortunately, the disease often returns and destroys the bone graft, so instrumentation or bulk allograft is usually employed.

Adamantinoma

- Adamantinoma is an exceedingly rare low-grade malignant fibrous tumor that almost always arises in the anterior cortex of the tibia in younger patients with closed growth plates. Radiographically, it is a bubbly, multiloculated lesion with sclerotic borders (Fig. 10-31). It has several different pathologic patterns, but cytokeratin is always expressed. It is a malignancy, so the patients have to be worked up for metastatic disease. Treatment is wide surgical excision only. A bulk allograft is often used for reconstruction.

Osteofibrous Dysplasia

- Osteofibrous dysplasia, also known as OFD or Campanacci disease, is a benign condition with a similar appearance to adamantinoma seen in the anterior cortex of the tibia in patients with open physes. Some experts believe it could represent a precursor

lesion to adamantinoma. It resembles fibrous dyplasia under the microscope, except the areas of dysplastic bone are rimmed by osteoblasts. Most cases are self-limited and stop growing at skeletal maturity, so watchful waiting is the treatment of choice.

Bone Cysts

- Bone cysts are benign, fluid-filled cavities that appear as radiolucent lesions on radiograph. MRI confirms the fluid nature and rules out a solid tumor.

Simple Bone Cyst

- A simple or unicameral bone cyst is a single-chambered, symmetric, and central lytic lesion seen in children and adolescents most commonly in the metaphysis of the proximal humerus just below the growth plate (although lesions in the proximal femur and about the knee occur). The lesion thins and expands the cortical bone, presenting with pain or a pathologic fracture (Fig. 10-32). A thin wafer of cortical

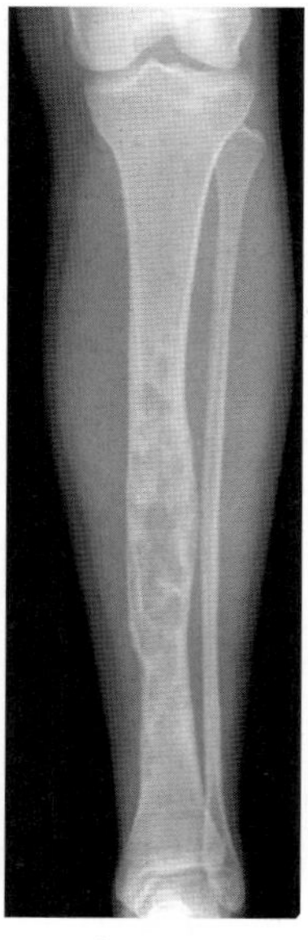

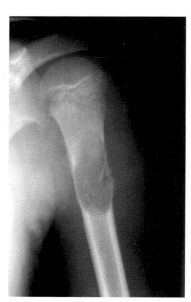

Figure 10-32. A pathologic fracture through a simpe bone cyst of the humerus. The wafer of cortical bone laterally is a "fallen leaf" sign.

Figure 10-31. An adamantinoma showing the expansile remodeling of the tibial cortex.

bone that fractures and floats to the bottom of the cyst is called a "fallen leaf" sign. In the proximal humerus, these fractures will heal with the cyst often recurring. Multiple fractures can lead to deformity. Treatment of proximal humerus lesions should begin with allowing fractures to heal followed by aspiration and injection of bone graft into the cyst. Sometimes, when the cyst has migrated away from the physis, intramedullary rods can be used to correct deformity or prevent further fractures. Because of the high stresses around the proximal femur, simple cysts in that area should be treated more aggressively with instrumentation.

Aneurysmal Bone Cyst

■ An aneurysmal bone cyst, or ABC, is a benign, eccentric, expansile, lytic lesion made up of multiple cavities filled with blood (Fig. 10-33). On MRI, the blood settles out and characteristic fluid-fluid levels are seen on T2-weighted images (Fig. 10-34). They most commonly occur around the knee but can also be seen in the posterior elements of the spine. ABCs can be locally aggressive and

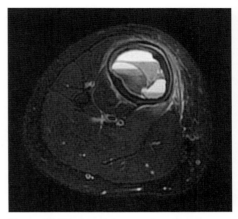

Figure 10-34. An axial magnetic resonance image of the cyst in Figure 10-33 shows the multiple septations and fluid-fluid levels.

mimic a telangiectatic osteosarcoma. Pathology should be carefully examined to rule out malignancy and a precursor lesion (such as chondroblastoma or chondromyxoid fibroma). Standard treatment is curettage and bone graft, but large lesions may need to be embolized as well.

Subchondral Cysts

■ Subchondral cysts are radiographically lucent lesions just below the joint surface that represent the collection of simple fluid through defects in the articular cartilage. The most common causes are osteoarthritis and posttraumatic. Treatment of large cysts may require curettage and bone grafting.

Epidermal Inclusion Cyst

■ An epidermal inclusion cyst can be seen in bone as a lytic lesion in the distal phalanges of the fingers and toes. There is normally a history of trauma, and theoretically epidermal tissue is introduced into the periosteum, where it proliferates into a cyst. These may present with pain or a fracture and can require curettage and bone grafting.

Intra-articular Tumors
Synovial Chondromatosis

■ Synovial chondromatosis is an intra-articular metaplastic disease in which

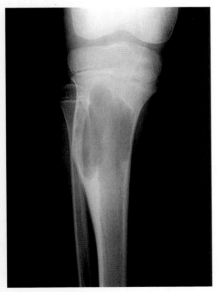

Figure 10-33. The eccentric, benign lucency of an aneurysmal bone cyst.

the synovial tissue forms multiple nodules of otherwise normal hyaline cartilage. These can be seen as a sea of calcified masses around a joint, with the knee being the most commonly affected (Fig. 10-35). The many loose bodies can damage the normal cartilage, so removal and synovectomy are the treatments of choice.

Pigmented Villonodular Synovitis

- Pigmented villonodular synovitis, or PVNS, is a benign, proliferative disease of the synovium. It can affect almost any joint, but it is most common in the knee of patients in their third or fourth decade of life. On MRI, due to the hemosiderin deposition in the tissue, the lesions have a characteristic low intensity on both T1- and T2-weighted images (Fig. 10-36). It can present as a focal, nodular mass or as a more diffuse, villous involvement of the entire joint. The nodular form is easily treated with excision, but the diffuse form can damage the joint and be challenging to treat (recurrence is common even after attempted total synovectomy).

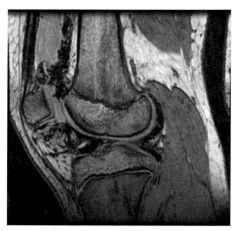

Figure 10-36. A sagittal magnetic resonance image of the knee joint demonstrating diffuse pigmented villonodular synovitis. The low-intensity areas represent the hemosiderin-rich tumor.

Eosinophilic Granuloma

- Eosinophilic grauloma (EG) is a benign, lytic bone lesion seen in children and adolescents, most commonly in flat bones and the diaphysis of long bones. It is often called the great imitator because of its varied appearance radiographically, but classically it is a well-defined "hole in bone" (Fig. 10-37). Histologically, eosinophils are usually seen along with larger histiocytic cells called Langerhans cells. EG can manifest as a systemic disease (Langerhans cell granulomatosis) and be seen in multiple bones and other organs. Treatment for bone disease can simply be steroid injection. Larger or unstable lesions may need curettage and fixation.

Soft Tissue Lesions

- The orthopaedic oncologist also treats soft tissue masses of the extremities and joints. There are many different benign and malignant soft tissue masses that may present in children and adults. These should be worked up with an MRI to gain as much knowledge about the actual tissue in addition to the anatomic location.
- Classically, a soft tissue sarcoma presents as an enlarging, painless

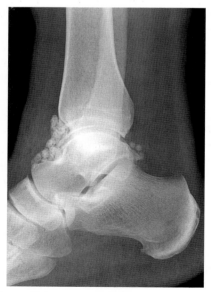

Figure 10-35. Synovial chondromatosis of the tibiotalar joint.

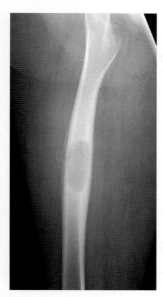

Figure 10-37. The "hole-in-bone" appearance of an eosinophilic granuloma of the femoral diaphysis with abundant periosteal reaction.

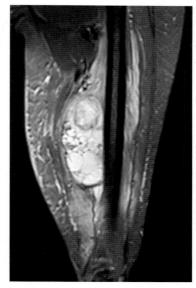

Figure 10-38. A T2-weighted magnetic resonance image of the thigh demonstrating the heterogenous, high-signal intensity of a soft tissue sarcoma.

mass in an older patient. The classic MRI findings of a soft tissue sarcoma (no matter what the histologic subtype) are intermediate intensity on T1-weighted images and bright and heterogeneous on T2-weighted images (Fig. 10-38). After being staged for metastatic disease with CT scans, these masses should be biopsied by or under the direction of the treating surgeon. Standard treatment is surgery and radiation therapy (it may be preoperative or postoperative depending on the tumor and surgeon preference). Chemotherapy is being studied as adjuvant treatment for soft tissue sarcomas and can be useful in some subtypes. Local recurrence rates for soft tissue sarcomas are low, but 5-year survival rates are poor, especially in patients with metastatic disease.

- Soft tissue masses in the extremities are most commonly benign, and there are many possible diagnoses. Lipomas, or benign fatty tumors, are exceedingly common and can be diagnosed from MRI alone before surgical resection. However, many benign soft tissue masses can have indeterminate MRI findings or even mimic a sarcoma. These masses should be referred to a treating surgeon for further treatment.

Splinting and Casting
Damond A. Cromer

11

INTRODUCTION

Splints and casts share a common purpose, which is to immobilize, protect, and/or counter a given musculoskeletal injury. The most notable difference between a splint and a cast, though, is that splints are designed to immobilize along three or fewer margins of an injured extremity, where casts immobilize circumferentially. Therein, splints are by property noncircumferential, which is often essential for the acute care of an injury, the aim being to adequately constrain an injury while still providing for any edema inherent to the acute inflammatory response thereof. Subsequently, casts are best used for the managed care of an injury, where edema has either resolved or is considered negligible to properly immobilizing the injury.

PEARLS OF SPLINTING AND CASTING

The following are some guidelines, tips, and recommendations for applying some of the more common extremity splints and casts. Bear in mind that these recommendations, although intended to suit most patients, should be adjusted accordingly. Children and smaller individuals will often be better fit in more narrow-width materials than described later, and likewise, larger width materials may better suit a larger individual. Common terms and considerations follow:

- The stockinette should fit the extremity without being too loose or tight.
- Cast/undercast padding should be appropriate to the diameter and length of the extremity.
- Plaster or synthetic (prefabricated) splint material should not overlap circumferentially but should be large enough to adequately maintain reduction of the injury.

- An elastic bandage or wrap should be appropriate to the diameter and length of the extremity.
- When wrapping the elastic bandage, be sure not to pull too much tension on the wrap or it could compromise circulation.
- When rolling the cast/undercast padding or synthetic cast tape, respectively, a 50% overlay technique is commonly employed (i.e., each new layer overlaps half the prior).
- When rolling the cast/undercast padding:
  - Pull just enough tension on the wrap so that it is taut but not so much that the material tears away.
  - The padding should be predominantly rolled from distal toward proximal.
  - Commonly, roll just enough padding to eliminate any residual shadow-effect (i.e., the padding should be relatively opaque versus the layers below, typically three layers thick)
- When ready to apply the splint:
  - Thoroughly wet the selected material with clean room-temperature water and squeeze out the excess water. A dry towel may be used to help absorb or damp dry the material as needed.
  - The warmer the water, the quicker the set time of the material; however, the heat released by the material also increases and this can be sufficient to cause skin burns or irritation.
  - If using plaster, keep in mind while measuring to fit the splint that plastic will shrink a bit when wet.
    - For the typical adult, a plaster splint will need to be between 10 and 15 layers thick for adequate stability.

- When ready to apply the cast:
  - Thoroughly wet the selected cast tape with clean room-temperature water and leave the material wet or lightly wring depending on time likely required for end application.
    - It is best to leave the material a bit saturated because any wringing will only quicken the set time of the material and care must be taken so that the material does not cure before the cast has finished being rolled in its entirety.
  - The warmer the water, the quicker the set time of the material as well, so follow the same guidelines.
  - Pay great care not to pull significant tension on the tape when wrapping the cast; simply unroll it onto the extremity to avoid compromising circulation.

SPLINTS
Upper Extremity Sugar Tong (Reverse) Splint: Figure 11-1, A
Common Indications
- Nondisplaced or minimally displaced fractures of the distal radius and ulna
- Maintaining reduced fractures of the distal radius
- Forearm fractures (radius or ulna shaft fractures)

Recommended Materials
- Stockinette: 2-inch width (1-inch width optional)
- Cast padding/Undercast padding: 3- and 4-inch width
- Plaster or synthetic (prefabricated) splint material: 3- or 4-inch width
- Elastic bandage/Wrap: 2-, 3-, and 4-inch width

Application
1) With the patient's arm flexed to approximately 90 degrees and their wrist at neutral, fit the 2-inch stockinette in length from just beyond the fingertips up to midway of the humerus. Cut a hole in the stockinette to adequately accommodate the thumb (Fig. 11-1, B).
   - The 1-inch width stockinette may be used specifically for the thumb to create a protective sleeve of padding by folding suitable length over on itself three times.

2) At the antecubital fossa, cut a slit in the stockinette (epicondyle to epicondyle), and pull the proximal portion of the stockinette to overlap the distal portion (or vice versa) (Figs. 11-1, C and 11-1, D).
3) Begin wrapping the padding at the metacarpal heads (MCHs) and proceed proximally with a 50% overlay. Figure-of-eight wrap around the elbow and apply ample padding around the bony prominences of the epicondyles. Continue wrap up to the midhumerus, but keep about 2 fingerbreadths distal to the stockinette edge (Fig. 11-1, E).
   - The 3-inch width padding works for wrapping the hand, wrist, and forearm, whereas the 4-inch width is suitable for wrapping from the forearm, elbow, and arm.
4) Measure so that the selected splint material fits as a "U" around the elbow and along the dorsal and volar sides of the arm all the way to the MCHs, respectively (Fig. 11-1, F).
5) Apply the splint material beginning on the volar side at the palmar crease of the hand, proximally toward the elbow, around the elbow, and back to just distal to the MCHs on the dorsal side of the hand. Any excess material can be trimmed away or folded back on itself.
   - Pay particular care to any material obstructing the thumb.
   - At the elbow, you may cut slits (ulnar toward radial) partway through the splint on both the volar and dorsal aspects, and overlap the wings of the splint material on itself to allow for a better mold around the elbow (Figs. 11-1, G and 11-1, H).
6) Pull the underlying stockinette and padding back over the splint at the distal and proximal ends, respectively (Fig. 11-1, I). This will protect and pad the patient from the edge of the splint at those areas.
7) Wrap the elastic bandage over the wet splint to just secure it in place. Wrap distal toward proximal; use a figure-of-eight wrap to cover around the elbow (Fig. 11-1, J).
8) The splint should be molded to maintain given reduction or with the wrist at neutral (functional) unless otherwise indicated.

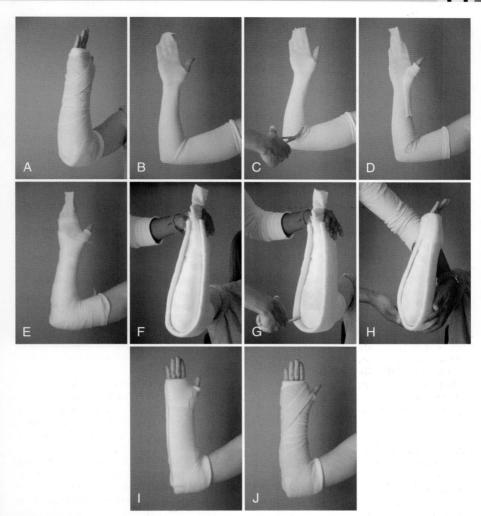

Figure 11-1. A, Upper extremity sugar tong (reverse) splint. **B,** Apply stockinette. **C,** Cut the stockinette and overlap at the antecubital fossa. **D,** Create a protective sleeve of padding over the thumb with the stockinette and fold over on itself. **E,** Apply casting padding. **F,** Apply splint and trim to fit. **G,** Cut slits in the splint at the elbow to create wings that overlap. **H,** Mold the wings around the elbow. **I,** Fold the ends of the stockinette back over the splint. **J,** Wrap elastic bandage over splint to secure in place.

Upper Extremity Long Arm Posterior Splint: Figure 11-2, A

Common Indications
- Distal humerus fractures
- Radial head/neck fractures
- Proximal ulna fractures
- Reduced elbow dislocations
- Elbow sprains/strains

Recommended Materials
- Stockinette: 2-inch width (1-inch width optional)
- Cast padding/Undercast padding: 3- and 4-inch width
- Plaster or fiberglass (prefabricated) splint material: 4- or 5-inch width
- Elastic bandage/Wrap: 2-, 3-, and 4-inch width

Application
1) With the patient's arm flexed to approximately 90 degrees and their wrist at neutral, fit the 2-inch stockinette in length from just beyond the fingertips up to (and with some gather at) the axilla. Cut a hole in the stockinette to adequately accommodate the thumb (Fig. 11-2, B).
- The 1-inch width stockinette may be used specifically for the thumb to create a protective sleeve of padding by folding suitable length over on itself three times.
2) At the antecubital fossa, cut a slit in the stockinette (epicondyle to epicondyle) and pull the proximal portion of the stockinette to overlap the distal portion (or vice versa) (Fig. 11-2, C).
3) Begin wrapping the padding at the MCHs and proceed proximally with a 50% overlay. Figure-of-eight wrap at the elbow, and apply ample padding around the bony prominences of the epicondyles. Continue wrapping up to the axilla (Fig. 11-2, D).
- The 3-inch width padding works for wrapping the hand, wrist, and forearm, whereas the 4-inch width is suitable for wrapping from the forearm, elbow, and arm.
4) Measure so that the selected splint material fits from the fifth MCH to the axilla.
5) Apply the splint material beginning on the ulnar side at the palmar crease along the fifth metacarpal of the hand, along the ulna, posteriorly along the elbow up just distal to the axilla. Any excess material can be trimmed away or folded back on itself (Fig. 11-2, E).
- Pay particular care to any material obstructing the axilla.
- At the elbow, you may cut partway through the splint on both the volar and dorsal aspects, and then overlap the wings of the splint material on itself to allow for a better mold around the elbow (Fig. 11-2, F).
6) Pull the underlying stockinette and padding back over the splint at the distal and proximal ends, respectively. This will protect and pad the patient from the edge of the splint at those areas.
7) Wrap the elastic bandage over the wet splint to just secure it in place. Wrap distal toward proximal; use a figure-of-eight wrap to cover around the elbow.
8) The splint should be molded to maintain given reduction and with the wrist in a functional position unless otherwise indicated.

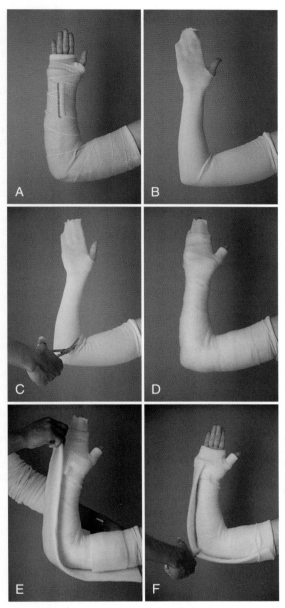

Figure 11-2. A, Upper extremity long arm posterior splint. **B,** Apply stockinette. **C,** Cut the stockinette and overlap at the antecubital fossa. **D,** Apply casting padding. **E,** Apply splint and trim to fit. **F,** Fold the ends of the stockinette back over the splint. Cut slits in the splint at the elbow to create wings that overlap to mold around the elbow.

Upper Extremity Volar Short Arm Splint: Figure 11-3, A

Common Indications
- Finger injuries
- Metacarpal injuries
- Carpal injuries (excluding occult scaphoid or trapezium fractures)
- Protection of lacerations of the hand/wrist/forearm
- Wrist sprains/strains

Recommended Materials
- Stockinette: 2-inch width (1-inch width optional)
- Cast padding/Undercast padding: 3-inch width
- Plaster or synthetic (prefabricated) splint material: 3- or 4-inch width
- Elastic bandage/Wrap: 2-inch and 3-inch width

Application
1) With the patient's wrist at neutral, fit the 2-inch stockinette in length from just beyond the fingertips up to the antecubital fossa. Cut a hole in the stockinette to adequately accommodate the thumb (Fig. 11-3, B).
   - If enclosing the fingers in the splint, place padding between each finger, respectively, to protect against skin maceration.
   - The 1-inch width stockinette may be used specifically for the thumb to create a protective sleeve of padding by folding suitable length over on itself three times (Fig. 11-3, C).
2) Begin wrapping the padding at the MCHs and proceed proximally with a 50% overlay. Continue wrapping up to the antecubital fossa (Figs. 11-3, D and 11-3, E).
   - If enclosing the fingers in the splint, alternatively begin wrapping the padding at the distal phalanges.
3) Measure so that the selected splint material fits in length from the MCHs to within about two to three finger-breadths (about 2 inches) of the antecubital fossa.
   - Start measuring from the distal phalanges if protecting for finger or metacarpal injuries.
4) Apply the splint material beginning on the volar side at the palmar crease of the hand, proximally toward the antecubital fossa. Any excess material can be trimmed away or folded back on itself (Fig. 11-3, F).
   - Pay particular care to any material obstructing the thumb or antecubital fossa.
5) Pull the underlying stockinette and padding back over the splint at the distal and proximal ends, respectively. This will protect and pad the patient from the edge of the splint at those areas (Fig. 11-3,G).
6) Wrap the elastic bandage over the wet splint to secure it in place. Wrap distal toward proximal.
7) The splint should be molded as to counter the given injury or with the wrist at neutral unless otherwise indicated.

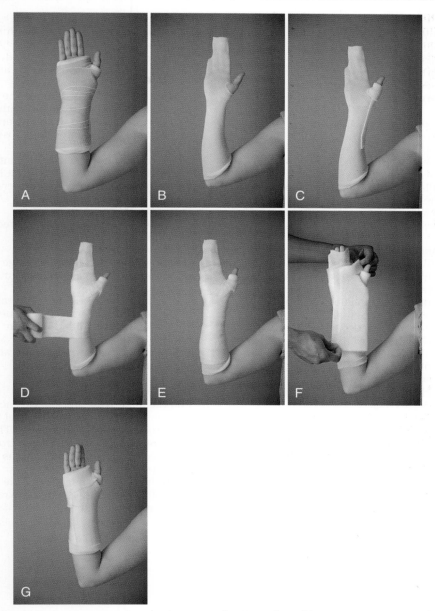

Figure 11-3. A, Upper extremity volar short arm splint. **B,** Apply stockinette. **C,** Create a protective sleeve of padding over the thumb with the stockinette and fold over on itself. **D,** Apply casting padding. **E,** Apply casting padding. **F,** Apply splint and trim to fit. **G,** Fold the ends of the stockinette back over the splint.

Upper Extremity Thumb Spica Splint: Figure 11-4, A

Common Indications
- Thumb injuries
- Wrist injuries (occult/suspected scaphoid or trapezium fractures)
- Wrist sprains/Strains

Recommended Materials
- Stockinette: 2-inch width (1-inch width optional but shown)
- Cast padding/Undercast padding: 3-inch width
- Plaster or synthetic (prefabricated) splint material: 3- or 4-inch width
- Elastic bandage/Wrap: 2- and 3-inch width

Application
1) With the patient's wrist at neutral, fit the 2-inch stockinette in length from just beyond the fingertips up to the antecubital fossa. Cut a hole in the stockinette to adequately accommodate the thumb (Fig. 11-4, B).
   - The 1-inch width stockinette may be used specifically for the thumb to create a protective sleeve of padding by folding suitable length over on itself three times (Fig. 11-4, C):
     - Interphalangeal joint (IP) free = If leaving the distal phalanx free, the collar should be just proximal to the distal interphalangeal joint (DIP).
     - IP joint included = If enclosing the distal phalanx, the collar should approach the thumb tip.

- Alternative to 1-inch stockinette, about three layers of 3-inch width cast/undercast padding may be wrapped circumferentially around the thumb (same considerations as earlier)
2) Begin wrapping the padding at the MCHs and proceed proximally with a 50% overlay. Continue wrapping up to just distal to the antecubital fossa (Figs. 11-4, D and 11-4, E).
3) Measure so that the selected splint material fits in length from the MCHs to within about two to three finger-breadths (about 2 inches) of the antecubital fossa.
4) Apply the splint material centered over the radial border of the thumb and forearm, beginning just proximal to the padded edge of stockinette (or cast/undercast padding) protecting the thumb proximally toward the antecubital fossa. Any excess material can be trimmed away or folded back on itself (Fig. 11-4, F).
   - Pay particular care to any material that would otherwise make the splint circumferential about the thumb.
5) Pull the underlying stockinette back just over the padding at the distal and proximal ends, respectively. This will protect and pad the patient from the edge of the cast at those areas (Fig. 11-4, G).
6) Wrap the elastic bandage over the wet splint to secure it in place. Wrap distal toward proximal.

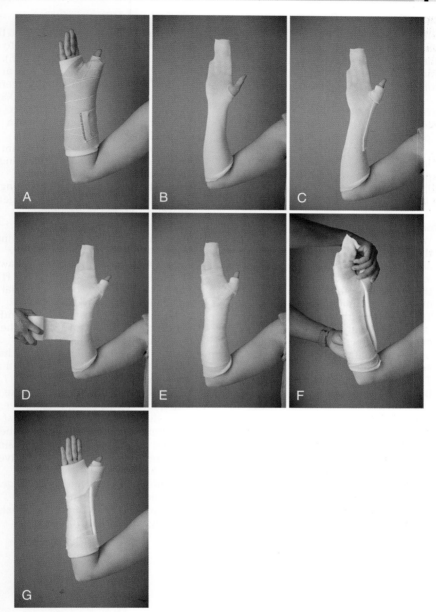

Figure 11-4. **A,** Upper extremity thumb spica splint. **B,** Apply stockinette. **C,** Create a protective sleeve of padding over the thumb with the stockinette and fold over on itself. **D,** Apply casting padding. **E,** Apply casting padding. **F,** Apply splint and trim to fit. **G,** Fold the ends of the stockinette back over the splint.

Upper Extremity Ulnar Gutter Splint: Figure 11-5, A

Common Indications
- Ring and small finger injuries
- Ring and small finger metacarpal injuries

Recommended Materials
- Stockinette: 2-inch width (1-inch width optional)
- Cast/Undercast padding: 3-inch width
- Plaster or synthetic (prefabricated) splint material: 4- or 5-inch width
- Elastic bandage/Wrap: 2- and 3-inch width

Application
1) With the patient's wrist at neutral, fit the 2-inch stockinette in length from about 1 inch beyond the fingertips up to the antecubital fossa. Cut a hole in the stockinette to adequately accommodate the thumb (Fig. 11-5, B).
   - The 1-inch width stockinette may be used specifically for the thumb to create a protective sleeve of padding by folding suitable length over on itself three times (Fig. 11-5, C).
   - The 1-inch width stockinette may also be used specifically for the ring and small fingers (instead of cast/undercast padding as described later) to create a similar sleeve of padding to capture both digits. In this case, fit the stockinette and roll the cast/undercast padding in the same manner as for the volar short arm splint, omitting the relevant steps that follow.
2) At the distal end of the stockinette, cut a slit in the stockinette longitudinally toward the web space between the long and ring fingers (Fig. 11-5, D).

3) Trim or fold a few layers of cast/undercast padding to place between the length of the ring and small fingers to prevent skin maceration (Fig. 11-5, E).
4) Begin wrapping the padding just at the tips of the ring and small fingers and proceed proximally with a 50% overlay. Continue wrapping up to just distal to the antecubital fossa (Figs. 11-5, F and 11-5, G).
5) Measure so that the selected splint material fits from the tip of the ring finger to the antecubital fossa.
6) Apply the splint material beginning on the ulnar side of the small finger (distally equal to the ring ginger) forming a "gutter" along the fifth metacarpal and the ulna proceeding toward the antecubital fossa. Any excess material can be trimmed away or folded back on itself (Fig 11-5, H).
   - Pay particular care to any material obstructing the antecubital fossa.
7) Pull the underlying stockinette and padding back over the splint at the distal and proximal ends, respectively. This will protect and pad the patient from the edge of the splint at those areas.
8) Wrap the elastic bandage over the wet splint to just secure it in place. Wrap distal toward proximal.
9) The splint should be molded at the fingers, hand, and wrist to maintain a given reduction or counter the given injury as indicated.
   - Commonly the ring and small fingers are molded fully extended in the intrinsic plus position (metacarpal phalangeal joints in 70 degrees of flexion, interphalangeal joints extended).

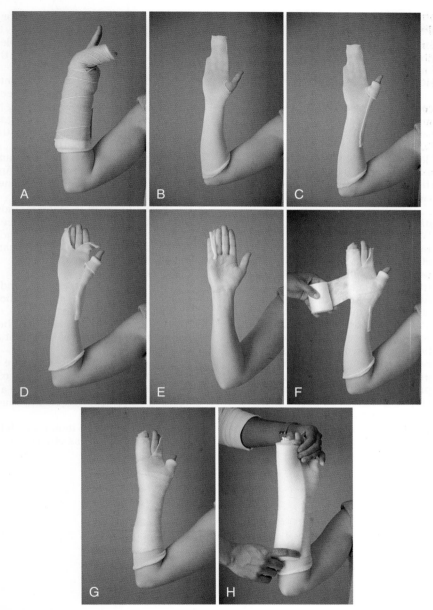

Figure 11-5. A, Upper extremity ulnar gutter splint. **B,** Apply stockinette. **C,** Create a protective sleeve of padding over the thumb with the stockinette and fold over on itself. **D,** Cut a slit in the stockinette between the long and ring fingers. **E,** Place some cast padding between the fingers to prevent skin maceration. **F,** Apply cast padding starting around the wrist and fingers. **G,** Continue cast padding proximally. **H,** Apply splint and trim to fit.

Lower Extremity Sugar Tong (Ankle-Stirrup/U) Splint:
Figure 11-6, A

Common Indications
- Ankle sprains/Strains
- Medial and lateral malleolus injuries

Recommended Materials
- Stockinette: 3-inch width
- Cast/Undercast padding: 4- and/or 6-inch width
- Plaster or synthetic (prefabricated) splint material: 3-inch width
- Elastic bandage/Wrap: 4- and 6-inch width

Application
1) With the patient's ankle at neutral (ankle dorsiflexed to approximately 90 degrees), fit the 3-inch stockinette in length distally from the MTHs up to the patella and popliteal fossa.
2) At the ankle joint, cut a slit in the stockinette (malleolus to malleolus) and pull the proximal portion of the stockinette to overlap the distal portion (or vice versa) (Fig. 11-6, B).
3) Begin wrapping the padding just proximal to the MTHs and proceed proximally with a 50% overlay. Figure-of-eight wrap at the ankle/heel and apply ample padding around the bony prominences of the malleoli. Continue wrapping up to the tibial tuberosity (Fig. 11-6, C).

- The 4-inch width padding works for wrapping the midfoot and ankle, whereas the 6-inch width is suitable for wrapping from the ankle up to the tibial tuberosity.
4) Measure so that the selected splint material fits as a "U" under the heel of the foot and up the ankle along the lateral and medial sides of the leg all the way to even with the level of the fibular head (Fig. 11-6, D).
5) Apply the splint material in the same manner used to measure above. Any excess material can be trimmed away or folded back on itself.
   - Pay particular care to any material obstructing the motion of the knee.
   - Center the splint on the lateral and medial sides of the leg and take care not to overlap the proximal ends (Fig. 11-6, E).
6) Pull the underlying stockinette and padding back over the splint at the distal and proximal ends, respectively. This will protect and pad the patient from the edge of the splint at those areas.
7) Wrap the elastic bandage over the wet splint to just secure it in place. Wrap distal toward proximal; use a figure-of-eight wrap to cover around the ankle and heel.
8) The splint should be molded with the ankle at neutral unless otherwise indicated.

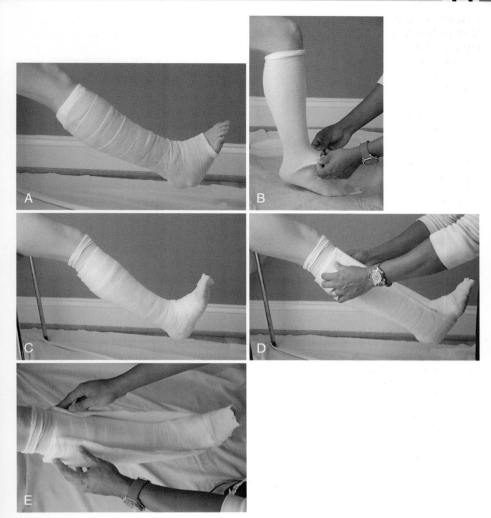

Figure 11-6. A, Lower extremity sugar tong (ankle stirrup/U) splint. **B,** Apply stockinette and create a fold over the anterior ankle. **C,** Apply cast padding. **D,** Apply splint and trim to fit. **E,** Center the splint on the lateral and medial sides of the leg and care not to overlap the proximal ends.

Lower Extremity Posterior Leg Splint: Figure 11-7, A

Common Indications
- Ankle sprains/Strains
- Ankle dislocations
- Achilles tendon ruptures
- Distal tibia and fibula fractures
- Tarsal injuries
- Metatarsal injuries

Recommended Materials
- Stockinette: 3-inch width
- Cast/Undercast padding: 4- and 6-inch width
- Plaster or synthetic (prefabricated) splint material: 4-inch width
- Elastic bandage/Wrap: 4- and 6-inch width

Application
1) With the patient's ankle at neutral (ankle dorsiflexed ≈ 90 degrees), fit the 3-inch stockinette in length about 1 inch distal to the hallux up to the patella and popliteal fossa.
   - In the case of an Achilles tendon injury, particularly, the foot should be kept in slight equinus (plantar flexion).
2) At the ankle joint, cut a slit in the stockinette (malleolus to malleolus) and pull the proximal portion of the stockinette to overlap the distal portion (or vice versa) (Fig. 11-7, B).
3) Begin wrapping the padding just distal to the MTHs and proceed proximally with a 50% overlay. Figure-of-eight wrap at the ankle and heel and apply ample padding around the bony prominences of the malleoli. Continue wrapping up to the tibial tuberosity (Figs. 11-7, C and 11-7, D).
   - The 4-inch width padding works for wrapping the foot and ankle, whereas the 6-inch width is suitable for wrapping the leg.
4) Measure so that the selected splint material fits in length posteriorly from the MTHs to the popliteal fossa.
5) Apply the splint material in the same manner used to measure above. Any excess material can be trimmed away or folded back on itself (Fig. 11-7, E).
   - Pay particular care to any material obstructing the motion of the knee or intruding the popliteal fossa.
   - At the heel, you may cut partway through the splint on both the lateral and medial aspects and then overlap the wings of the splint material on itself to allow for a better mold around calcaneus (Fig. 11-7, F).
6) Pull the underlying stockinette and padding back over the splint at the distal and proximal ends, respectively. This will protect and pad the patient from the edge of the splint at those areas.
7) Wrap the elastic bandage over the wet splint to just secure it in place. Wrap distal toward proximal; use a figure-of-eight wrap to cover around the ankle and heel.
8) The splint should be molded to maintain the patient's ankle at neutral unless otherwise indicated.

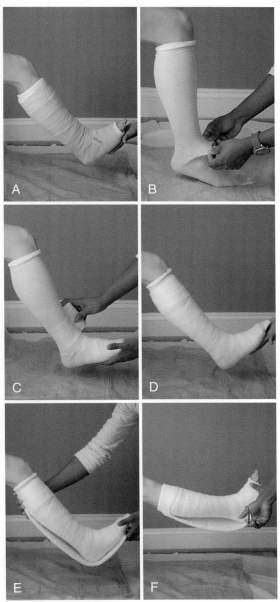

Figure 11-7. A, Lower extremity posterior leg splint. **B,** Apply stockinette and create a fold over the anterior ankle. **C,** Apply cast padding. **D,** Apply cast padding with ankle in neutral. **E,** Apply splint and trim to fit. **F,** Fold the ends of the stockinette back over the splint and cut splint to create wings that mold around the ankle.

Lower Extremity Long Leg Splint: Figure 11-8, A

Common Indications
- Knee injuries
- Unstable tibia and fibula fractures

Recommended Materials
- Stockinette: 4-inch width
- Cast/Undercast padding: 4- and 6-inch width
- Plaster or synthetic (prefabricated) splint material: 4- or 5-inch width
- Elastic bandage/Wrap: 4- and 6-inch width

Application
1) With the patient's ankle at neutral (ankle dorsiflexed ≈90 degrees) and the knee just slightly flexed (≈15 degrees), fit the 4-inch stockinette in length about 1 inch distal to the hallux up to (and with some gather at) the groin (Fig. 11-8, B).
2) At the ankle joint, cut a slit in the stockinette (malleolus to malleolus) and pull the proximal portion of the stockinette to overlap the distal portion (or vice versa).
3) Begin wrapping the padding just distal to the MTHs and proceed proximally with a 50% overlay. Figure-of-eight wrap about the ankle and heel and apply ample padding around the bony prominences of the malleoli. Likewise, use ample padding on the bony prominences of the knee. Continue wrapping up to the groin (Figs. 11-8, C and 11-8, D).

- The 4-inch width padding works for wrapping the distal portion, whereas the 6-inch width is suitable for the proximal portion.
4) Measure so that the selected splint material fits in length posteriorly from the MTHs to the gluteal sulcus.
5) Apply the splint material in the same manner used to measure above. Any excess material can be trimmed away or folded back on itself (Fig. 11-8, E).
   - Pay particular care to any material obstructing the motion of the leg or intruding the groin or buttock.
   - At the heel, you may cut partway through the splint on both the lateral and medial aspects and then overlap the wings of the splint material on itself to allow for a better mold around the calcaneus.
6) Pull the underlying stockinette and padding back over the splint at the distal and proximal ends, respectively. This will protect and pad the patient from the edge of the splint at those areas.
7) Wrap the elastic bandage over the wet splint to just secure it in place. Wrap distal toward proximal; use a figure-of-eight wrap to cover around the ankle and heel.
8) The splint should be molded to maintain the patient's ankle at neutral and knee slightly bent unless otherwise indicated.

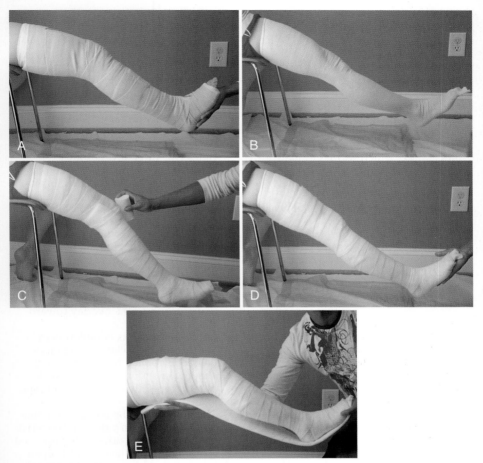

Figure 11-8. A, Lower extremity long leg splint. **B,** Apply stockinette. **C,** Apply cast padding. **D,** Apply cast padding with ankle in neutral. **E,** Apply splint and trim to fit.

CASTS
Short Arm Cast: Figure 11-9, A

Common Indications
- Metacarpal fractures
- Carpal fractures (*excluding* scaphoid or trapezium fractures)
- Distal radius and ulna fractures
- Management of soft tissue injuries affecting the hand or wrist

Recommended Materials
- Stockinette: 2-inch width (1-inch width optional but shown)
- Cast padding/Undercast padding: 3-inch width
- Synthetic (fiberglass, polyester) cast tape: 3-inch width

Application
1) With the patient's wrist at neutral, fit the 2-inch stockinette in length from just beyond the fingertips up to the antecubital fossa. Cut a hole in the stockinette to adequately accommodate the thumb (Fig. 11-9, B).
- The 1-inch width stockinette may be used specifically for the thumb to create a protective sleeve of padding by folding suitable length over on itself three times (Fig. 11-9, C).
2) Begin wrapping the padding at the MCHs and proceed proximally with a 50% overlay. Continue wrapping up to just distal to the antecubital fossa (Figs. 11-9, D and 11-9, E).
3) Pull the underlying stockinette back just over the padding at the distal and proximal ends, respectively. This will protect and pad the patient from the edge of the cast at those areas (Fig. 11-9, F).
4) Begin wrapping the cast tape at the wrist joint (Fig. 11-9, G). One wrap circumferentially around to anchor is suitable before proceeding distally to fit the tape proper about the hand/palm. At the first web space, cut proportionately through the width of the tape proximal toward distal, laying the remaining width through web space and the newly cut ends dorsal and volar about the base of the thumb, respectively (Fig. 11-9, H). Roll the tape circumferentially en route just proximal to the base of the thumb to overlay both of the cut ends. Fit the tape through the web space in this manner two additional times (for three layers total).
- Keep the tape proximal to the padded edge of stockinette (i.e., proximal to the distal palmar crease and proximal to the MCHs dorsally).
5) Continue wrap proceeding proximally with a 50% overlay up toward the antecubital fossa, but keep about one fingerbreadth distal to the padded edge of stockinette (Fig. 11-9, I).
6) Roll the tape three times around the proximal end before proceeding back distally with a 50% overlay toward the wrist.
- Roll the tape to its completion or cut the roll free when enough tape has been applied to eliminate any shadow effect or noticeable weak points (typically three layers of tape is ideal)
7) The cast should be molded to counter the given injury or with the wrist at neutral unless otherwise indicated.
- Continually rub the cast with open hands to help laminate and smooth the layers until the cast has set firm with care not create any undue indentations or pressure points.
  - Avoid using fingertips while molding.
- Be sure to apply a careful interosseous mold about the distal radius/ulna by sandwiching the palms dorsally and volarly, respectively, with adequate pressure.
  - This is particularly important when casting fractures in children.

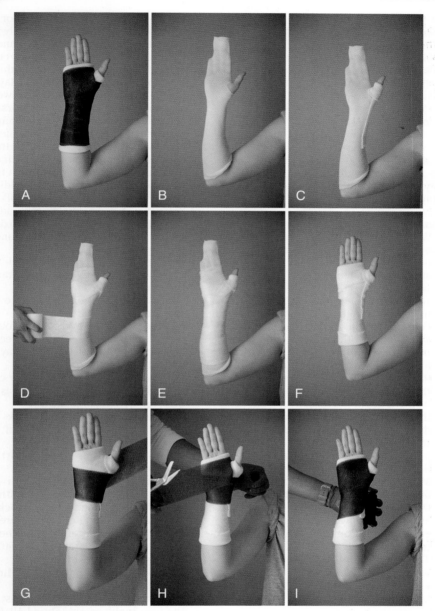

Figure 11-9. A, Short arm cast. **B,** Apply stockinette. **C,** Create a protective sleeve of padding over the thumb with the stockinette and fold over on itself. **D,** Apply cast padding. **E,** Apply cast padding. **F,** Fold the ends of the stockinette back over the cast padding. **G,** Begin wrapping the cast tape at the wrist. **H,** Partially cut the cast tape from proximal to distal and place between the first web space and repeat two additional times. **I,** Continue wrapping cast tape proximally.

Long Arm Cast: Figure 11-10, A

Common Indications
- Distal humerus fractures
- Radius and ulna shaft fractures
- Proximal radius and ulna fractures
- Distal radius and ulna fractures in children

Recommended Materials
- Stockinette: 2-inch width (1-inch width optional but shown)
- Cast padding/Undercast padding: 3- and 4-inch width
- Synthetic (fiberglass, polyester) cast tape: 3- and 4-inch width

Application
1) With the patient's elbow flexed to approximately 90 degrees and his or her wrist at neutral, fit the 2-inch stockinette in length from just beyond the fingertips up to (and with some gather at) the axilla. Cut a hole in the stockinette to adequately accommodate the thumb (Fig. 11-10, B).
- The 1-inch width stockinette may be used specifically for the thumb to create a protective sleeve of padding by folding suitable length over on itself three times.
2) At the antecubital fossa, cut a slit in the stockinette (epicondyle to epicondyle) and pull the proximal portion of the stockinette to overlap the distal portion (or vice versa) (Fig. 11-10, C).
3) Begin wrapping the padding at the MCHs and proceed proximally with a 50% overlay. Figure-of-eight wrap at the elbow, and apply ample padding around the bony prominences of the epicondyles. Continue wrapping up to the axilla (Fig. 11-10, D).
- The 3-inch width padding works for wrapping the hand, wrist, and forearm, whereas the 4-inch width is suitable for wrapping from the forearm, elbow, and arm.
4) Pull the underlying stockinette back just over the padding at the distal and proximal ends, respectively. This will protect and pad the patient from the edge of the cast at those areas (Fig. 11-10, E).
5) Begin wrapping the 3-inch width cast tape at the wrist joint. One wrap circumferentially around to anchor is suitable before proceeding distally to fit the tape properly about the hand and palm. At the first web space, cut proportionately through the width of the tape proximal toward distal, laying the remaining width through web space and the newly cut ends dorsal and volar about the base of the thumb, respectively. Roll the tape circumferentially en route just proximal to the base of the thumb to overlay both of the cut ends. Fit the tape through the web space in this manner two additional times (for three layers total).
- Keep the tape proximal to the padded edge of stockinette (i.e., proximal to the distal palmar crease and proximal to the MCH dorsally)
6) Continue wrap proceeding proximally with a 50% overlay up toward the antecubital fossa, but keep about one fingerbreadth distal to the antecubital fossa.
7) Roll the tape three layers thick around the proximal forearm before proceeding back distally with a 50% overlay toward the wrist (Fig. 11-10, F).
- Roll the tape to its completion or cut the roll free when enough tape has been applied to eliminate any shadow effect or noticeable weak points (typically ≥ three layers of coverage ideal).
- The cast should resemble a short arm cast at this point.
8) Begin wrapping the 4-inch width cast tape about two fingerbreadths distal to the padded edge of stockinette at the axilla. Roll circumferentially three layers thick around before proceeding distally with a 50% overlay toward the elbow.
9) Figure-of-eight wrap the elbow three times, and overlap at least half width the still wet end of the cast at the proximal forearm (Fig. 11-10, G). Ensure adequate coverage at the elbow (three or more layers) before proceeding proximally with a 50% overlay toward the axilla.
- Roll the tape to its completion or cut the roll free when enough tape has been applied to eliminate any shadow effect or noticeable weak

points (typically three or more layers of coverage is ideal).

10) To further unify the distal and proximal portions of the cast, wrap another 3-inch width cast tape beginning at the distal end capturing the hand (one layer as earlier) before proceeding proximally with a 50% overlay to the proximal end at the axilla (one layer).

- Cut the roll free or optionally roll the tape to its completion with a 50% overlay proceeding distally again toward the hand and wrist.

11) The cast should be molded to counter the given injury or with the

wrist at neutral unless otherwise indicated.

- Continually rub the cast with open hands to help laminate and smooth the layers until the cast has set firm with care not to create any undue indentations or pressure points.
  - Avoid using fingertips while molding.
- Be sure to apply a careful interosseous mold about the distal radius/ulna by sandwiching the palms dorsally and volarly, respectively, with adequate pressure.
  - This is particularly important when casting fractures in children.

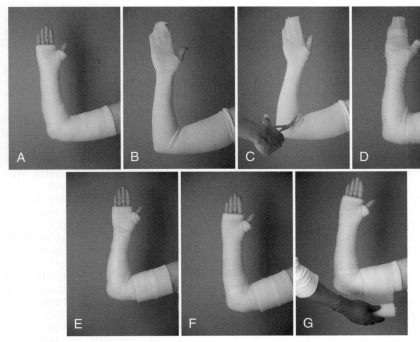

Figure 11-10. A, Long arm cast. **B,** Apply stockinette. **C,** Cut the stockinette and overlap at the antecubital fossa. **D,** Apply cast padding. **E,** Fold the ends of the stockinette back over the cast padding. **F,** Apply cast tape from distal to proximal. Partially cut the cast tape from proximal to distal and place between the first web space and repeat two additional times. **G,** Apply the cast tape proximally and use a figure-of-eight around the elbow.

Thumb Spica Cast:
Figure 11-11, A

Common Indications
- Thumb fractures
- Thumb sprains/strains
- Scaphoid or trapezium fractures (*including* occult or suspected fractures)
- Management of some wrist sprains/strains

Recommended Materials
- Stockinette: 2-inch width (1-inch width optional but shown)
- Cast padding/Undercast padding: 3-inch width
- Synthetic (fiberglass, polyester) cast tape: 3-inch width

Application
1) With the patient's wrist at neutral, fit the 2-inch stockinette in length from just beyond the fingertips up to the antecubital fossa. Cut a hole in the stockinette to adequately accommodate the thumb (Fig. 11-11, B).
   - The 1-inch width stockinette may be used specifically for the thumb to create a protective sleeve of padding by folding suitable length over on itself three times (Fig. 11-11, C):
     - IP free = If leaving the distal phalanx free, the collar should be just proximal to the DIP.
     - IP joint included = If enclosing the distal phalanx, the collar should approach the thumb tip.
   - Alternative to 1-inch stockinette, about three layers of 3-inch width cast/undercast padding may be wrapped circumferentially around the thumb (same considerations as mentioned earlier).
2) Begin wrapping the padding at the MCHs and proceed proximally with a 50% overlay. Continue wrapping up to just distal to the antecubital fossa (Figs. 11-11, D and 11-11, E).
3) Pull the underlying stockinette back just over the padding at the distal and proximal ends, respectively. This will protect and pad the patient from the edge of the cast at those areas (Fig. 11-11, F).

4) Begin wrapping the 3-inch width cast tape at the wrist joint. One wrap circumferentially around to anchor is suitable before proceeding distally to fit the tape proper about the thumb, hand, and palm.
5) To fit the tape around the thumb, roll the tape to the dorsal-radial border of the thumb and approaching the first web space, cut partially through the width (proximal toward distal) to just fit the tape around the proximal phalanx segment of the thumb (or distal phalanx segment additionally if IP joint is included). Continue through and around the respective phalanx segment(s) circumferentially back to the dorsal-radial border of the thumb again. Fit the tape around the thumb in this manner two additional times (for three layers total) (Figs. 11-11, G and 11-11, H).
   - Keep the tape just proximal to the padded edge of stockinette (or cast/undercast padding) protecting the thumb.
6) To fit the tape about the hand and palm, from the thumb roll toward the first web space, cut proportionately through the width of the tape proximal toward distal, laying the remaining width through the web space and the newly cut ends dorsal and volar about the base of the thumb, respectively (Fig. 11-11, I). Roll the tape circumferentially en route just proximal to the base of the thumb to overlay both of the cut ends. Fit the tape through the web space in this manner two additional times (for three layers total).
   - Keep the tape proximal to the padded edge of the stockinette (i.e., proximal to the distal palmar crease and proximal to the MCH dorsally).
   - When fitting the tape through the web space and about the thumb as described earlier, be sure to overlay the proximal-most portion of tape of the thumb spica.
7) Continue wrap proceeding proximally with a 50% overlay up toward the

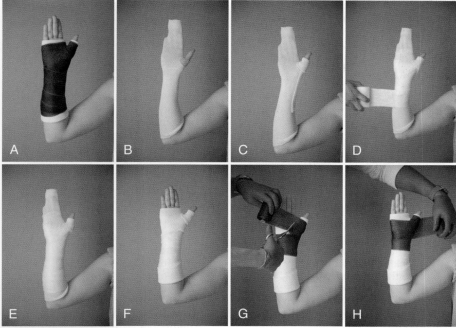

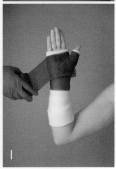

Figure 11-11. A, Thumb spica cast. **B,** Apply stockinette. **C,** Create a protective sleeve of padding over the thumb with the stockinette and fold over on itself. **D,** Apply cast padding. **E,** Apply cast padding. **F,** Fold the ends of the stockinette back over the cast padding. **G,** Apply the cast tape starting at the wrist. Wrap from the dorsal-radial thumb toward the first web space. Cut the cast tape from proximal to distal in order to cover the proximal phalanx when placed into the first web space. **H,** Repeat two additional times around the thumb. **I,** To fit the tape over the hand and palm, cut the tape from proximal to distal and lay into the first web space so that the newly cut ends surround the thumb.

antecubital fossa, but keep about one fingerbreadth distal to the padded edge of the stockinette.

8) Roll the tape three times around the proximal end before proceeding back distally with a 50% overlay toward the wrist.

- Roll the tape to its completion or cut the roll free when enough tape has been applied to eliminate any shadow effect or noticeable weak points (typically three layers of tape is ideal).

9) The cast should be molded to counter the given injury or with the wrist and thumb at neutral unless otherwise indicated.

- Continually rub the cast with open hands to help laminate and smooth the layers until the cast has set firm, taking care to not create any undue indentations or pressure points.
  - Avoid using fingertips while molding.
- Be sure to apply a careful interosseous mold about the distal radius/ulna by sandwiching the palms dorsally and volarly, respectively, with adequate pressure.
  - This is particularly important when casting fractures in children.

Outrigger (Routinely Ulnar Gutter) Cast: Figure 11-12, A

Common Indications
- Ring and small finger fractures
- Ring and small finger metacarpal fractures

Recommended Materials
- Stockinette: 2-inch width (1-inch width optional but shown)
- Cast padding/Undercast padding: 3-inch width
- Synthetic (fiberglass, polyester) cast tape: 3-inch width

Application

1) With the patient's wrist at neutral, fit the 2-inch stockinette in length from about 1 inch beyond the fingertips up to the antecubital fossa. Cut a hole in the stockinette to adequately accommodate the thumb (Fig. 11-12, B).
   - The 1-inch width stockinette may be used specifically for the thumb to create a protective sleeve of padding by folding suitable length over on itself three times (Fig. 11-12, C).
2) At the distal end of the stockinette, cut a slit in the stockinette longitudinally toward the web space between the long and ring fingers (Fig. 11-12, D).
3) Trim and fold a few layers of cast/undercast padding to place between the length of the ring and small fingers to prevent skin maceration (Fig. 11-12, E).
   - These fingers can (optionally) be secured to one another via buddy-tape to further stabilize the injury.
4) Begin wrapping the padding just at the tips of the ring and small fingers and proceed proximally with a 50% overlay (Figs. 11-12, F and 11-12, G). Continue wrapping up to just distal to the antecubital fossa.
5) Pull the underlying stockinette back just over the padding at the distal and proximal ends, respectively. This will protect and pad the patient from the edge of the cast at those areas (Fig. 11-12, H).
6) Begin wrapping the 3-inch width cast tape at the wrist joint (preferably starting on the volar surface rolling radial toward ulnar). One wrap circumferentially around to anchor is suitable before proceeding distally.

7) To fit the tape about the respective phalanges, angle and roll the tape to the dorsal aspect of the phalanges, even with the radial border of the ring finger cut at a slight angle partially through the width (proximal toward distal) to just fit the tape through the long and ring finger web space and around the ring and small finger phalanx segment(s) (Fig. 11-12, I). Continue through and around the respective phalanx segment(s) circumferentially back to the dorsal-radial border of the ring finger again. Fit the tape around the phalanges in this manner two additional times (for three layers total).
   - Keep the tape just proximal to the padded edge of stockinette (or cast/undercast padding), protecting the phalanges.
   - Tuck or trim any tape that would intrude the long and ring finger web space or distal palm, respectively.
8) To fit the tape about the hand, from the phalanges roll toward the first web space, cut proportionately through the width of the tape proximal toward distal, laying the remaining width through web space and the newly cut ends dorsal and volar about the base of the thumb, respectively. Roll the tape circumferentially en route just proximal to the base of the thumb to overlay both of the cut ends. Fit the tape through the web space in this manner two additional times (for three layers total).
9) Continue wrap proceeding proximally with a 50% overlay up toward the antecubital fossa, but keep about one fingerbreadth distal to the padded edge of stockinette.
10) Roll the tape three times around proximal end before proceeding back distally with a 50% overlay toward the wrist.
    - Roll the tape to its completion or cut the roll free when enough tape has been applied to eliminate any shadow effect or noticeable weak points (typically three layers of tape is ideal).
11) The cast should be molded to counter the given injury, commonly with the wrist in moderate extension and the ring and small fingers molded

fully extended in the intrinsic plus position (metacarpal phalangeal joints in about 70 degrees of flexion) unless otherwise indicated.

■ Continually rub the cast with open hands to help laminate and smooth the layers until the cast has set firm, taking care to not create any undue indentations or pressure points.

• Avoid using fingertips while molding.

■ Be sure to apply a careful interosseous mold around the distal radius/ulna by sandwiching the palms dorsally and volarly, respectively, with adequate pressure.

• This is particularly important when casting fractures in children.

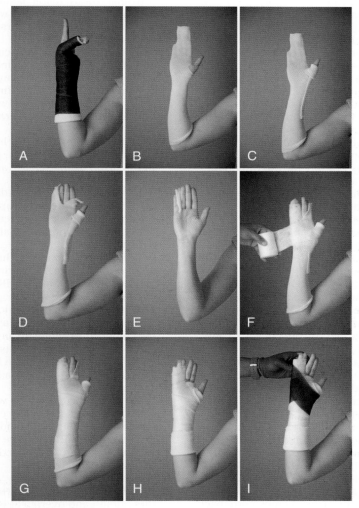

Figure 11-12. A, Outrigger (ulnar gutter) cast. **B,** Apply stockinette. **C,** Create a protective sleeve of padding over the thumb with the stockinette and fold over on itself. **D,** Cut a slit in the stockinette between the long and ring fingers. **E,** Place some cast padding between the fingers to prevent skin maceration. **F,** Apply cast padding starting around the wrist and fingers. **G,** Continue the cast padding proximally. **H,** Fold the ends of the stockinette back over the cast padding. **I,** Begin wrapping the cast tape at the wrist and angle toward the fingers. Wrap around the fingers, cutting the cast tape from proximal to distal to fit between the long and ring finger web space.

Muenster Cast: Figure 11-13, A

Common Indications
- Distal radius and ulna fractures
- Radius and ulna shaft fractures

Recommended Materials
- Stockinette: 2-inch width (1-inch width optional but shown)
- Cast padding/Undercast padding: 3- and 4-inch width
- Synthetic (fiberglass, polyester) cast tape: 3- and 4-inch width

Application
1) With the patient's elbow flexed to approximately 90 degrees and his or her wrist at neutral, fit the 2-inch stockinette in length from just beyond the fingertips up to midway of the humerus. Cut a hole in the stockinette to adequately accommodate the thumb (Fig. 11-13, B).
   - The 1-inch width stockinette may be used specifically for the thumb to create a protective sleeve of padding by folding suitable length over on itself three times (Fig. 11-13, C).
2) At the antecubital fossa, pull the proximal portion of the stockinette to overlap the distal portion to create a measurable fold (tongue) to be used subsequently.
   - The tongue should resemble a crescent that extends from epicondyle to epicondyle (as shown in preceding figure).
3) Begin wrapping the padding at MCHs and proceed proximally with a 50% overlay. Figure-of-eight wrap at the elbow and apply ample padding around the bony prominences of the epicondyles. Continue wrapping up to the midhumerus, but keep about two fingerbreadths distal to the stockinette edge (Fig. 11-13, D).
   - The 3-inch width padding works for wrapping the hand, wrist, and forearm, whereas the 4-inch width is suitable for wrapping from the forearm, elbow, and arm.
4) Pull the underlying stockinette back just over the padding at the distal end. This will protect and pad the patient from the edge of the cast at that area (Fig. 11-13, E).

- The underlying stockinette at the proximal end will be pulled back over for padding at that end subsequently.
5) Begin wrapping the 3-inch width cast tape at the wrist joint. One wrap circumferentially around to anchor is suitable before proceeding distally to fit the tape proper about the hand. At the first web space, cut proportionately through the width of the tape proximal toward distal, laying the remaining width through the web space and the newly cut ends dorsal and volar about the base of the thumb, respectively. Roll the tape circumferentially en route just proximal to the base of the thumb to overlay both of the cut ends. Fit the tape through the web space in this manner two additional times (for three layers total) (Fig. 11-13, F).
   - Keep the tape proximal to the padded edge of the stockinette (i.e., proximal to the distal palmar crease and proximal to the MCHs dorsally).
6) Continue wrapping, proceeding proximally with a 50% overlay up toward the antecubital fossa but keeping about one fingerbreadth distal to the antecubital fossa.
7) Roll the tape three layers thick around the proximal forearm before proceeding back distally with a 50% overlay toward the wrist.
   - Roll the tape to its completion or cut the roll free when enough tape has been applied to eliminate any shadow effect or noticeable weak points (typically ≥ 3 layers of coverage ideal)
   - The cast should resemble a short arm cast at this point.
8) Begin wrapping the 4-inch width cast tape just distal to the cast/undercast padding at the midhumerus. Roll circumferentially three layers total around before proceeding distally with a 50% overlay toward the elbow.
9) Figure-of-eight wrap about the elbow three times, and overlap at least one-half width (2 inches) the still wet end of the cast at the proximal forearm. Ensure adequate coverage about the elbow (three or more

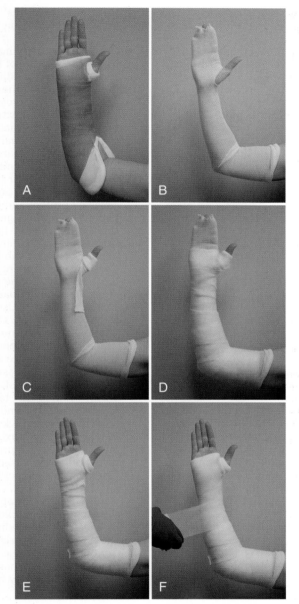

Figure 11-13. A, Muenster cast. **B,** Apply stockinette. **C,** Create a protective sleeve of padding over the thumb with the stockinette and fold over on itself. **D,** Apply cast padding. **E,** Fold the ends of the stockinette back over the cast padding. **F,** Apply cast tape from distal to proximal. Partially cut the cast tape from proximal to distal and place between the first web space and repeat two additional times.

layers) before proceeding proximally with a 50% overlay toward the mid-humerus (Fig. 11-13, G).

■ Roll the tape to its completion or cut the roll free when enough tape has been applied to eliminate any shadow effect or noticeable weak points (typically three or more layers of coverage is ideal).

■ The cast should resemble a shortened long arm cast at this point.

10) The cast should be molded to counter the given injury or with the wrist at neutral unless otherwise indicated.

■ Continually rub the cast with open hands to help laminate and smooth the layers until the cast has set firm, taking care to not create any undue indentations or pressure points.

• Avoid using fingertips while molding.

■ Be sure to apply a careful interosseous mold around the distal radius/ulna by sandwiching the palms dorsally and volarly, respectively, with adequate pressure.

• This is particularly important when casting fractures in children.

11) Once the cast has set firm, tailor the proximal portion using an oscillating cast saw (Figs. 11-13, H and 11-13, I). Remove the areas otherwise obstructing the extension and flexion of the elbow while still leaving the portions that reduce the pronation and supination of the wrist.

■ Ergo, the cast should ultimately curve around two to three fingerbreadths proximal to the lateral and medial epicondyles, respectively, scoop down (distal) just proximal to the olecranon posteriorly, with an appropriate two to

three fingerbreadths' notch extending along the length of the proximal radius anteriorly.

■ Remove the overlying cast with care to remove as little of the underlying cast/undercast padding as possible.

12) Cut a slit through the middle of the anterior cast/undercast padding proximal to distal extending to the notch at the proximal forearm. Fold the padding proximal to distal to rim the proximal margins of the cast, and pull the underlying stockinette taut back over the padding and the cast at the proximal end. This will protect and pad the patient from the edge of the cast at those areas (Fig. 11-13, J).

■ The tongue of stockinette (created in Step 2 earlier) can be accessed once the cast/undercast padding has been slit and the proximal stockinette pulled back over the cast as described. Use this tongue to further tailor the stockinette/padding about the notch by pulling it taut distally, the ends of which will be fixed in place subsequently when overlaid by cast tape.

13) To complete the cast, wet another 3-inch width of cast tape and begin wrap at the distal end capturing the hand (one layer thick as earlier) before proceeding proximally with a 50% overlay to the proximal end to just capture the unsecured stockinette (one layer thick) (Figs. 11-13, K and 11-13, L).

■ Cut the roll free or optionally roll the tape to its completion with a 50% overlay proceeding distally again toward the wrist and hand.

14) Continually rub the cast with open hands to help laminate and smooth the layers until they have set firm.

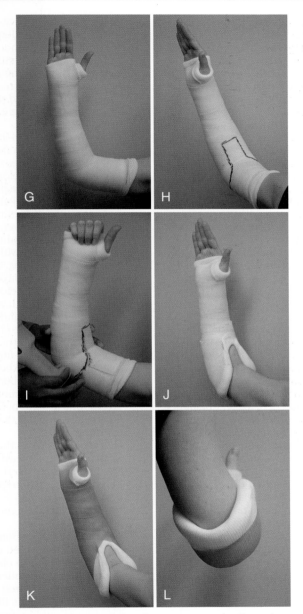

Figure 11-13—cont'd. G, Continue wrapping the cast tape proximally up the arm and use a figure-of-eight around the elbow. Allow to set with the elbow in the desired position. **H,** Draw lines around the elbow to guide cutting. **I,** Cut the splint using an oscillating cast saw. **J,** Fold the ends of the stockinette back over the cut end of the cast. **K,** Apply another layer of cast tape from distal to proximal and lay over the ends of the stockinette. **L,** Posterior view of completed cast.

Short Leg Non–Weight-Bearing Cast: Figure 11-14, A

Common Indications
- Ankle sprains/Strains
- Ankle dislocations
- Achilles tendon ruptures
- Distal tibia and fibula fractures
- Tarsal fractures
- Metatarsal fractures

Recommended Materials
- Stockinette: 3-inch width
- Cast/Undercast padding: 4- and/or 6-inch width
- Synthetic (fiberglass, polyester) cast tape: 3- and 4-inch width
- Self-adhering orthopaedic foam: 4-inch width
  - If self-adhering foam is unavailable, about five layers of 4-inch width cast/undercast padding may be substituted.

Application
1) With the patient's ankle at neutral (ankle dorsiflexed to approximately 90 degrees) fit the 3-inch stockinette in length about 1 inch distal to the hallux up to the patella and popliteal fossa.
   - In the case of an Achilles tendon injury, particularly, the foot should be kept in moderate equinus (plantar flexion).
2) At the ankle joint, cut a slit in the stockinette (malleolus to malleolus) and pull the proximal portion of the stockinette to overlap the distal portion (or vice versa) (Fig. 11-14, B).
3) Begin wrapping the padding just distal to the MTHs and proceed proximally with a 50% overlay. Use a figure-of-eight wrap about the ankle and heel and apply ample padding around the bony prominences of the malleoli. Continue wrapping up to the tibial tuberosity (Figs. 11-14, C and 11-14, D).
4) Fit and apply the self-adhering orthopaedic foam (or cast/undercast padding) to extend anteriorly from just distal to the MTHs up to the tibial tuberosity (centered directly over the foot/shin). Additionally, apply a section of foam just even with the tibial tuberosity yet extending laterally from fibular head to proximal-medial tibia. Lastly, apply a section

of foam posteriorly at the heel with length and width adequate to protect the Achilles tendon insertion.
5) Pull the underlying stockinette back just over the padding at the distal and proximal ends, respectively. This will protect and pad the patient from the edge of the cast at those areas (Fig. 11-14, E).
6) Begin wrapping the 4-inch width cast tape just proximal to the ankle joint. One wrap circumferentially around to anchor is suitable before proceeding distally to fit the tape properly around the foot and ankle. Figure-of-eight wrap the ankle three times, and ensure adequate coverage around the heel (three or more layers) before proceeding distally with a 50% overlay toward the MTHs (Fig. 11-14, F).
7) Roll the tape three layers thick around the MTHs before proceeding back proximally with a 50% overlay toward and/or beyond the ankle joint. Roll the tape to its completion.
8) Begin wrapping another 4-inch width cast tape about two fingerbreadths distal to the padded edge of stockinette at the tibial tuberosity/popliteal fossa. Roll circumferentially three layers total around before proceeding distally with a 50% overlay toward the ankle.
9) Figure-of-eight wrap the ankle and further overlap at least the midfoot. Ensure adequate overlay around the heel and ankle before proceeding proximally with a 50% overlay back toward the tibial tuberosity and popliteal fossa.
   - Roll the tape to its completion or cut the roll free when enough tape has been applied to eliminate any shadow effect or noticeable weak points (typically three or more layers of coverage is ideal).
10) The cast should be molded to maintain the patient's ankle at neutral unless otherwise indicated.
    - Continually rub the cast with open hands to help laminate and smooth the layers until the cast has just set firm, taking care to not create any undue indentations or pressure points.
      - Avoid using fingertips while molding.

- Shape and mold to accommodate the malleoli and Achilles tendon insertion.
11) To further unify the distal and proximal portions of the cast, wrap another 4-inch width of cast tape (or 3-inch width, alternatively) beginning at the distal end (one layer) before proceeding proximally with a 50% overlay to the proximal end at the tibial tuberosity and popliteal fossa (one layer).
    - Cut the roll free or optionally roll the tape to its completion with a 50% overlay proceeding distally again toward the foot and ankle.
12) Continually rub the cast with open hands to help laminate and smooth the layers until the cast has set firm.

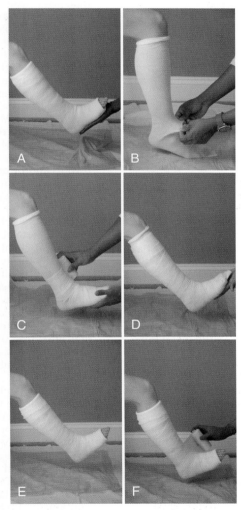

Figure 11-14. A, Short leg non–weight-bearing cast. **B,** Apply stockinette and create a fold over the anterior ankle. **C,** Apply cast padding. **D,** Apply cast padding with the ankle in neutral. **E,** Fold the ends of the stockinette back over the cast padding. **F,** Apply cast tape from distal to proximal and use a figure-of-eight around the ankle.

Short Leg Walking Cast:
Figure 11-15, A

Common Indications
- Ankle sprains/Strains
- Ankle dislocations
- Distal tibia and fibula fractures
- Tarsal fractures
- Metatarsal fractures

Recommended Materials
- Stockinette: 3-inch width
- Cast/Undercast padding: 4- and 6-inch width
- Synthetic (fiberglass, polyester) cast tape: 3- and 4-inch width
- Synthetic (prefabricated) splint material: 3- or 4-inch width
- Self-adhering orthopaedic foam: 4-inch width
  - If self-adhering foam is unavailable, about five layers of 4-inch width cast/undercast padding may be substituted.

Application
1) With the patient's ankle at neutral (ankle dorsiflexed ≈ 90 degrees), fit the 3-inch stockinette in length about 1 inch distal to the hallux up to the patella and popliteal fossa.
   - Casting the ankle at neutral (even minute dorsal flexion) is essential for the walking cast to allow proper balance and toe-off.
2) At the ankle joint, cut a slit in the stockinette (malleolus to malleolus) and pull the proximal portion of the stockinette to overlap the distal portion (or vice versa) (Fig. 11-15, B).
3) Begin wrapping the padding just distal to the MTHs and proceed proximally with a 50% overlay. Figure-of-eight wrap the ankle and heel and apply ample padding around the bony prominences of the malleoli. Continue wrapping up to the tibial tuberosity (Figs. 11-15, C and 11-15, D).
4) Fit and apply the self-adhering orthopaedic foam (or cast/undercast padding) to extend anteriorly from just distal to the MTHs up to the tibial tuberosity (centered directly over the foot and anterior tibia). Additionally, apply a section of foam just even with the tibial tuberosity yet extending laterally from fibular head to

proximal-medial tibia. Lastly, apply a section of foam posteriorly at the heel with length and width adequate to protect the Achilles tendon insertion.
5) Pull the underlying stockinette back just over the padding at the distal and proximal ends, respectively. This will protect and pad the patient from the edge of the cast at those areas (Fig. 11-15, E).
6) Begin wrapping the 4-inch width cast tape just proximal to the ankle joint. One wrap circumferentially around to anchor is suitable before proceeding distally to fit the tape properly around the foot/ankle. Figure-of-eight wrap the ankle three times, and ensure adequate coverage about the heel (three or more layers) before proceeding distally with a 50% overlay toward the MTHs (Fig. 11-15, F).
7) Roll the tape three times thick around the MTHs before proceeding back proximally with a 50% overlay toward and/or beyond the ankle joint. Roll the tape to its completion.
8) Begin wrapping another 4-inch width cast tape about two finger-breadths distal to the padded edge of stockinette at the tibial tuberosity and popliteal fossa. Roll circumferentially three layers total around before proceeding distally with a 50% overlay toward the ankle.
9) Figure-of-eight wrap the ankle and further overlap at least the midfoot. Ensure adequate overlay around the heel and ankle before proceeding proximally with a 50% overlay back toward the tibial tuberosity and popliteal fossa.
   - Roll the tape to its completion or cut the roll free when enough tape has been applied to eliminate any shadow effect or noticeable weak points (typically three or more layers of coverage is ideal.)
10) The cast should be molded to maintain the patient's ankle at neutral as indicated (Fig. 11-15, G).
   - Continually rub the cast with open hands to help laminate and smooth the layers until the cast has set firm, taking care to not create any undue indentations or pressure points.
     - Avoid using fingertips while molding.

11) Measure so that the selected splint material fits double the length of the patient's foot from the MTHs to the heel. Remove the splint material from any protective sleeve it may be contained in, fold the splint over on itself, and subsequently trim it to roughly proportion the sole of the patient's foot. Hold this in place (Fig. 11-15, H).

12) To further unify the distal and proximal portions of the cast and to tie in the newly made cast sole, wrap another 4-inch width of cast tape (or 3-inch width alternatively) beginning at the distal end (one layer) before proceeding proximally with a 50% overlay to the proximal end at the tibial tuberosity and popliteal fossa (one layer) (Fig. 11-15, I).

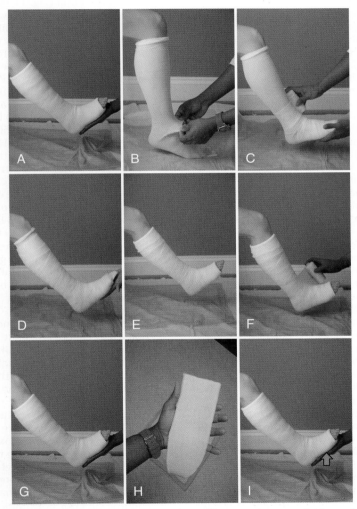

Figure 11-15. A, Short leg walking cast. **B,** Apply stockinette and create a fold over the anterior ankle. **C,** Apply cast padding. **D,** Apply cast padding with the ankle in neutral. **E,** Fold the ends of the stockinette back over the cast padding. **F,** Apply cast tape from distal to proximal and use a figure-of-eight around the ankle. **G,** Allow to set with the ankle in neutral. **H,** Splint material, doubled over and trimmed. **I,** Apply splint material to dorsum of foot and secure with another layer of cast tape around the foot and ankle.

■ Cut the roll free or optionally roll the tape to its completion with a 50% overlay proceeding distally again toward the foot/ankle.

13) Continually rub the cast with open hands to help laminate and smooth the layers until the cast has set firm.

Long Leg Cast: Figure 11-16, A

Common Indications
■ Unstable tibia/Fibula fractures

Recommended Materials
■ Stockinette: 4-inch width
■ Cast/Undercast padding: 4- and/or 6-inch width
■ Synthetic (fiberglass, polyester) cast tape: 3- and 4-inch width
■ Self-adhering orthopaedic foam: 4-inch width is commonly suitable
  • If self-adhering foam is unavailable, about five layers of 4-inch width cast/undercast padding may be substituted.

Application
1) With the patient's ankle at neutral (ankle dorsiflexed to approximately ≈90 degrees) and the knee just slightly flexed (≈15 degrees), fit the 4-inch stockinette in length about 1 inch distal to the hallux up to (and with some gather at) the groin (Fig. 11-16, B).
2) At the ankle joint, cut a slit in the stockinette (malleolus to malleolus) and pull the proximal portion of the stockinette to overlap the distal portion (or vice versa).
3) Begin wrapping the padding just distal to the MTHs and proceed proximally with a 50% overlay. Figure-of-eight wrap the ankle and heel and apply ample padding around the bony prominences of the malleoli. Likewise, amply pad the bony prominences of the knee. Continue wrapping up to the groin (Figs. 11-16, C and 11-16, D).
4) Pull the underlying stockinette back just over the padding at the distal and proximal ends, respectively. This will protect and pad the patient from the edge of the cast at those areas (Fig. 11-16, E).

5) Fit and apply the self-adhering orthopaedic foam (or cast/undercast padding) to extend anteriorly from just distal to the MTHs up to the tibial tuberosity (centered directly overtop the foot and anterior tibia). Additionally, apply a square section of foam over each condyle. Lastly, apply a section of foam posteriorly at the heel with length and width adequate to protect the Achilles tendon insertion (Fig. 11-16, F).
6) Begin wrapping the 4-inch width cast tape just proximal to the ankle joint. One wrap circumferentially around to anchor is suitable before proceeding distally to fit the tape properly around the foot and ankle. Figure-of-eight wrap the ankle three times, and ensure adequate coverage around the heel (three or more layers) before proceeding distally with a 50% overlay toward the MTHs (Fig. 11-16, G).
7) Roll the tape three layers thick around the MTHs before proceeding back proximally with a 50% overlay toward and/or beyond the ankle joint. Roll the tape to its completion.
8) Begin wrapping another 4-inch width cast tape about two to three fingerbreadths distal to the padded edge of stockinette at the groin and gluteal sulcus. Roll circumferentially three layers thick around before proceeding distally with a 50% overlay toward the knee.
9) Figure-of-eight wrap the knee three times and ensure adequate overlay around the knee and popliteal fossa before proceeding proximally with a 50% overlay back toward the groin and gluteal sulcus. Roll the tape to its completion.
10) Begin wrapping another 4-inch width cast tape to quickly capture the ankle joint before proceeding proximally with a 50% overlay capture the knee.
■ Roll the tape to its completion or cut the roll free when enough tape has been applied to eliminate any shadow effect or noticeable weak points along the length of the entire cast (typically three or more layers of coverage is ideal).

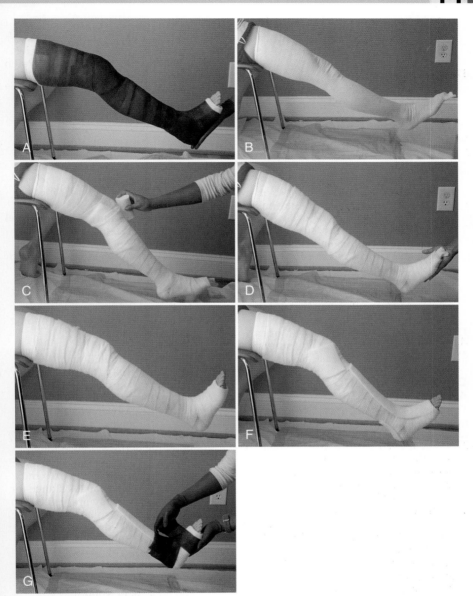

Figure 11-16. A, Long leg cast. **B,** Apply stockinette. **C,** Apply cast padding. **D,** Keep the ankle in neutral. **E,** Fold the ends of the stockinette back over the cast padding. **F,** Apply self-adhering orthopaedic foam padding to the anterior foot, ankle, and tibia, bilateral knee condyles, and the posterior heel. **G,** Apply cast tape from distal to proximal and use a figure-of-eight around the ankle.

11) The cast should be molded to maintain the patient's ankle at neutral and knee slightly bent unless otherwise indicated.
   ■ Continually rub the cast with open hands to help laminate and smooth the layers until the cast has just set firm, taking care to not create any undue indentations or pressure points.
      • Avoid using fingertips while molding.
12) To further unify the distal and proximal portions of the cast, wrap another 4-inch width of cast tape (or 3-inch width alternatively) beginning at the distal end (one layer) before proceeding proximally with a 50% overlay to the proximal end at the groin and gluteal sulcus (one layer). Use a subsequent roll if necessary.
   ■ Cut the roll free or optionally roll the tape to its completion with a 50% overlay proceeding distally again toward the foot and ankle.
13) Continually rub the cast with open hands to help laminate and smooth the layers until the cast has set firm.

CRUX OF SPLINTING AND CASTING

The effect of the splint or cast is ultimately as dependent on the compliance of the patient as its proper application. Essential to complete application of the splint or cast, the patient's care instructions on discharge should include the following:
■ Keep the splint or cast and the skin around the edges clean and dry:
   • When showering or bathing: Roll up a small towel and wrap it around your arm or leg, just about the splint or cast (do not tuck the towel into the splint or cast) and tape the towel into place. Place an arm or leg into a bag. Tape the bag into place.
   • Protect the splint or cast from getting wet during rain.
   • A wet splint or cast must be changed within 24 hours to prevent skin breakdown.

■ Do not put anything down inside of your splint or cast:
   • No powder, spray, lotion, water or liquids, or foreign objects to scratch under the splint or cast
■ Do not pull out the padding.
■ Do not remove the splint or cast.
■ Regular activities should include upper/lower extremity range of motion and edema control:
   • Move all joints/appendages not immobilized by the splint/cast.
   • Massage fingers/toes from the tips toward extremity several times daily as needed.
   • Elevate the extremity above the level of your heart (20 to 30 minutes, several times daily), especially whenever any of the following symptoms occur:
      • Increased swelling
      • Increased pressure
      • Increased tightness of cast
      • Increased thumping or throbbing
      • Increased pain, tingling, or numbness
      • Decreased circulation at the end of the extremity (fingers/toes)
■ Use a marker to circle any drainage from wounds on the outside of splint or cast. Report any changes in the amount of drainage.
■ A splint or cast is meant to be snug and immobilize the involved joint; however, it should not cut off or decrease circulation to the extremity.
■ Report or seek medical assistance for any of the following symptoms within 24 hours of cast or splint application:
   • Increase in pain, pressure, swelling, tingling, or numbness that cannot be controlled with elevation and movement (range of motion)
   • An increase in drainage, foul odor, fever, nausea, or vomiting
   • Any splint or cast that gets wet, cracked, broken, or too loose
   • Any pain related to rubbing or sores caused by rubbing

Wound Care 12
Shruti Tannan and Adam Katz

WOUNDS
Fundamentals of Wound Healing
- The wound healing process is like a symphony, requiring many integral components to work together toward a common goal—healing a wound.
- Normal wound healing begins with the initial platelet plug in the inflammatory phase, to a proliferative collagen-producing phase and an ultimate remodeling phase, which can last up to 1 year. Platelets, neutrophils, macrophages, and fibroblasts interact via multiple cytokines and cell signaling pathways to coordinate the transition from one phase to another.
- The arrest of a wound in one of those states, as well as prevention of progress to the next phase, may result in a nonhealing wound. As part of a surgical team, it is helpful to recognize potential challenges to normal wound healing and prepare patients for delayed wound healing or refer them promptly when indicated.

Principles of Wound Care
History
- Identify any comorbid medical conditions or medications that could delay normal wound healing:
- Medical Conditions
  - Diabetes
  - Vascular disease
  - Smoking
  - Malnutrition
  - Radiation history (at location of wound)
  - Autoimmune disorders
- Obtain a history of taking anticoagulants (aspirin, clopidogrel, coumadin) and the reason for taking them.

- Medications
  - Immunosuppression (for transplant recipients, autoimmune diseases)
  - Prednisone (steroids)
  - Chemotherapy
- Clarify the Wound Etiology or Mechanism of Injury
1) Is it acute or chronic?
   - If chronic, how long has the wound been there, and what has been tried before?
2) Was the offending agent contaminated or relatively clean?

Physical Examination
- Inspect the Wound for Injury to Neurovascular or Tendinous Structures
- Inspect the Wound for Hemostasis, Exposed Bone, or Hardware if Postsurgical

Acute Wounds
- Inspect the wound for the degree of contamination (e.g., road rash, grass, dirt).
- Determine if there is actual tissue loss versus the appearance of a "gaping wound" because the wound margins are pulled in opposite directions.
  - This helps distinguish wounds with sharply cut margins that can be reapproximated from ones with skin and soft tissue loss that can be treated with local wound care acutely.
- Determine if there is a skin avulsion or a flap of skin detached from underlying structures but attached to intact skin along one margin.
  - If so, then assess the viability of the skin by checking for capillary refill in the flap or seeing if it bleeds after a pinprick from an 18-gauge needle.

Chronic Wounds
- Is the wound clean or does it have necrotic debris? Is there evidence of infection?
- Is the patient sensate in the anatomic location of the wound (i.e., plantar ulcer with lack of plantar sensation)?
- Does the patient have palpable pulses in the extremity with the wound?
- Is there exposed bone (or tendon)? If so, osteomyelitis must be considered.

Principles of Wound Care: Treatment
Acute Wounds
Irrigation and Débridement
1) Irrigate the wound with sterile normal saline with a device producing 7 to 15 pounds per square inch (psi) of pressure. Examples include commercially available pulse lavage devices and a 30-mL syringe attached to an 18-gauge angiocatheter.
2) Débride the wound of any contaminants such as grass and gravel. Minimize actual excision of tissue in the acute setting, and only débride obviously nonviable tissues.

Closure
- To minimize scarring, close acute wounds on extremities (excluding the hand and fingers) in layers.
  - Use monofilament suture for contaminated wounds to minimize bacterial seeding of braided suture (see later section on Sutures).
  - Avoid tension-creating techniques (vertical and horizontal mattress suture repair) because these are more likely to cause necrosis of the skin edges.
  - Approximate muscle with strong absorbable monofilament suture that will last around 90 days (e.g., PDS suture).
  - Approximate dermis with absorbable monofilament suture that will last around 40 days (e.g., Monocryl).
  - Approximate skin with permanent monofilament suture that will be removed in 1 to 2 weeks (e.g., Prolene, Nylon).
  - Wounds on the hand, fingers, and plantar foot should be closed in one layer only, with permanent monofilament suture taking bites through the epidermis and dermis.

Chronic Wounds
- Treatment is based on the etiology of the chronicity of the wound. Identify (on the basis of the history) the main etiology for the delayed wound healing.
  - Treat contaminated wounds with mechanical débridement in the office or enzymatic débridement or dressings that will débride the wound (normal saline wet-to-dry dressing changes twice daily). Chemicals such as Dakin solution should not be used for more than 48 hours because they can be toxic to healthy tissues.
  - Treat pressure ulcers with appropriate orthotics for pressure offloading or total contact casts if the patient is a candidate.
  - Treat arterial ulcers with referrals to vascular surgery for evaluation of inflow.
  - Treat diabetic ulcers with education (inspecting footwear and regular extremity examinations) and adequate glucose control.
  - Treat venous ulcers with graduated compression and edema control with an Unna boot, compression stockings, and elevation.
  - Infected wounds need operative débridement and appropriate antibiotic therapy.
- Many commercially available products are available for wound care, which is as much an art as it is a science. Fundamentally the provider must determine if the wound needs débridement or if it needs a moist environment with adjuncts to allow proper healing.
  - The ideal wound healing environment is slightly moist to encourage epithelialization. Topical antimicrobials (e.g., polysporin, bacitracin) or hydrogels are helpful when applied with a gauze dressing changed once a day.
  - More frequent dressing changes are helpful when trying to débride the wound with dressing changes (as in normal saline wet-to-dry dressing changes).

- Refer your patient to a dedicated wound care specialist if you are not seeing improvement in the wound.

Negative Pressure Therapy for Wounds
- Wound vac therapy effectively decreases wound surface area and increases blood flow to promote healing in clean wounds.
- Wounds should be clean, without exposed vital structures, before placement of this dressing. Often this is best accomplished in the operating room, and the dressing is then changed every other day.

Hyperbaric Oxygen for Wounds
- This can be a useful adjunct to healing certain chronic wounds. Consider a referral to your local hyperbaric medicine specialist for chronic wounds with a history of radiation or for wounds that you suspect are associated with impaired oxygen delivery.

Suggested Readings
Broughton G II, Janis JE, Attinger CE: Wound healing: an overview, *Plast Reconstr Surg* 117:1e–S, 2006.
Fan K, Tang J, Escandon J, Kirsner RS: State of the art in topical wound-healing products, *Plast Reconstr Surg* 127:44S, 2011.

SUTURES
Suture Material
Absorbable or Permanent
- Use absorbable suture for wounds under less tension and permanent suture for wounds under greater tension.
- If using absorbable suture, pick one that will lose strength at the same time the wound is expected to heal and recover that strength.

Monofilament or Braided
- Monofilament suture slides easily through tissues and has fewer potential small spaces for serving as a nidus for opportunistic microorganisms; thus, it is more appropriate for closure of the contaminated wound.

Size
- The numeric designation is based on breaking strength, not diameter.

- Use the smallest possible size that is strong enough to close the wound.

Needle
Taper or Cutting Needle
- A taper needle is more appropriate for tendons, muscles, and deep tissues.
- A reverse cutting needle is more appropriate for skin closure.

Commonly Used Absorbable Suture
Vicryl
- Braided
- Loses all of its strength by 2 weeks
- Good for closing deeper tissues

Monocryl
- Monofilament
- Loses all of its strength by 3 weeks
- Good for closing deeper tissues, especially in contaminated wounds

PDS
- Monofilament
- At 6 weeks, 25% still remains
- Good for closing fascia, muscle, and other deep tissues

Commonly Used Permanent Suture
Nylon
- Monofilament

Prolene
- Monofilament
- Both Nylon and Prolene have similar applications: skin closure and tendon repairs. It is often a matter of personal preference as to the choice of one over another.
- Permanent skin suture should be removed as soon as the wound is ready to prevent unsightly cross-hatched scars (7 to 14 days depending on the patient and anatomic site).

Suture Technique
General Principles
- For percutaneous suturing:
1) Always enter the skin with the needle perpendicular to the skin.
2) The distance from the entry of the needle to the wound on one side of the wound should equal the distance

of the needle entry to exit on the other side of the wound.

3) The depth of the needle penetration should be equivalent on both sides of the wound to prevent the creation of a shelf, or mismatched wound margins.

4) Maximize eversion of the wound margins to facilitate optimal appearance of the ultimate scar.

- Strength layers include dermis and fascia. Sutures in subcutaneous fat will not hold tension and will not minimize scarring, but careful placement of buried approximating sutures in the fascia and dermis will result in finer scars.

- Regardless of the technique, if percutaneous sutures remain in place for too long, they will result in a scar with crosshatching or have a so-called "railroad track" appearance. Prevent this with timely removal of sutures. Placement of a deep, buried layer of dermal approximating suture allows expedient removal of percutaneous epidermal sutures.

- Practice atraumatic tissue handling (e.g., avoid pinching skin with forceps) to optimize the appearance of the scar and minimize damage to tissues being repaired.

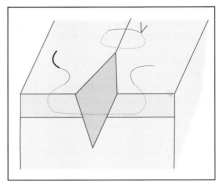

Figure 12-1. Simple interrupted suture.

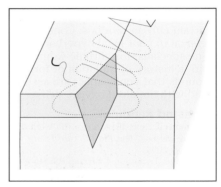

Figure 12-2. Simple running suture.

Simple Interrupted: Figure 12-1

- *Technique:* With wrist pronated, enter the skin with the needle perpendicular to the skin and wound. Then supinate and travel across the wound, taking equal bites on either side of the wound edge, and grasp the needle. When viewed in cross section the bite should look like a pear, wider in the dermis and narrower in the epidermis to optimize the final appearance of the scar. The knot is secured after the needle passes through both sides of the wound.

- *Common Uses*
  - Percutaneous skin closure
  - Fascial reapproximation

Simple Running: Figure 12-2

- *Technique:* See earlier description for a simple interrupted suture. The difference is that after the first bite, the

needle is left attached to the suture end and continuously used from one wound margin to the other with a knot secured at the beginning and one secured at the end of the area to be approximated.

- *Common Uses*
  - Percutaneous skin closure, not recommended for wounds under great tension.

Vertical Mattress: Figure 12-3

- *Technique:* Also called "far-far-near-near stitch." See earlier description for a simple interrupted suture. After taking the first bite in the deeper layer, the needle is reversed and the "near-near" bite is taken. This is a smaller bite (both in depth and distance to the wound), taken in the opposite direction

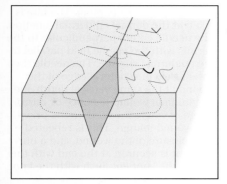

Figure 12-3. Vertical mattress suture.

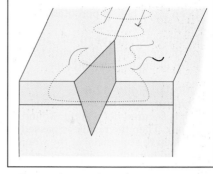

Figure 12-4. Horizontal mattress suture.

as the first bite. The knot is secured on the side of the wound. The knot should be secured away from any potentially compromised tissue (e.g., the knot is not secured on the same side as a flap of skin).

■ *Common Uses*
- A vertical mattress suture should not be commonly used in the acute setting because this technique can strangulate tissue if the wound is under great tension.
- This is an effective technique for eversion of skin edges when the wound is under minimal tension.

Horizontal Mattress: Figure 12-4
■ *Technique:* See earlier technique for a simple interrupted suture. Before tying the knot, the needle is brought back in the reverse direction across the wound. The second entry point is made after traveling parallel to the wound the same distance as the previous exit point was from the wound edge. The needle is then passed as a simple interrupted suture in the reverse direction and secured on the side of the wound. The knot should be secured away from any potentially compromised tissue (e.g., the knot is not secured on the same side as a flap of skin).
■ *Common Uses*
- Should not be commonly used in the acute setting because this technique can strangulate tissue if the wound is under great tension.

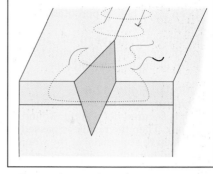

Figure 12-5. Deep dermal buried suture.

- This is an effective technique for eversion of skin edges when the wound is under minimal tension.

Buried Deep Dermal: Figure 12-5
■ *Technique:* Enter the wound from a deep aspect, not the epidermis. With the needle perpendicular to the dermis, the dermis is entered and the wrist is supinated. The needle should exit just deep to the dermal-epidermal junction and travel across the wound. Enter the other side of the wound at the same level as the exit on the opposite side (just below the dermal-epidermal junction). Supinate and then exit in the deep dermis across from the entry point on the other side. The knot is secured deep in the wound, and the tails of the knot are cut flush with the knot.

■ **Common Uses**
  • Deep layer before percutaneous skin closure
  • Effective technique to take tension off of the epidermal closure to optimize ultimate scar outcome

Subcuticular: Figure 12-6
■ **Technique:** A buried deep dermal stitch is secured deep in the wound at the apex. Then the needle is passed from deep to superficial at the wound apex, and horizontal bites are taken (in contrast to all the previous bites

described in this chapter). The bite is taken at the dermal-epidermal junction. The needle enters perpendicular to the dermis with the needle held parallel to the epidermal surface. The needle then enters the contralateral edge of the wound at the same vertical depth and longitudinal wound distance or mirror image of where it exited on the previous wound margin. This is repeated until closure of the wound, and a buried knot is secured at the end with the tails of the knot cut flush with the knot.
■ **Common Uses**
  • Skin closure in areas of minimal tension, in combination with buried deep dermal stitches.

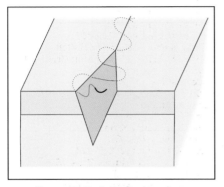

Figure 12-6. Subcuticular suture.

Suggested Readings

Ethicon: *Knot tying manual,* Somerville, NJ, 2005, Ethicon.
Ethicon: *Wound closure manual,* Somerville, NJ, 2005, Ethicon.
Vasconez HC, Habash A: Plastic and reconstructive surgery. In Doherty GM, editor: *Current diagnosis & treatment: surgery,* ed 13, New York, 2010, McGraw-Hill.
Weitzul S, Taylor RS: Suturing technique and other closure materials. In Robinson JK, editor: *Surgery of the skin,* ed 2, Saint Louis, 2010, Elsevier.

Index